RENEWALS 458-4574

DATE DUE

GAYLORD			PRINTED IN U.S.A.

Fundamentals of
Genetic Epidemiology

Monographs in Epidemiology and Biostatistics
Edited by Jennifer L. Kelsey, Michael G. Marmot, Paul D. Stolley,
Martin P. Vessey

MONOGRAPHS IN EPIDEMIOLOGY AND BIOSTATISTICS   VOLUME 22

Fundamentals of Genetic Epidemiology

Muin J. Khoury, M.D., Ph.D.
Deputy Chief, Birth Defects and
Genetic Diseases Branch
National Center for Environmental Health
Centers for Disease Control
Atlanta, Georgia

Terri H. Beaty, Ph.D.
Professor, Department of Epidemiology
Johns Hopkins University
School of Hygiene and Public Health
Baltimore, Maryland

Bernice H. Cohen, Ph.D., M.P.H.
Professor, Department of Epidemiology
Johns Hopkins University
School of Hygiene and Public Health
Baltimore, Maryland

New York   Oxford
OXFORD UNIVERSITY PRESS
1993

Oxford University Press

Oxford   New York   Toronto
Delhi   Bombay   Calcutta   Madras   Karachi
Kuala Lumpur   Singapore   Hong Kong   Tokyo
Nairobi   Dar es Salaam   Cape Town
Melbourne   Auckland   Madrid

and associated companies in
Berlin   Ibadan

Library of Congress Cataloging-in-Publication Data
Khoury, Muin J.
Fundamentals of genetic epidemiology / Muin J. Khoury,
Terri H. Beaty, Bernice H. Cohen.
p.   cm.   Includes bibliographical references and index.
ISBN 0-19-505288-9
1. Genetic epidemiology.
2.   Hereditary Diseases—epidemiology.
I. Beaty, Terri H.   II. Cohen, Bernice H.   III. Title.
[DNLM: 1. Epidemiologic Methods.   QZ 50 K45f]
RB155.K49   1992   616′.042—dc20
DNLM/DLC for Library of Congress   92-16492

*This work was not written as part of Dr. Khoury's
official duties at the Centers for Disease Control.

19   18   17   16   15   14   13   12   11

Printed in the United States of America
on acid-free paper

Preface

This book was designed to describe and delineate an emerging field: genetic epidemiology. With increasing evidence of the importance of genetic factors and genetic-environmental interactions in the etiology and pathogenesis of human diseases, it is important to begin integrating research methods of traditional epidemiology with those of human genetics. Our task was not simple given the rapid methodologic advances in human genetics. The explosion of molecular genetic technology, the ongoing progress of the human genome project, and the advances in statistical genetic methods will continue to influence genetic epidemiology for years to come. Although presently no book can be considered the definitive treatise on the field, we have attempted to provide a balanced presentation and to combine important principles of epidemiology and genetics in the study of human disease.

The book contains a background section on important genetic and epidemiologic methods and approaches (chapters 2 and 3). While limiting this section to a concise overview, we feel it is necessary because epidemiologists and geneticists tend to come from different worlds and speak different languages. The book is then divided into a section on population studies (chapters 4 and 5) and a section on family studies (chapters 6 through 9). In both sections, we outline the available methods for studying the distribution and determinants of genetic traits and disease endpoints, as well as the various approaches in investigating the role of genetic factors in disease etiology. Lastly, we consider the applications of the emerging field of genetic epidemiology in both clinical medicine and public health (chapter 10).

Clearly, as new methods and more refined techniques are developed, the field of genetic epidemiology will evolve; yet the need to recognize the role of both genetic and environmental factors in disease control and prevention will not diminish. We hope that both the methodology and the philosophy of this book's approach to genetic epidemiology will prove useful to teachers, students, researchers, and other health professionals in developing strategies for disease prevention and health promotion.

September, 1992   *MJK*
                                                                      THB
                                                                      BHC

Acknowledgments

We wish to thank several individuals who have read and commented on parts of the manuscript including Melissa Austin, Gary C. Chase, Earl L. Diamond, J. David Erickson, W. Dana Flanders, Kung-Yee Liang, Patricia P. Moll, and Beth Newman. In addition, we thank Mrs. Mary E. Wollett for her technical skills in compiling the manuscript. Without her patience and diligence, the project could never have been completed.

Contents

Fundamentals of
Genetic Epidemiology

1

Scope and Strategies of
Genetic Epidemiology

1.1. INTRODUCTION

In the mid-1980s a new discipline emerged, an offspring that resulted from many years of interaction between genetics and epidemiology. This new field, called *genetic epidemiology*, focuses on the role of genetic factors and their interaction with environmental factors in the occurrence of disease in human populations. The growth of genetic epidemiology has been enhanced by remarkable advances in molecular biology that have expanded our understanding of genetic diseases at the molecular level and have had numerous applications to the classification, diagnosis, prognosis, and treatment of many Mendelian disorders. The study of genetic variation at the molecular level promises to contribute to the understanding of the etiology and pathogenesis of the major chronic diseases that appear to have a genetic component, such as coronary heart disease, cancer, and birth defects (Bishop, 1984; Slamon, 1987; Gibbs and Caskey, 1989; Holtzman, 1989; Taylor, 1989). These prospects are being nurtured by the initiation of the Human Genome Project, a long-term scientific effort whose goal is to map and sequence the entire human genome (McKusick, 1989; Antonorakis, 1990; Watson, 1990; Watson and Cook-Dugan, 1991). Accompanying this progress, however, are growing concerns regarding the ethical implications of genetic testing and the potential misuse of information about each person's genetic constitution (Holtzman, 1989; McKusick, 1989; Suzuki and Knudston 1989; Chapman, 1990; Huggins et al., 1990; Fost, 1992).

1.2. HISTORICAL PERSPECTIVES

Before discussing the scope and strategies of genetic epidemiology, we will first briefly review relevant historical developments of human genetics and epidemiology as two separate entities and their gradual rapprochement. Certainly, no scientific discipline evolves in isolation, and there are many instances of shared aims and techniques in genetics and epidemiology. In general, however, these two fields have considered questions of human disease from quite different perspectives.

1.2.1. Historical Development of Human Genetics

The history of human genetics can be viewed as the concurrent development of, and sometimes contest between, two paradigms: Mendel's concept of discrete genes and Galton's biometric approach (Vogel and Motulsky, 1986). Mendel's experiments in plant hybridization, first published in 1865, led to the concept that a fundamental unit of inheritance, the *gene*, followed predictable patterns of transmission across generations. On the other hand, Galton's work on hereditary talent and character (Galton, 1865) paved the way for the development of statistical genetics, which based inferences concerning the inheritance of a trait on statistical analysis of groups of relatives. Originally, the biometric approach was applied exclusively to quantitative traits (such as height and weight), and the Mendelian approach was applied primarily to qualitative traits. Eventually, the two approaches have converged in application, if not outlook, and modern human genetics relies heavily on both.

One of the first historical milestones in medical genetics was the application of Mendel's paradigm to alkaptonuria, an inborn error of metabolism (Garrod, 1902). Bernstein's application of the Mendelian approach to antigens of the ABO blood group system began the documentation of polymorphic genetic traits, that is, where multiple allelic forms of a single gene exist at high frequencies in the population (Bernstein, 1931). In the 1940s and 1950s, improvement in biochemical methods enhanced understanding of the gene at the biochemical level and revealed how genes function to code for proteins, both enzymes and nonenzyme structural gene products. Such work has further documented the immense genetic variation among individuals in populations (Harris, 1969). Some of this variation appears to be related to disease processes.

Since the mid-1970s, powerful techniques for the analysis and manipulation of the DNA itself (Watson et al., 1983; Weatherall, 1985) have revealed greater detail about the structure of genes, as well as the extent of genetic variability in populations. As it became possible to examine the molecular structure of genes, earlier concepts regarding its structure and function had to be modified and expanded (Weatherall, 1985). A major discovery that resulted from this new molecular technology was the enormous variation at the DNA level that exists among individuals. This variation is obviously inherited, but often appears phenotypically silent and is frequently not directly expressed in any gene product (Weatherall, 1985; Cooper and Clayton, 1988). DNA markers are extremely useful in mapping and linkage analysis and have been used in the presymptomatic diagnosis of single-gene disorders, such as Huntington's disease (Gusella et al., 1983), as well as in identifying previously unknown gene products involved in genetic diseases such as Duchenne's muscular dystrophy and cystic fibrosis.

At the statistical level, the pioneering works of Hardy and Weinberg at the turn of this century (Hardy, 1908) served as the foundation of population genetics. Between 1910 and 1930, the works of Haldane, Fisher, and Wright were instrumental in providing a mathematical framework for the behavior of genes in populations. These ideas collectively founded the discipline of population genetics, which is primarily concerned with factors that affect the distribution of genes in populations. Moreover, many of these same early researchers were also responsible for the growth of the field of statistical genetics. At first, these techniques were considered inappropriate for single-gene traits, and there was an early split between supporters of Mendel and followers of Galton. In 1918, Fisher proposed a model that could bridge the gap between the Galtonian and the Mendelian approaches by noting that correlations in continuous traits between relatives could be the result of the combined action of a large number of independently segregating genes, termed *polygenes*, each of which exerts a small, equal, and direct effect on the observed continuous phenotype. This polygenic component could be easily measured using the statistical principles of analysis of variance or of correlation. The techniques of path analysis developed by Sewall Wright (1934) have experienced a renaissance since Rao and colleagues (1974) showed how familial correlations could be partitioned into genetic and cultural factors shared among relatives. The concept of a genetic basis for correlation was also applied to discrete traits (such as diseases) by Falconer (1960), who proposed that risk of a disease could be considered as an unobserved continuous trait, and that data on disease frequency in the population and in relatives of affected individuals could be used to estimate correlations in unobserved risk or liability.

After 1960, there was an expansion in the statistical tools available to test genetic hypotheses and fit genetic models. Segregation analysis was originally designed to estimate the proportion of affected offspring for a given genetic model in sibships only. A number of methods were proposed to correct for biases under various ascertainment schemes. Morton and others extended the classical segregation analysis of sibships to the analysis of nuclear families (parents and offspring in two-generation pedigrees). Aided by advances in computer technology, the 1970s and 1980s witnessed the development of more general algorithms for extending segregation analysis to pedigrees of arbitrary structure, including complex genealogies (Elandt-Johnson, 1970; Elston and Stewart, 1971; Morton and MacLean, 1974; Lange and Elston, 1975; Cannings et al., 1978; Lalouel and Morton, 1981; Hasstedt, 1982; Lalouel et al., 1983; Bonney, 1986; Demenais, 1991). These advances in segregation analysis led to the development of models of inheritance that allow for explicit testing of a single-gene model versus the more descriptive polygenic model (Morton and MacLean, 1974; Lalouel et al., 1983). The statistical techniques of segregation analysis, variance components analysis (Lange et al., 1976), and path analysis (Hanis et al., 1983; Rao et al., 1983) have also found increasing applications in the analysis of pedigree data and have become the analytic cornerstone of genetic epidemiology.

At the same time, linkage analysis of genetic markers and disease became an active area in human genetics (Morton, 1955). Substantial progress has been made in the statistical techniques of linkage analysis (Conneally and Rivas, 1980; Ott, 1985). Continuing advances in computer modeling have allowed the merging of the methods of segregation and linkage analyses into a more complete genetic analysis of pedigree data (Bonney et al., 1986).

1.2.2. Historical Development of Epidemiology

Although during the past 50 years epidemiology has matured to the point where it is regarded as a separate scientific discipline (Lilienfeld, 1978), many feel it is still in an early stage (Rothman, 1986). Epidemiologists often disagree on the definition of epidemiology itself (Lilienfeld, 1978; Rothman, 1986) and on the basic terminology for measures of disease frequency such as incidence (Elandt-Johnson, 1975). Nevertheless, in the last 20 years there has been an enormous development of epidemiologic concepts, tools and applications. As summarized by Lilienfeld and Lilienfeld (1980) and by MacMahon and Pugh (1970), the history of epidemiology can be viewed as the development of two broad concepts: the role of the environment (broadly defined) in causing human disease, and the epidemiologic approach to disease and to inference about biologic causation.

The concept that the environment is important in determining human disease is an ancient one, dating back almost 2000 years to Hippocrates' *Treatise on Airs, Waters, and Places* (Adams, 1939). Since world history had been dominated across the ages by infectious disease, a major concern of epidemiologists has been the investigation and the control of epidemics (Last, 1986a). Snow's epidemiologic work on the mode of transmission of cholera via drinking water in London in the 1850s (Snow, 1936) occurred about 30 years before the cholera vibrio organism was isolated and identified (Last, 1986b). Despite major victories in the control of infectious diseases (such as smallpox eradication), the role of infections in human disease has not been eliminated. Legionnaires' disease, toxic shock syndrome, the emergence of antibiotic resistant strains of bacteria, nosocomial infections, and the acquired immunodeficiency syndrome are sharp reminders of the importance of infectious agents in causing human illness (Evans and Brachman, 1986). In addition to infectious agents, epidemiologists have become increasingly interested in a wide spectrum of noninfectious environmental factors in disease etiology (Lilienfeld, 1973) including radiation, air pollution, chemical toxic sites, drug use, cigarette smoking, alcohol ingestion, coffee consumption, and nutritional factors.

The development of epidemiologic concepts and methods for the study of disease etiology can be traced to William Farr in the early nineteenth century. Farr defined many epidemiologic concepts widely used today such as the person-years approach, dose-response effects, disease prevalence, and herd immunity (Lilienfeld and Lilienfeld, 1980). He also set up one of the first modern vital statistics systems in Europe (Farr, 1975). Epidemiologic reasoning about biologic transmission of disease was used by Snow in his studies of the cholera epidemic in London (Snow, 1936).

In the twentieth century, epidemiologists increasingly have addressed the complex etiology of chronic diseases, such as coronary heart disease and cancer, as these diseases emerged as leading causes of mortality and morbidity in many populations (Lilienfeld, 1973). Gradually, the approach of counting and describing the distribution of disease in populations by place, time and persons evolved into an "inductive science, concerned not merely with describing the distribution of disease, but equally or more, with fitting it into a consistent philosophy" (Frost, 1941). Epidemiologists began "to elucidate the etiology of a specific disease by combining epidemiologic data with information from other disciplines, such as genetics, biochemistry, and microbiology" (Lilienfeld and Lilienfeld, 1980). Large-scale population-based cohort studies such as the Framingham study (Dawber, 1980) contributed to the growth of epidemiology. Recent decades have been marked by the development of causal theories and quantitative methods (Greenland, 1987b; Susser, 1991), the refinement of the case-control approach to identify causes of disease (Schlesselman, 1982; Rothman, 1986), and the increasingly sophisticated use of statistical models (Breslow, 1980; Thomas, 1988; Prentice and Farewell, 1986; Kahn and Sempos, 1989). Epidemiology has expanded to include the design of clinical trials (Meinert, 1986); record linkage studies (Kurland and Molgaard, 1981; Baldwin et al., 1987); the use of laboratory methods to measure exposures more adequately and to define biomarkers for disease, exposure, and susceptibility (Hulka and Wilcosky, 1988; National Research Council, 1989; Loomis and Wing, 1990); surveillance for environmental hazards; and health risk assessment (Gordis, 1988c). Amid all these advances, the primary objective of epidemiologic studies remains "to provide the basis for developing and evaluating preventive procedures and public health practices" (Lilienfeld and Lilienfeld, 1980). As stated by Last (1986), "Epidemiology is not merely the abstract, academic study of disease and health-related phenomena. . . . Control of disease, prevention of disability, impairment, and premature death are the raison d'être of epidemiology."

1.2.3. The Rapprochement Between Genetics and Epidemiology

The rapprochement between genetics and epidemiology was made slowly by epidemiologically oriented geneticists and by genetically oriented epidemiologists. Both groups have realized the importance of genetic factors in human disease and the need to merge genetic and epidemiologic methodologies in the study of such factors. In 1954, Neel and Schull (1954) provided the first account of "genetics and epidemiology" in a textbook of human genetics. They presented, in simple terms, "the manner in which genetic concepts must be an integral part of the armamentarium of the modern epidemiologist." Referring to the field of "epidemiological genetics," they introduced four main criteria that can be used in epidemiologic studies to infer the influence of genetic factors in the etiology of a disease:

   i) the occurrence of disease in definite numerical proportions among individuals related by descent,
   ii) failure of the disease to spread among relatives,
   iii) onset of disease at a characteristic age without a known precipitating event, and
   iv) greater concordance of the disease in identical than in fraternal twins.

These criteria represented an early attempt to incorporate genetic concepts into epidemiologic studies.

In 1965, the proceedings of a conference on genetics and the epidemiology of chronic diseases was published (Neel et al., 1965). Genetically determined polymorphic systems were found to be associated with numerous diseases (e.g., the α_1-antitrypsin genotype and pulmonary emphysema). Blood group-disease associations were reported (Clarke, 1961; Mourant et al., 1978). In the 1970s, a wave of publications on HLA-disease associations invaded the medical literature (Dausset and Svejgaard, 1977). In spite of many documented associations between various diseases and genetic markers (including blood groups and HLA types), the biologic significance of many such associations remains ill-defined. Moreover, most common disorders exhibit evidence of familial aggregation with or without a documented relationship to any genetic marker (MacMahon, 1978).

In the 1960s and 1970s, geneticists began to appreciate the role of numerous single-gene mutations that affect both the nature and the rate of drug metabolism, and the discipline of "pharmacogenetics" emerged (Vessel, 1979). That drug reactions provide a model for genetically determined differential susceptibility to disease was pointed out by Motulsky in a symposium on genetic polymorphisms and geographic variation in disease (Motulsky, 1962), providing another example of an early dialogue between genetics and epidemiology. Since then, it has become increasingly apparent that much genetically determined biochemical variability may go unrecognized and remains relatively innocuous unless the individual is exposed to some critical environmental agent. The environmental agent could be drugs, dietary factors, environmental chemicals, and so on. The exposure may be acute (e.g., hemolytic crisis) or prolonged (e.g., cigarette smoking) leading to gradual buildup or deterioration (e.g., atherosclerosis, chronic obstructive lung disease). With the burgeoning knowledge of these relationships, the discipline of pharmacogenetics has expanded to become "ecogenetics," where a wide range of genetically mediated differential susceptibilities to environmental agents (as well as to drugs) are considered (Brewer, 1971; Omenn and Motulsky, 1978; Calabrese, 1984; Omenn, 1988; Motulsky, 1991).

With the rapid growth of statistical techniques in human genetics and with advances in computer technology, increasingly complicated mathematical models have been used in the genetic analysis of common diseases. A notable application of the new tools was summarized in two workshops on the genetic epidemiology of coronary heart disease (Sing and Skolnick, 1979; Rao et al., 1984) that brought together geneticists and epidemiologists for discussions of common issues and interests. Nevertheless, several researchers have questioned the true integration of disciplines. While Morton and Chung (1978) stated that genetic epidemiology "represents the efforts of geneticists to become epidemiologists", Feinleib (1984) suggested that "many epidemiologists are trying to become geneticists." An unfortunate prototype of the genetic epidemiologist has been a "geneticist prone to accept epidemiology only on his or her own terms" (Schull and Weiss, 1980).

At the same time, many epidemiologists have begun to recognize the importance of genetics in epidemiology. In a chapter on "genetics and epidemiology" written in their textbook of epidemiology, MacMahon and Pugh (1970) stated that "genetics and epidemiology have much in common," and that "genes being a major determinant of disease frequency, must be considered in the development of any hypothesis explaining epidemiologic observations." They pointed out that both fields rely on data collection from large populations, use similar mathematical and statistical tools, and overlap considerably in their interest in certain types of investigations, such as the twin method. Almost ten years before, Abraham Lilienfeld had noted that "for the geneticist and the epidemiologist alike, family studies may provide one of the best means of studying genetic-environmental interactions in disease" (Lilienfeld, 1961). He also cautioned, however, that "even though familial aggregation is observed, it is necessary to decide whether such aggregation is a result of genetic or environmental factors or both" (Lilienfeld, 1965), and advocated careful consideration of environmental factors that aggregate in families before implicating genetic mechanisms. In a classic study of familial aggregation of medical school attendance, Lilienfeld (1959) found that a characteristic such as being a student at the University of Buffalo Medical School was consistent with a simple Mendelian model. He attributed the failure of rejecting a single-gene hypothesis to the lack of power of statistical tests used with small sample sizes. A more recent analysis of this same question of power to discriminate between genetic and nongenetic causes of behavioral traits (such as attendance in medical school) underscores the limitations of even sophisticated analytic models (McGuffin and Huckle, 1990).

1.2.4. The Birth of Genetic Epidemiology

During the past decade, genetic epidemiology has become established as an entity distinct from both genetics and epidemiology. To our knowledge, Morton and Chung first used the term "genetic epidemiology" to describe this new field (Morton and Chung, 1978), although other terms have been proposed, such as "epidemiological genetics" (Neel and Schull, 1954), and "clinical population genetics" (Vogel and Motulsky, 1986). A literature search reveals that before 1977 the term "genetic epidemiology" was virtually nonexistent in titles of published articles. After 1977, an increasing number of journal articles on the "genetic epidemiology of" various conditions could be found. Despite some concern about the new field representing a unidirectional input from geneticists (Schull and Weiss, 1980), about the "lack of appreciation for the importance of epidemiologic principles" (Ward, 1979), and about the indiscriminate use of statistical models without regard to the underlying biologic nature of the disease (Murphy, 1978; Ward, 1979; Motulsky, 1984), genetic epidemiology is alive and thriving, as evidenced by an increasing number of books and articles (Morton, 1982; Philippe, 1982; Morton et al., 1983; Roberts, 1983; King et al., 1984; Rao, 1984; Khoury et al., 1986; Morton 1986; Thompson, 1986; Bishop et al., 1987; Harper 1988; Schull and Hanis, 1990).

1.3. DEFINITION AND SCOPE OF GENETIC EPIDEMIOLOGY

Since the field of genetic epidemiology can be considered the offspring of two parent disciplines, it is not surprising to find a wide spectrum of activities, interests, and philosophies among those active in the field.

1.3.1. What is Genetic Epidemiology?

Researchers have still not fully agreed on the definition and the scope of genetic epidemiology. Several definitions that have appeared in the literature are listed in Table 1–1. One that is often cited comes from Morton and Chung, who referred to two main components of genetic epidemiology: (1) the

Table 1–1. Some definitions of genetic epidemiology

N. E. Morton and C. S. Chung (1978): "A science that deals with the etiology, distribution, and control of disease in groups of relatives, and with inherited causes of disease in populations."

R. Ward (1979): "The primary objective of the genetic epidemiologist will be to identify the genetic contribution to the etiological pathway."

B. H. Cohen (1980): Genetic epidemiology is defined "as examining the role of genetic factors, along with the environmental contributors to disease, and at the same time, giving equal attention to the differential impact of environmental agents, nonfamilial as well as familial, on different genetic backgrounds."

P. Phillippe (1982): "Genetic epidemiology studies the interaction between genetic and environmental factors at the origin of disease."

M.C. King et al. (1984): "Genetic epidemiology is the study of how and why diseases cluster in families and ethnic groups."

D.C. Rao (1984): "Genetic epidemiology is an emerging field with diverse interests, one that represents an important interaction between the two parent disciplines: genetics and epidemiology. Genetic epidemiology differs from epidemiology by its explicit consideration of genetic factors and family resemblance; it differs from population genetics by its focus on disease; it also differs from medical genetics by its emphasis on population aspects."

D.F. Roberts (1985): argues the distinction of genetic epidemiology from epidemiology in general. Genetic epidemiology "is not merely the application of the central concept of epidemiology, the study of the distribution of disease in space and time, to genetic disease. Instead, in genetic epidemiology, the concept is extended to include the additional variables of the genetic structure of the population, with the object of elucidating the etiology of disease in which there may be a genetic component."

E.A. Thompson (1986a): "Genetic epidemiology is the analysis of the familial distributions of traits, with a view to understanding any possible genetic basis."

study of the etiology of disease among groups of relatives to unravel the causes of family resemblance and (2) the study of inherited causes of disease in populations (Morton and Chung, 1978). Two other definitions seem to restrict genetic epidemiology mainly to the analysis of familial aggregation (King et al., 1984; Thompson, 1984), whereas others stress the role of genetic epidemiology in studying genetic-environmental interactions in disease etiology (Cohen, 1980; Philippe, 1982). Alternatively, Roberts (1985) emphasizes the importance of the underlying genetic structure of a population in determining disease and other physiologic processes that could be considered within the range of normal human variation.

Thus, it is not surprising to find that the kinds of studies that are included under the rubric "genetic epidemiology" tend to differ in scope and applications. By reviewing papers in the journal *Genetic Epidemiology*, and reports using the term "genetic epidemiology" in their titles, one finds heavy emphasis on the genetic analysis of pedigree data (segregation or linkage analysis), often from ill-defined populations (e.g., Go et al., 1983; King et al., 1983; Tiwari et al., 1984; Williams and Anderson, 1984; Horn and Morton, 1986). This emphasis on statistical genetic analysis by researchers in the field has raised the issue as to whether genetic epidemiology may be just another name for statistical genetics (Chakraborty and Szathmary, 1985). As indicated by Ward (1979), "there is a general complaint that all too often, the underlying biologic nature of the disease is ignored in favor of the development of a specific model of analysis." Motulsky (1984) has expressed the concern that the field may lead to "the erection of barriers and consolidation of a self-contained group of research workers using complex statistical models understandable to this group alone who do not communicate with biologic and medical workers in the relevant fields."

1.3.2. Nature of Genetic Involvement in Disease

It is important to consider briefly how geneticists and epidemiologists have envisioned the spectrum of disease etiology. Geneticists have viewed disease etiology as ranging from totally genetic causation (point mutations) to totally environmental causation (such as a plane crash). From a genetic viewpoint, Ward (1979) discussed six categories of disease causation that span the range of this spectrum (see Table 1–2):

1. *Single-gene causation:* The disease is caused by single-gene mutation leading to a disturbed protein function and to phenotypic manifestations resulting from disruption in cell and organ function.
2. *Chromosomal causation:* Alterations in chromosome numbers or morphology at the germinal or the somatic cell levels lead to clinical disease.
3. *Multifactorial causation with "high heritability"*: This is an arbitrary classification of disorders where genetic factors are believed to play a major role either in the disease or its precursors. The group may include, for example, some birth defects, such as neural tube defects and oral clefts, where multiple studies have repeatedly shown familial ag-

Table 1–2. The range of the etiology spectrum from a genetic viewpoint

Category	Examples
Single-gene	Inborn errors of metabolism such as phenylketonuria and galactosemia
Chromosomal	Down syndrome, cri-du-chat syndrome
Multifactorial	
High heritability	Isolated birth defects, such as cleft lip and palate, neural tube defects
Low heritabilty	Coronary heart disease, chronic obstructive pulmonary disease
Infectious	Bacterial, viral, and fungal infections
Environmental	Radiation, injuries

Adapted from *Ward (1979)*.

gregation, but no simple Mendelian basis had been shown to be responsible for the disease, and there are few apparent environmental risk factors.

4. *Multifactorial causation with "low heritability"*: This is another arbitrary group of disorders where certain environmental factors are known to be related to the development of disease, but consistent familial aggregation is observed that is independent of such environmental factors. This group may include, for example, coronary heart disease and chronic obstructive pulmonary disease.

5. *Infectious causes*: This group encompasses a wide variety of disorders caused by infectious agents (bacteria, viruses, parasites).

6. *Environmental causes*: This group involves disorders caused by defined environmental agents such as chemicals, radiation, physical agents, and injury.

In a similar conceptual context, epidemiologists' ideas of disease etiology have also been expressed in terms of complicated interaction among the agent, the host (recognizing the role of constitutional factors that are often genetic), and the environment, the trio known as the "epidemiologic triangle" (Mausner and Kramer, 1985). Disease is viewed as the result of a chain of events that comprise an intricate "web" of external causal events and internal pathogenetic mechanisms (MacMahon and Pugh, 1970).

Despite the appeal of any simple etiologic classification of disease, it is becoming more apparent that most diseases are not purely genetic or environmental in etiology, but depend on a complex interaction of the two. Even with "infectious" and "environmental" etiology, differential genetic susceptibility may be involved in determining the ultimate clinical manifestation. Moreover, within the etiologic category of "totally genetic," there could be considerable environmental influence on disease occurrence. Environmental mutagenic agents, such as radiation, drugs, or infections, can affect the frequency of single-gene disorders in populations. Also, many single-gene conditions do not manifest clinically at all unless triggered by specific environmental exposures, for example, glucose-6–phosphate dehydrogenase deficiency and other ecogenetic traits (Omenn and Motulsky, 1978; Calabrese, 1984). Another example of the interplay between single-gene disease and environment is the effect of maternal phenylketonuria (PKU) on pregnancy outcomes, where elevated phenylalanine levels during pregnancy of a woman with PKU can irreversibly damage a genetically normal fetus because of the abnormal intrauterine milieu created by the maternal genotype (Lenke and Levy, 1980).

Furthermore, chromosomal abnormalities, traditionally the domain of the geneticist, often entail complex environmental components that can be documented only by epidemiologic studies (e.g., the relationship of Down syndrome to advanced maternal age). Major advances have also been achieved in the field of cancer cytogenetics, where specific patterns of chromosomal abnormalities can be found in a variety of cancers (Yunis, 1983), although the precise pathogenic mechanisms for these changes are not yet well understood. Even more intriguing is the observation that environmental agents (such as retroviruses) often may be incorporated into the genome and operate as part of the genetic constitution of the cell. Insight into the relationship among viruses, oncogenes, and chromosomal changes in cancer pathogenesis is only beginning to unfold (Brugge et al., 1991, Littlefield, 1984; Taylor, 1989). Thus, the increasing recognition of genetic-environmental interactions in the etiology of almost all diseases has contributed not only to the expansion of the scope of both genetics and epidemiology, but provided the foundations of the new discipline of genetic epidemiology.

1.3.3. Scope of Genetic Epidemiology

It is clear from the above discussion that genetic epidemiology may be best viewed as the study of the role of genetic factors and their interaction with environmental factors in the occurrence of disease in human populations. Environmental factors are broadly defined as exogenous factors—chemical, physical, infectious, and nutritional. Genetic epidemiology is closely related to the biomedical sciences and to the field of public health. Its broad goal is to understand the role of genetic factors in the etiology of disease in human populations with the ultimate objective of disease control and prevention. From that perspective, available study designs (e.g., family studies, inbreeding studies, population surveys), and statistical techniques (e.g., segregation analysis, linkage analysis) should be considered the means rather than the end. Family studies represent one of several available study methods to explore the role of genetic factors in disease. Their design should follow sound epidemiologic guidelines as to case definition, sample representativeness, ascertainment methods, data collection pertaining to disease and exposures, and appropriate methods of analysis (Dorman et al., 1988). For example, if segregation analysis is performed on pedigrees of patients with a certain disorder, and evidence for a particular model of inheritance is seen, it is still difficult to make broad inferences about the underlying population if such pedigrees were not collected in a systematic and unbiased fashion. If the study sample was restricted to high-risk families or to referred patients from one specialty clinic, it may be difficult to generalize findings to the population at large. Although such evidence for genetic control may be extremely useful for further biologic research, it does not in itself provide answers concerning the contribution of genetic factors to the etiology of the disease in the population. Furthermore, statistical evidence in the form of a goodness of fit to a particular model from pedigree data remains tentative until specific and measurable genetic factors are documented, using molecular or biochemical methods. Studies of individual pedigrees or groups of pedigrees point to the fundamental distinction between genetic epidemiology and genetic analysis. While genetic analysis is a component of genetic epidemiology, genetic epidemiology is not limited to genetic analysis of family data. Thus, the relationship between genetic epidemiology and statistical genetics can be viewed as similar to the relationship between epidemiology and biostatistics. Although epidemiology relies heavily on the use of statistical techniques to plan, execute, and analyze etiologic studies, epidemiology and biostatistics have remained complementary but not synonymous over their history.

Accordingly, Figure 1–1 illustrates the scope of genetic epidemiology as the interface of genetic and environmental interaction in disease. Mutations are the basis for genetic variation in populations. Mutation can be broadly defined to include any alteration in the genetic material, including simple base substitutions (point mutations), rearrangement of genes, gross duplications or deletions of genetic material, and derangements of the entire chromosomal complement (e.g., aneuploidy). Mutations can occur in both germ cells and somatic cells, and both are influenced by environmental factors. Although somatic mutations may play an important role in both physiologic and pathologic processes and the occurrence of disease such as cancer (Omenn, 1983, 1988; Dulbecco, 1986), only germ-cell mutations can be transmitted across generations and contribute to the genetic constitution of the population and to the evolutionary process as a whole. The frequency of specific genotypes, the survival of germ-cell mutations in subsequent generations, and the frequency of the new mutation in a particular generation are determined by a balance between the occurrence and recurrence of such mutations (possibly influenced by environmental factors) and other dynamic population processes, such as selection, chance fluctuations, and mating patterns.

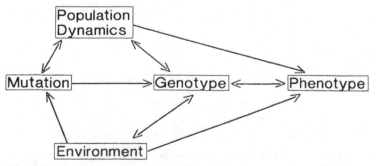

Figure 1–1. Scope of genetic epidemiology.

Diseases and other clinical phenotypes occur in relation to genetic factors in three ways that are not necessarily mutually exclusive:

1. The new mutation can be directly deleterious to the individual. This category includes numerous single-gene dominant disorders (such as achondroplasia and Marfan's syndrome) and chromosomal abnormalities (such as Down syndrome).
2. The new mutation may be deleterious, but could remain hidden over several generations. For example, in classic Mendelian autosomal recessive diseases such as the inborn errors of metabolism (e.g., galactosemia, phenylketonuria), the disease phenotype ensues only when individuals inherit two deleterious alleles, that is, one from each parent. This is obviously related to the dynamics and genetic structure of the population and will reflect inbreeding and the effective population size.
3. The mutation may be deleterious only when it interacts with other genetic and/or environmental factors.

Here, one can briefly contrast the scope of genetic epidemiology with those of traditional epidemiology and population genetics. While traditional epidemiology focuses on the relationship between the environment and the occurrence of disease (although recognizing the importance of the host and its genetic constitution), population genetics is largely devoted to predicting the consequences of population structure, selection, and mutation on genetic traits but is not restricted to questions of disease (Rao, 1984). Genetic epidemiology, on the other hand, includes the fundamental interaction between genetic variation (and its determinants) with the environment in the occurrence of disease. Such interaction transcends the cross-sectional view of any one generation (the focus of traditional epidemiology), and its effects may be observed longitudinally in the evolution of populations.

1.4. STRATEGIES OF GENETIC EPIDEMIOLOGY

The research strategies of genetic epidemiology include population and family study approaches that provide parallel and often overlapping methodologies for studying the role of genetic factors in disease (Table 1–3). Two broad but overlapping groups of studies are available: (1) descriptive studies, that involve the characterization of the distribution of genetic traits and diseases in populations or families, and (2) analytic studies, that involve the characterization of the determinants of the distribution of genetic traits and their role in health and disease in populations and families. The following is a brief overview of both population and family study approaches in genetic epidemiology. These topics are discussed in greater depth in subsequent chapters.

1.4.1. Population Study Approaches

An overview of population studies in genetic epidemiology is given in Figure 1–1. Population studies in genetic epidemiology include two facets: (1) the

Table 1–3. Population and family study approaches in genetic epidemiology

Approach	Population studies	Family studies
Descriptive	Distribution of genetic traits and disease in populations	Genetic traits and disease distribution in families
Analytic	Risk factors associated with the frequency of genetic traits in populations	Risk factors that may cause familial aggregation
	Role of genetic factors in disease etiology	Specific genetic mechanisms in families

study of the distribution and determinants of observable genetic traits in populations, and (2) the study of the role of genetic factors, many of which are not directly observable, in disease processes and other physiologic variations.

Study of Genetic Traits

Here, the term "genetic trait" (i.e., genetically determined trait) includes observable phenotypic traits, such as classic single-gene disorders, chromosomal abnormalities, and any genetically determined characteristic regardless of their association with disease phenotypes. Table 1–4 describes two broad

Table 1–4. Various strategies of population studies in genetic epidemiology

Aspects	Examples
Epidemiology of genetic traits	
Descriptive studies of the distribution of genetic traits	Estimation of mutation rate for achondroplasia Frequency of blood groups antigens, HLA haplotypes, sickle cell allele, cystic fibrosis in various populations
Analytic studies of the determinants of genetic traits	
New mutations	The effects of advanced maternal age on the frequency of maternally derived trisomy 21 cases.
Genetic traits	The effects of inbreeding and founder effect on the occurrence of autosomal recessive diseases
Epidemiologic study of genetic factors in disease	
Study of specific genetic traits in disease occurrence	HLA and disease associations; pharmacogenetic traits, (e.g., acetylator phenotype in bladder cancer, debrisoquine hydroxylation in lung cancer)
Analytic studies of unspecified genetic factors	Migrant studies Effects of inbreeding and racial admixture

types of population studies of genetic traits. The first consists of descriptive studies of the distribution of genetic traits in populations, in which the traditional epidemiologic questions of time, place, and person are applied to specific genetic traits. Examples of relevant questions are as follows: What is the frequency of achondroplasia at birth in a certain population, and can one estimate mutation rates for this autosomal dominant condition? What is the prevalence of certain blood group alleles and HLA antigens in different populations? What are the geographic differences in the frequency of a genetic trait?

The second type of population investigation of genetic traits consists of analytic studies of factors that influence the distribution of genetic traits in populations. Here the questions relate to why and how, and attempt to examine risk factors that may be involved in the occurrence of new mutations and in the distribution of existing genetic traits in populations. The distinction between new and existing genetic traits is important when searching for causative factors. New genetic traits in the offspring derive from mutations that occur in the parental germ cells such as chromosomal abnormalities and many single-gene mutations. The analytic strategy for studying such traits should include the evaluation of parental risk factors and environmental exposures. Two examples pertinent to the occurrence of new mutations are as follows: (1) Are there parental occupational exposures that affect the risk of certain chromosomal abnormalities or new dominant mutations? (2) What is the impact of advanced maternal age on the risk of maternal nondisjunction leading to Down's syndrome?

On the other hand, many genetic traits, such as autosomal recessive disorders, have been transmitted over one or more generations. The analytic strategy involves the evaluation of numerous social, demographic, cultural, and medical factors that can affect the transmission of these traits over generations, for example, the study of inbreeding, racial admixture, migration, and reproductive isolation. Traditionally, these types of studies fall into the realm of population genetics, but they can also have public health implications. The combination of epidemiologic approaches and the methods of population genetics can lead to a better understanding of the distribution and determinants of genetic traits in populations (see Chapter 4).

Some examples of analytic studies are also given in Table 1-4, and address such questions as the following: Why is the frequency of sickle cell allele higher in certain African populations than in other geographic areas? Why is the frequency of the Ellis-van Creveld syndrome high in the Old Order Amish in Lancaster County, Pennsylvania (McKusick, 1978)? These questions may seem trivial now because their answers have largely been worked out. For the sickle cell trait, the well-recognized explanation involves the selective forces which apparently operated in the presence of endemic falciparum malaria where a selective advantage in heterozygotes allowed rapid increases in the frequency of the recurring sickle cell mutation (see Chapter 4). For the Ellis-van Creveld syndrome, the answer appears to lie in the founder effect and genetic drift that can occur in small isolated populations (McKusick, 1978). For the vast majority of genetic traits, however, the complex interactions between the genetic structure of populations and forces of the environment remain largely unexplored.

Study of the Role of Genetic Factors in Disease

Using population studies, epidemiologic approaches can be applied to evaluate the role of genetic factors in disease occurrence (see Chapter 5). Genetic factors could be observed genetic traits (e.g., HLA, blood groups, DNA markers), or unobserved forces that are a function of the population structure. These include inbreeding effects on morbidity and mortality (e.g., Schull and Neel, 1965), racial admixture and outcrossing (Morton, 1967), migrant studies, and the study of the role of genetic drift in disease in small isolates (McKusick, 1978; Chakraborty and Szathmary, 1985).

While some genetic traits are always associated with a clinical phenotype and therefore can be considered the disease itself, other traits represent genetic variation present in normal individuals (e.g., blood group antigens, HLA antigens) which may confer increased susceptibility to certain diseases. One example of a disease genotype is trisomy 21, which has the clinical manifestations of Down syndrome. This example illustrates how classification of disease endpoints is heavily dependent on the status of biologic knowledge. Before chromosome studies were available, the clinical phenotype of Down syndrome, or mongolism was the only available endpoint for study. Our current knowledge of Down syndrome, based on available cytogenetic and molecular methods, not only permits discrimination between trisomy 21 and other chromosomal abnormalities in Down syndrome (e.g., translocation), but also permits classifying most cases by parental origin of the trisomy and its meiotic stage. The early epidemiologic studies of Down syndrome (Lilienfeld, 1969; Janerich and Bracken, 1986) can now be extended to the study of the epidemiology of sex- and stage-specific nondisjunction errors in the transmission of chromosome 21. This may lead to the identification of different risk factors and, thus, possibly to different prevention and intervention strategies.

For disorders of complex etiology such as many chronic diseases, however, specific observed genetic traits may be only one of several factors associated with the etiology of disease, and not all individuals with the specific genotype will develop clinical disease. For example, α_1-antitrypsin deficiency, due to homozygosity for the *PiZ* allele, is only one of possibly many causes of chronic obstructive pulmonary disease (COPD) (reviewed by Tockman et al., 1985). In this instance, the frequency of the *PiZ* allele in various populations should be considered along with other risk factors in studying the genetic epidemiology of COPD. Another example is the association between HLA-B27 and ankylosing spondylitis. Here, although most cases of the disease are associated with the HLA-B27 antigen, only a small fraction of individuals with HLA-B27 ever develop the disease (Ahearn and Hochberg, 1988). Thus, it is important in this situation to study the pathogenesis and natural history of disease in persons with HLA-B27, along with the interaction between HLA-B27 and other genetic or environmental factors that contribute to the development of this disease.

1.4.2. Family Study Approaches

The study of familial aggregation is a central theme in genetic epidemiology (King et al., 1984), and has been the focus of most of the methodological and statistical efforts. As pointed out by King et al. (1984), genetic epidemiology addresses three sequential questions in family studies:

1. Do diseases cluster in families?
2. Is familial clustering related to common environmental exposure, biologically inherited susceptibility, or cultural inheritance of risk factors?
3. How is genetic susceptibility inherited?

Unequivocally, these are three key questions in family study approaches in genetic epidemiology and are addressed in greater detail in Chapters 6 through 9. Here, a summary of the epidemiologic and genetic methodologies that can be applied in family studies is presented (Table 1–5).

Classically, the first question is approached epidemiologically, either by looking at disease frequency in relatives of cases and controls, or by comparing disease frequency in relatives of cases with that in the general population and computing some measure of relative risk (see Chapter 6). The occurrence of a high degree of familial aggregation (i.e., a high relative risk), however, does not prove the existence of a genetic mechanism nor does a low relative risk preclude a genetic mechanism. Infectious diseases frequently cluster in families (Susser, 1985; Susser and Susser 1987a, 1987b); and some noninfectious diseases may cluster because of similar life-styles and cultural patterns. On the other hand, single-gene disorders can also give low relative risks at certain gene frequencies (Weiss et al., 1982). Incomplete penetrance in a genetic form of the disease can further undermine the use of the case-control approach to measure familial aggregation (Majumder et al., 1983; Khoury et

Table 1–5. Strategies of family studies in genetic epidemiology

	Study approaches	
Question	*Epidemiologic*	*Genetic*
Does the disease or trait cluster in families?	Comparison of disease frequency in relatives of affected individuals with the general population or with disease frequency in relatives of unaffected individuals	
What are the causes of familial aggregation?	Search for known risk factors shared among relatives	Heritability analysis (variance components, path analysis) to estimate the overall role of genetic factors
What is the genetic model of inheritance?		Segregation and linkage analyses in pedigrees

Adapted from King et al. (1984).

al., 1990), as unaffected controls may carry the disease genotype without expressing it, and therefore have relatives at high risk. Under these conditions, tests for specific modes of inheritance may be compromised by misclassification (Chapter 6).

The second question is addressed by using both genetic and epidemiologic approaches that could be applied to quantitative and qualitative traits. Epidemiologic methods can be used to determine whether the familial aggregation has a nonMendelian basis, such as clustering by calendar year versus age at onset, birth order, and/or birth interval effects (Susser, 1985; Susser and Susser 1987a). An example of nonMendelian clustering is the occurrence of neural tube defects among siblings of cases, which shows a decline with increasing intervals from the birth of the index case (Yen and MacMahon, 1968). Epidemiologic methods can also be used to determine whether the increased risk of disease among relatives remains after controlling for potentially confounding factors. In various studies of COPD (Cohen et al., 1978; Cohen, 1980) and coronary heart disease (ten Kate et al., 1982), examination of numerous variables indicates that the increased risk among relatives cannot be accounted for by other factors, and investigators are left with the inference that the increased risk may be due to genetic factors (although unmeasured environmental factors cannot be completely ruled out). One proposed extension of this approach involves separating familial aggregation into indirect and direct components. In a study of COPD, it was postulated that if first-degree relatives of COPD patients tended to smoke more than first-degree relatives of controls and smoking per se was related to COPD, then smoking could be an indirect cause of familial aggregation (Khoury et al., 1985a). In this study, several indirect components of familial aggregation in COPD were detected. Nevertheless, a residual (direct) component was still significant after adjustment for all available intermediate factors. While this direct component could be genetic or environmental in nature, the absence of this component when spouses were examined, in contrast to its presence in sibs, strongly suggests the involvement of genetic factors.

The second question posed by King et al. (1984) can also be approached by using genetic methods. The multifactorial model of inheritance is the common framework for these analyses. This model, discussed in detail in Chapter 7, uses statistical methods of analysis of variance and path analysis to infer the degree of genetic control in either quantitative or qualitative traits. Briefly, the multifactorial model states that the phenotype is a linear function of independent, unobservable genetic and environmental factors, but it sheds little light on biologic mechanisms for either the genetic or environmental factors. Because relatives share genes in a predictable fashion and may also share environments in some defined manner, the covariance or correlation among relatives can be separated into components attributable to genetic differences and components attributable to environmental differences. When the phenotype is discrete (i.e., affected versus nonaffected), the statistical model assumes that an underlying continuous trait (termed *liability*) dictates risk of disease, and the analysis is then designed to estimate the correlation in this liability among relatives (Curnow and Smith, 1975; Elston,

1981). A crucial limitation of this model, however, is its inability to separate genetic sources of correlation in liability from environmental sources. If environmental factors influencing liability are also shared among relatives, the estimate of heritability will be inflated (See chapter 7).

When dealing with quantitative measures of risk factors for common diseases (e.g., lipid levels associated with heart disease), this same linear multifactorial model proves quite useful. Here the statistical models take on the form of a classic random effects analysis of variance model, and variance components due to genetic factors and a number of specified nongenetic shared environments can be estimated. Although long used for fixed samples of relatives (twins, full sibs, etc.), this approach can also be used on pedigrees of arbitrary structure (Lange et al., 1976). Fixed effects (such as sex-specific means, linear effects of covariates, or even genetic markers) may be included in the model, and the effects of shared environments may follow a predetermined pattern or may be time dependent (Hopper and Mathews, 1983).

The commonly used alternative to variance components models is path analysis (Wright, 1934), which also is based on the multifactorial linear model and can estimate "components of correlation." Although a single phenotypic trait in nuclear families does not provide a sufficient number of observed correlations for separating genetic from environmental factors, Rao and colleagues (1974) proposed that an index of environmental factors influencing the trait be used as a second phenotype to provide more observed correlations among members of a nuclear family. This approach has been widely applied to a number of phenotypic traits associated with common diseases (Rao, 1990), and allows the role of genetic factors to be estimated while adjusting for correlations due to specified patterns of shared environments among relatives.

The difficulty in discriminating between genetic and environmental causes of familial aggregation of diseases or traits under the multifactorial model of inheritance partly arises from the imbalance in the specification of the underlying mechanisms. While the genetic component of the multifactorial model is well understood in terms of both the biologic mechanism and its statistical implications, the environmental component is left entirely to the speculation of the investigator. Within the constraints of the statistical model, the effects of various shared nongenetic factors can be estimated (shared sib or parent-offspring environments, time-dependent environments, or culturally transmitted environments); however, these comprise only a few of the possible shared environmental factors and were chosen because of their statistical tractability rather than any underlying biologic mechanism. The goal of the general multifactorial model remains to quantitate the importance of genetic factors in the presence of an arbitrary nongenetic alternative.

If both evidence of familial aggregation and genetic control are suggested for a disease or quantitative phenotype, the third question is to identify the responsible genetic mechanism. For this purpose, the techniques of segregation analysis are useful to test for Mendelian transmission of the phenotypes (discrete or quantitative) in pedigree data (covered in detail in Chapter 8). These methodologies yield maximum likelihood estimators for key genetic parameters (Elston and Stewart, 1971; Cannings et al, 1978; Hasstedt, 1982). The parameters include transmission probabilities, gene frequencies, and penetrance parameters in Mendelian models; heritability, sample means and variances in polygenic models; and both types of parameters in what is termed the "mixed model" (Morton, 1982, 1983). The value of this latter mixed model is that it allows specific tests of hypotheses to discriminate between a single-locus model and polygenic inheritance. The disadvantage of the mixed model is that all environmental sources of correlation are lumped into a single polygenic component that can overestimate the role of genetic factors (see Chapter 8).

If a single-locus model is found to explain the distribution of a disease or trait in families best, the possibility still remains that a nongenetic mechanism may be the true etiologic agent, and it is merely mimicking a genetic mechanism as illustrated by Lilienfeld (1959) and McGuffin and Huckle (1990). This is especially true when the families are small. The final bit of statistical evidence for Mendelian inheritance can come from demonstrating genetic linkage with a known genetic marker, using statistical methods and other mapping strategies (see Chapter 9). The likelihood of a nongenetic mechanism cosegregating with a genetic marker (e.g., blood types, HLA types, or DNA marker) seems remote enough to justify classifying a disease as Mendelian, even in the absence of direct biochemical evidence of the gene product, if the answers to all of the three key questions consistently point to a genetic etiology, and particularly if evidence for linkage is found.

1.5. GENETIC EPIDEMIOLOGY AND DISEASE CONTROL AND PREVENTION

As indicated previously, genetic epidemiology plays a significant role in the practice of public health and the delivery of intervention and prevention strategies. While the subject is considered further in Chapter 10, an overview is presented here of four areas that have long been of interest to geneticists and epidemiologists alike.

1.5.1. Disease Surveillance and Registries

The interest in keeping records of individuals with specific diseases is shared by epidemiologists and geneticists for the purposes of health-care delivery, resource allocation and research (Robertson, 1983). An additional goal of disease registries is to monitor the occurrence of various conditions (such as cancer and birth defects; genetic indices such as sister chromatid exchange) that serve as early signals for possible detrimental effects of environmental factors. For example, birth defect registries have been useful in obtaining epidemiologic data on the occurrence of various malformations, monitoring for potential environmental teratogens, and conducting follow-up etiologic and family studies (Holtzman and Khoury, 1986; Cordero, 1992). Disease registries have been constructed using record linkage procedures on individuals and families (Baldwin et al, 1987; Newcombe, 1987). A further development in genetic epidemiology has been the use of family-based registries that record health events in either nuclear families or population-based genealogies (Fineman and Jorde, 1980; Schull and Weiss, 1980). Such genealogical registries provide a powerful tool for studying the genetic transmission of specific disease processes and for examining genetic-environmental interaction in disease.

1.5.2. Disease Intervention

A significant requisite in the development and evaluation of therapeutic regimens for disease intervention has been the rapidly expanding field of clinical trials where epidemiologic methods are applied in experimental settings (Meinert, 1986). Unfortunately, in many double-blind studies designed to test the value of new therapies, the importance of differential genetic susceptibility to drug effects and reactions has not been given adequate consideration. Despite numerous reports from pharmacogenetic studies demonstrating individual differences in the way drugs are handled and metabolized in the body and their possible implication in disease processes (e.g., Cartwright et al., 1982; Caparoso et al., 1989a; Lennard et al., 1990), such problems are rarely considered in the clinical trials literature. With the accumulating advances in the field, and the increasing scope and complexity of clinical trials, it has become clear that such knowledge needs to be recognized and incorporated into the design of clinical trials as well as their interpretation.

Intervention studies in classic genetic diseases (e.g., low phenylalanine diet in phenylketonuria and thyroid hormone treatment in congenital hypothyroidism) also might benefit from epidemiologic methods in their design, conduct, and analysis. In a disorder of less defined etiology, both geneticists and epidemiologists have joined efforts in studying whether periconceptual multivitamin supplementation can prevent the recurrence of neural tube defects in families with an already affected child (Laurence et al., 1981; Wald and Polani, 1984), and in studying the occurrence of neural tube defects in the general population (Mulinare et al., 1988: Mills et al., 1989; Milunsky et al., 1989). The initial report of the clinical trial by Smithells et al. (1981) drew much criticism because of deficiencies in its design (Edwards, 1981; Holmes-Snedle et al, 1982), underscoring the importance of epidemiologic principles in such studies. More recently, the protective effect of periconceptual folic acid in preventing the recurrence of neural tube defects has been unequivocally documented using a controlled clinical trial (MRC, 1991).

1.5.3. Disease Prevention

Screening, counseling, prenatal diagnosis and carrier detection are several of the strategies applied in the prevention of genetically mediated conditions. While the use of these procedures is clearly recognized for many Mendelian conditions, their application in common diseases is not well established. The methodologies of genetic epidemiology can be applied in the area of disease prevention. Combining information about risk factors (both genetic and environmental) in populations and within families to delineate genetic-environmental interactions can be most useful in devising prevention strategies that target appropriate "high risk" groups (see Chapter 10). For example, there has been a growing interest in applying genetic screening in the workplace for the purpose of detecting hypersusceptible workers (Calabrese, 1981; Omenn, 1982; Office of Technology and Assessment, 1983; Holtzman, 1989). While only a few genetic markers have been considered for screening purposes (Omenn, 1982), more will become available in the near future as a result of improved genetic technology (Holtzman, 1989). Epidemiologic principles should be applied to evaluate the usefulness of a specific genetic marker for screening purposes considering the frequency of the marker, the relationship between the marker and the disease, and the disease frequency in the population (Newill et al., 1986). In addition, ethical, social, and political issues must be addressed in the evaluation of any genetic screening program (Holtzman, 1989; Suzuki and Knudston, 1989). The applications of genetic epidemiology in disease prevention are further discussed in Chapter 10.

1.5.4. The Impact of Disease in Populations

Finally, the impact of genetically mediated disease in the population, in terms of morbidity, hospitalizations, mortality, handicap, and cost to society, is also of mutual interest to geneticists and epidemiologists. To assess the effects of genetic diseases on the population, several investigators have previously quantitated the proportion of hospital admissions due to single-gene, chromosomal, and multifactorial diseases (reviewed by Porter, 1982). Most studies have found that a substantial proportion of pediatric admissions are due to genetic factors, although epidemiologic considerations that pertain to the nature of the studied hospital (teaching versus primary care hospitals) must be taken into account. Much work remains to be done to assess the impact of genetic factors in common diseases on the public's health. This could be best accomplished by combining information on genetic risk factors with the application of epidemiologic measures of risk assessment.

1.6. CONCLUDING REMARKS

This chapter has outlined the scope of genetic epidemiology and pointed out that genetic epidemiology extends beyond genetics and epidemiology. Genetic epidemiology must approach disease causation in an integrated fashion by addressing the interaction of "nature and nurture" rather than pursuing "nature versus nurture." The strategies of genetic epidemiology include both population and family studies. Population studies include (1) the study of the distribution and determinants of genetic traits as endpoints, and (2) the study of the role of both specific and nonspecific genetic factors in disease processes. Family studies include (1) the evaluation of familial clustering of disease, (2) the search for genetic and environmental causes for such clustering, and

(3) the application of statistical techniques to test for specific genetic mechanisms. In addition, it is noted that genetic epidemiology is as much involved in disease prevention as are its two parent disciplines. As genetic epidemiology seeks to unravel the role of specific genetic and environmental factors in disease etiology, it must incorporate such findings into the development of intervention and prevention strategies.

Throughout the book, the need to apply both genetic and epidemiologic concepts and methods to the study of disease processes in human populations is emphasized. Unlike other fields of epidemiology (such as chronic disease epidemiology), where the etiology of specific diseases is studied by using epidemiologic methods, genetic epidemiology is unique in that it brings to epidemiology its own methods of studying biologic mechanisms of disease, as well as a host of analytic techniques. Finally, the continued growth of genetic epidemiology will depend not only on further developments in statistical techniques, but also on multidisciplinary collaboration with researchers in other biologic disciplines. Such an interaction is crucial to understanding the role of genetic and environmental factors in disease processes in terms of basic biologic mechanisms.

2

Fundamental Genetic Concepts and Approaches

2.1. INTRODUCTION

To understand the role of genetic factors in the occurrence of disease in human populations, it is important to have a basic knowledge of the structure and function of the genetic material as well as the principles underlying its transmission in families and populations. Only a brief outline of genetics is presented here; the reader is referred to several excellent textbooks for more details (Hartl, 1983; Thompson and Thompson, 1986; Vogel and Motulsky, 1986; Levitan, 1988; Sutton, 1988; Gelehter and Collins, 1990). In the past 15 years there has been remarkable progress in human genetics. Today we can examine the genetic material directly, and, consequently, we have a better understanding of the structure and function of genes. This information permits greater insight into the role of genes in disease processes in both individuals and populations.

2.2. THE GENETIC MATERIAL

Although cell biologists in the late 1800s suspected that the colored material in the cell nucleus (termed *chromatin*) carried the genetic material of the cell, it was not until the beginning of the twentieth century that the *chromosomes* (colored bodies) were actually described. The chromatin encapsulated in the nucleus is a complex of polymers of deoxyribonucleic acid (*DNA*) and basic proteins called *histones*.

2.2.1. Chromosomes

Human nuclear DNA is organized into 22 pairs of autosomal chromosomes and 2 sex-specific chromosomes (called X and Y) that become visible microscopically only during cell division. Since humans are diploid, there are two copies of each autosome in the cell nucleus; each parent donates one of each pair. Each chromosome is composed of two arms separated by a centromere; by convention the shorter arm is denoted p and the longer arm is denoted q. Before the development of staining techniques that revealed distinct bands along the chromosomal arms, chromosomes could be grouped only by their size and the relative length of the two arms. Three types of chromosomes were noted in humans: *metacentric*, where the arms are of approximately equal length, *submetacentric*, where the centromere is not centrally located and one arm is shorter than the other, and *acrocentric*, where one chromosomal arm is extremely short. Each species has a characteristic chromosomal complement with both the number and structure of the chromosomes varying across species, but constant within species (except for pathologic conditions).

Figure 2–1 is a diagram of 24 types of human chromosomes: 22 autosomes and the two sex chromosomes, X and Y. The 46 chromosomes of the normal human complement are composed of 22 pairs of homologous autosomes present in all individuals, and one pair that varies between males and females. Normally, females carry two medium-sized submetacentric X chromosomes (and thus are the *homogametic* sex), while males carry only one X chromosome and one small acrocentric Y chromosome (and thus are the *heterogametic* sex).

In most cell divisions, the duplicated nuclear material divides into daughter cells by a process called *mitosis*, the only cell division process for all *somatic* cells. In reproductive or *germinal* cells, a different process, called *meiosis*, occurs. The behavior of a hypothetical chromosome pair in mitosis and meiosis is illustrated in Figures 2–2 and 2–3, respectively. The fundamental difference between these two types of cell division is that mitosis exactly replicates the entire genetic complement in each daughter cell, with no changes in chromosome number or arrangement, while meiosis results in a systematic reduction of the usual diploid number (46 or 23 pairs for humans) into haploid daughter cells with 23 chromosomes, each having one member of each pair. Thus, when two haploid gametes (sperm and ova) fuse to form a new zygote, the original diploid complement of 46 chromosomes is restored. Moreover, in meiosis, there is *independent assortment* of chromosomes of maternal and paternal origin within each of the 22 homologous pairs of autosomes, as well as *random assortment* of the sex chromosomes into the resulting haploid daughter cells that will go on to develop into gametes. Along with the *genetic recombination* due to *crossing over* between loci located along the length of the chromosomes, this random assortment or independent segregation of homologous chromosomes guarantees a large number of different combinations of genetic traits at each generation.

2.2.2. Genes

While nuclear DNA is organized into these separate and distinct chromosomes, the basic unit of hereditary information is the gene or locus, which codes for some gene product (an enzyme or a structural protein). The tra-

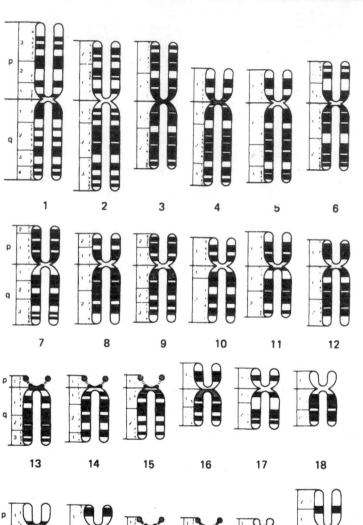

Figure 2–1. Diagrammatic representation of human chromosomes showing G-banding patterns for 22 autosomes and sex-specific chromosomes (X and Y) [From Moody (1975), p. 297.]

ditional diagram of the gene as an uninterrupted sequence of DNA is overly simplistic, as eukaryotic genes are composed of lengths of DNA in which the coding sequences (*exons*) are interrupted by *intervening sequences* (IVS or *introns*). Although these introns are initially transcribed to messenger RNA (*mRNA*), they are not present in the mature mRNA delivered to the cyto-

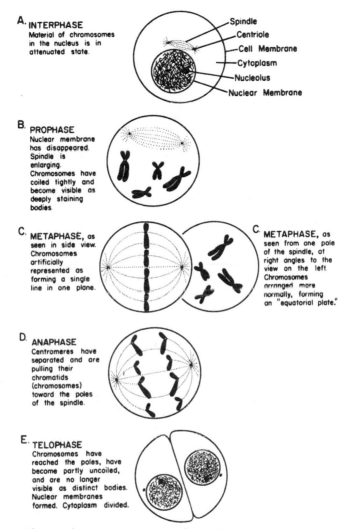

A. **INTERPHASE**
Material of chromosomes
in the nucleus is in
attenuated state.

Spindle
Centriole
Cell Membrane
Cytoplasm
Nucleolus
Nuclear Membrane

B. **PROPHASE**
Nuclear membrane
has disappeared.
Spindle is
enlarging.
Chromosomes have
coiled tightly and
become visible as
deeply staining
bodies.

C. **METAPHASE,** as
seen in side view.
Chromosomes
artificially
represented as
forming a single
line in one plane.

C. **METAPHASE,** as
seen from one pole
of the spindle, at
right angles to the
view on the left.
Chromosomes
arranged more
normally, forming
an "equatorial plate."

D. **ANAPHASE**
Centromeres have
separated and are
pulling their
chromatids
(chromosomes)
toward the poles
of the spindle.

E. **TELOPHASE**
Chromosomes have
reached the poles, have
become partly uncoiled,
and are no longer
visible as distinct bodies.
Nuclear membranes
formed. Cytoplasm divided.

Figure 2–2. Phases of mitosis. [From Moody (1975), p. 297.]

plasm and are thus never translated into protein sequences, that is, they are
not part of the final gene product. Small flanking regions of DNA at both
ends of the gene are important in the initiation and control of transcription,
and mutations in these regions can affect how the gene functions. While the
molecular structure of a gene is quite complex, it is important to remember
that the genes (even large ones) can still be thought of as discrete units located
at specific sites along a chromosome, that is, the terms *gene* and *locus* can
be used interchangeably.

At a given locus, many different forms of a gene representing individual
mutations may exist, and these are termed *alleles*. Each person carries two
copies of every autosomal gene, and these alleles may or may not be different.
Heterozygous individuals have two different alleles, while *homozygous* in-

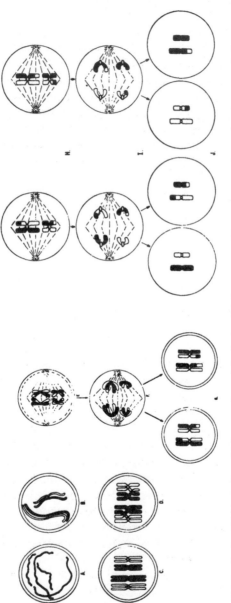

Figure 2–3. Phases of meiosis: prophase I includes (A) leptotene, (B) zygotene, (C) pachytene, (D) diakineses. The first division concludes with (E) metaphase I, (F) anaphase I, and (G) telophase I; resulting in two germ cells with completely duplicated haploid sets of chromosome. The second division is essentially a mitotic division with prophase II followed by metaphase II (H), anaphase II (I), and telophase II (J). [From Fraser and Nora (1975), pp. 14–15.]

dividuals have two copies of the same allele. Females also carry two alleles at all loci on the X chromosome, but males are *hemizygous* for every locus on both the X and Y chromosomes. It is important to note that more than one molecular event (i.e., more than one mutation) can give rise to a new allelic variant; this is especially true for alleles resulting in the absence of a functional gene product, sometimes termed *null alleles*. Thus, there may be more than one allelic form of the same genetic disease resulting from a deficiency of a given gene product. Furthermore, some alleles lead to partial deficiencies or to production of an altered gene product. Consequently, there is wide variation in the phenotypic expression of genetic traits: some alleles are associated directly with disease processes, while others contribute to the "normal" genetic variation seen in all human populations. Many genes have one or several alleles represented at high frequencies in populations, and such loci are said to be *polymorphic*. Typically, a *polymorphism* exists when the most frequent allele has a frequency of less than 0.99 in a population.

Although disease alleles can attain polymorphic frequencies under certain circumstances, many polymorphic loci represent neutral *genetic markers*, including antigenically defined blood groups (e.g., ABO and Rh blood groups), enzyme variants (usually detected by electrophoresis), and other cellular antigens (e.g., the immunologically defined HLA antigens). Genetic markers not causally related to any disease can still be extremely useful if *genetic linkage* or *cosegregation* can be demonstrated between the marker locus and a locus controlling a disease. While many marker alleles represent altered gene products, there is also variability outside the formal coding regions of the genes. Such genetic variability can be detected by looking at the DNA itself. These *DNA polymorphisms* are measured as differences in the lengths of fragments of DNA digested by restriction endonucleases (enzymes that cleave the DNA at specific nucleotide sequences). Two main classes of DNA polymorphisms can be detected. The first class is termed restriction fragment length polymorphisms (*RFLPs*), where a mutation occurs at the recognition site for a restriction enzyme (usually a small sequence of four to six nucleotides), resulting in two allelic forms: one where the site is recognized (and thus cleaved) and one where it is not. The second class of DNA polymorphisms reflect variation in the number of tandem repeats of small sequences of DNA (usually three to six nucleotides) in noncoding regions. There is considerable variation in the number of these short repeated segments of DNA among individuals, and thus many allelic forms termed variable number of tandem repeats (VNTR) exist in populations. Similar to these VNTR alleles, there is also variability in the number of single nucleotides that can serve as genetic markers in regions immediately adjacent to exons.

2.3. THE GENETIC MATERIAL IN DISEASE

Because genes specify the coding of proteins that in turn constitute the structural and functional building blocks of the human organism, any alteration in the genetic material that leads to a disturbance in the structure and/or function of a vital protein (enzyme or structural protein) can result in disease. *Mutation* is broadly defined as any change in the genetic material, and thus many mutations will disrupt the structure and function of gene products. Mutations can range from single-base substitutions in the DNA up to and including alterations involving large chromosomal segments. Mutations can occur in both somatic and germinal cells, but only germinal mutations are heritable and transmitted to subsequent generations. Mutations also provide the genetic variability upon which natural selection operates to produce changes in the genetic structure of populations over time. Factors that affect the occurrence of mutations and interact with the environment, as well as the genetic structure of the population in producing disease, are central to the study of genetic epidemiology.

2.3.1. Germinal Mutations

Only mutations in germinal cells can be transmitted to offspring, and only germinal mutations are subject to the evolutionary pressures of natural selection. In this section, the two main types of germinal mutations are reviewed: mutations involving individual genes and chromosomal mutations.

Gene Mutations

Mutations can occur in exons, introns, the regulatory sequences surrounding coding regions, and in noncoding regions of the DNA. The impact of mutations on the structure of the resulting proteins can range from nil to total disruption of the functional gene, leading to deficiency of the final gene product. Single base substitutions do not always lead to changes in the amino acid sequence of the gene product because the genetic code is degenerate, i.e., more than one triplet of bases can code for the same amino acid. However, a single base substitution causing premature termination of transcription results in the absence of a functional gene product. Depending on the ultimate role of the gene product, this can lead to disease. A classic example of *base substitution* or *point mutation* is that of sickle cell hemoglobin, in which a single base change leads to substitution of glutamic acid by valine in the sixth amino acid of the β-globin chain of the hemoglobin molecule. This single amino acid difference leads to an altered hemoglobin molecule (*S* hemoglobin) with different electrophoretic mobility and altered response to some physiologic conditions. This leads to the clinical manifestation of sickle cell disease in persons homozygous for the *S* allele.

Insertion or deletion of one or two nucleotides results in *frameshift mutations*, because the genetic code is read in triplets, and such mutations will alter the reading frame of all the remaining DNA in the coding sequence. Frameshift mutations can also cause premature termination of translation if they result in converting a codon into the stop signal for translation. Conversely, a frameshift mutation may alter an existing stop signal and, therefore, may result in an altered gene product where codons beyond the usual exon are translated. Analysis of variant hemoglobins has provided several examples of such mutations involving the stop codon (e.g., hemoglobin Constant Spring has a β-globin chain with six additional amino acids, while hemoglobin McKees Rock has a β-globin chain with two fewer amino acids) (Vogel and Motulsky, 1986).

Mutations can also occur in regulatory DNA sequences outside the exons, and in sequences critical for proper splicing of the mRNA before its translation into the protein gene product. Such mutations in regulatory sequences can alter the usual process of transcription and translation, leading to abnormal rates of production of an otherwise normal gene product. For example, the many β-thalassemia mutations reflect defects in gene regulation (Orkin and Kazazian, 1984).

When considering the overall impact of mutations on the occurrence of disease, it is important to establish the mode of expression of a mutant allele. If the phenotype (e.g., a disease or trait) is altered by a mutant allele, in both the homozygous and the heterozygous states, the disease or trait is said to be *dominant*. If the phenotype is altered only in the homozygous state, the disease or trait is said to be *recessive*. When both alleles in heterozygotes are fully expressed, that is, the heterozygote is phenotypically distinct from the two homozygotes, the trait is said to be *codominant*. Dominance and recessivity are merely relative concepts, however, and depend on the level of the phenotypic analysis. For example, in the case of sickle cell hemoglobin, heterozygous individuals have both normal and sickle cell hemoglobin detectable by electrophoresis, and heterozygotes can even produce sickling of the red blood cells if exposed to low oxygen pressures. Thus, the sickle cell allele can be described as codominant at the biochemical and physiologic levels. However, sickle cell disease (manifesting as severe anemia accompanying repeated sickling crises) occurs only in homozygotes, since the presence of one-half the usual amount of normal hemoglobin in heterozygotes compensates for the abnormal sickle cell hemoglobin. Thus, sickle cell disease is autosomal recessive.

The variety of known single-gene disorders (autosomal dominant, autosomal recessive, and X-linked) has been cataloged and periodically updated by V. A. McKusick (1990). The number of such diseases, both confirmed and suspected, has grown remarkably over time and includes more than 4000 conditions. These diseases are referred to as *Mendelian* disorders because they follow Mendel's laws for single gene transmission in families (see section 2.4.1). In general, Mendelian disorders, considered individually, are quite rare. Some have been reported only in isolated families, while others are present mainly in small isolated populations or their descendants. A few genetic disorders have reached substantial frequencies in certain populations, and these represent situations where the allele for a recessive disease may be associated with a selective advantage in the heterozygote. For example, sickle cell anemia represents a major public health burden in many West African populations, and the thalassemias are a major public health problem in certain Mediterranean populations. Both situations are thought to reflect an increased fitness of the heterozygote in the presence of endemic malaria.

Chromosome Mutations

Chromosomal mutations include abnormalities of chromosome number and aberrations of chromosome structure, and they represent a form of genetic disease distinct from the Mendelian diseases. Numerical abnormalities include (1) those that lead to multiples of the entire haploid complement of chromosomes (*polyploid*), such as *triploidy* (69 chromosomes or 3 haploid sets) and *tetraploidy* (96 chromosomes or 4 haploid sets), and (2) those that lead to a number that is not a simple multiple of the haploid set, referred to as *aneuploidy*. Polyploidy in humans is generally lethal. Aneuploidies usually involve only one chromosome and can involve an extra chromosome or *trisomy* (e.g., trisomy 21 in Down syndrome), or the deletion of one chromosome or *monosomy* (e.g., Turner syndrome or 45,X). Aneuploidy generally results from a failure of chromosomes to separate at one of the two meiotic divisions, termed *nondisjunction*. Nondisjunction may occur at the first division, where two homologous chromosomes fail to segregate, or at the second division, where the two replicated copies of a single chromosome fail to separate. In either case, one or more gametes contain an extra chromosome, while other gametes have one too few. Whenever nondisjunction occurs in a mitotic division, the resulting line of daughter cells will have different chromosomal complements, and the individual is said to be *mosaic*.

Recent improvements in the techniques of chromosome banding have led to better identification of chromosome structure and the detection of *heteromorphisms* (variants in the banding patterns of the separate chromosomes), *fragile sites* (unstained gaps in otherwise normal appearing chromosomes), and better delineation of minute chromosomal alterations and rearrangements of chromosomal segments that are important in certain diseases. Aberrations of chromosome structure can involve *deletions*, *duplications*, and *rearrangements* of parts of chromosomes. Rearrangements can involve inversions of segments of a single chromosome or *translocations*, in which there is an exchange of large lengths of DNA between two nonhomologous chromosomes.

Chromosomal aberrations usually lead to more severe phenotypic disturbances than do single-gene mutations because they involve many genes and often result in multiple congenital anomalies. Human polyploidy is usually incompatible with life, and affected fetuses frequently are spontaneously lost early in gestation. The toll of chromosomal abnormalities on prenatal loss is extremely high. Studies of spontaneous abortuses show that 50% or more have some form of chromosomal abnormalities, while only 0.5% to 1% of live-born infants are affected (Kline et al., 1989). On the other hand, some chromosomal abnormalities may be quite subtle (e.g., deletions of a small part of one arm or tiny rearrangements). Such abnormalities may involve only a few genes and can be transmitted in families like single-gene disorders, usually with a dominant expression of the affected phenotype, but there may be considerable variation in its expression. With the advent of high-resolution banding, several apparent single-gene disorders have recently been found to involve minute chromosomal deletions (e.g., deletion of 15q11 in the Prader-Willi syndrome, and 11p13 in aniridia-Wilms tumor syndrome). Thus, the boundary between single-gene and chromosomal mutations has recently become blurred, and this overlap is likely to increase.

2.3.2. Somatic Mutations

Gene and chromosome mutations can also occur in somatic cells. Although these are not heritable, mounting evidence suggests that they play an important role in the pathogenesis of human disease, notably cancer. For example, in many types of cancer, several consistent chromosomal changes have been observed. One example is that of the translocation between chromosomes 9 and 22 observed in chronic myelogenous leukemia (the so-called Philadelphia chromosome).

In addition to chromosomal changes in neoplasia, recently a group of cellular genes called *oncogenes* have been shown to have increased activity in some cancers. Transforming viruses act by incorporating segments of host oncogenes into their own genome, where they play a role in neoplastic transformation of host cells. In addition to retroviral involvement, oncogenes may be important in the genesis of cancer by other mechanisms (e.g., point mutations, increased gene dosage by gene amplification, and DNA or chromosomal rearrangements). In Burkitt's lymphoma, where a translocation between chromosomes 8 and 14 is frequently seen in tumor cells, the *c-myc* oncogene has been located to a particular break-point on chromosome 8 (8q24). Translocation transfers the oncogene *c-myc* to the immunoglobulin heavy-chain region on chromosome 14, where it may influence the highly active immunoglobulin gene complex involved in the genesis of the lymphoma. The relationship among cancer, viruses, chromosomes, and oncogenes is only beginning to unravel.

2.4. THE GENETIC MATERIAL IN FAMILIES

Recent advances in human genetics have altered the concept of the structure of genes. Furthermore, evidence from other species raises the possibility that transposition of genetic material, gene conversions, amplification, and imprinting may underlie some diseases previously thought to follow simple Mendelian inheritance. Nevertheless, the principles of Mendelian transmission, both in families and in populations, still hold, and these serve as the cornerstone of genetic analysis.

2.4.1. Mendelian Principles

The first cohesive explanation of the inheritance of discrete traits was developed by Gregor Mendel in 1865. From his breeding experiments with pea plants, Mendel developed the concept that pairs of unobserved "factors" were responsible for physical traits in individuals, and single members of these pairs were transmitted unaltered from parent to offspring. Mendel's results are summarized into two basic principles: (1) the principle of *segregation* of alleles, and (2) the principle of *independent assortment*.

The principle of segregation treats the gene as the unit of heredity. While Mendel had no physical evidence for genes, he hypothesized that each individual carried pairs of genetic "factors," having received one member of each pair from the father and one from the mother. When an individual contributed a "factor" to the next generation, a random process determined which member of the parental pair went to any given offspring.

Mendel used a simple experimental design, where pure breeding lines were crossed and their resulting progeny were interbred to show that each of seven phenotypic traits consistently followed a regular pattern in subsequent generations. It was this reappearance of both forms of the trait that led Mendel to conclude that the underlying "factor" was passed unaltered and in a random fashion to offspring. The Punnett square in Figure 2–4 is a useful tool for illustrating the expected probabilities.

After carefully documenting this pattern for seven different phenotypic traits, Mendel considered two phenotypic traits simultaneously and showed that combinations of two phenotypes were consistent with complete independence between the underlying "factors" controlling the different traits. The number of phenotypic combinations increased of course, but the regularity of the segregation was maintained, and the observed frequencies of the phenotypic classes were consistent with simple multiplication of probabilities. In essence, when dealing with 2 independent genes, there are 4 possible gametes, and the Punnett square expands to a 4×4 matrix. In general, if there are n distinct and independent genes, each with 2 alleles, there are 2^n possible gametes and 3^n possible genotypes. The exact number of phenotypic combinations will, however, depend on the dominance relationship between alleles controlling any given trait.

Because of the profound nature of Mendel's work, it was not widely understood and accepted for over 30 years. The fundamental difficulty was that Mendel could offer no observable biologic basis for his proposed mechanism. All his observations clearly pointed to segregation of "factors," but there was no physical evidence for these "factors." By the 1840s cytologists had already suggested that the contents of the cell nucleus carried the hereditary material as the chromosomes appearing in mitotic cell division. But mitosis offered no confirmation of Mendel's work because this is the mech-

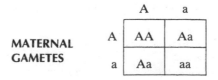

Figure 2–4. Punnett square showing genotypes possible for a single Mendelian locus with two alleles.

anism of cell division that exactly preserves the entire genetic constitution of the cell. However, in 1902 two workers (Walther Sutton and Theodor Boveri) independently published papers describing the parallels between Mendel's laws and the behavior of chromosomes during meiosis, the mechanism of cell division necessary for sexual reproduction. They pointed out that if one substitutes the term "chromosome" for Mendel's general term "factor," the terms segregation and independent assortment perfectly describe the movement of chromosomes in meiosis.

2.4.2. Patterns of Single Locus Inheritance

Mendelian principles have been successfully applied to the study of transmission of single-gene traits and diseases in families. This section briefly reviews the patterns of single-locus inheritance observed in families. Formal statistical methods that test for segregation in families are presented in Chapter 8. Summarized here are the simplest mechanisms for transmission of single-gene traits or disorders (terms that may be used interchangeably) in families.

There are four major types of single-locus Mendelian transmission: autosomal dominant (AD), autosomal recessive (AR), X-linked recessive (XR), and X-linked dominant (XD). Table 2–1 lists several prominent features of these four mechanisms that can be used to discriminate among competing hypotheses for individual pedigrees (diagrams of extended families). Family data generally are collected as pedigrees, although sibships or other fixed structure groups of relatives can also be used to test specific hypotheses about genetic control. The term pedigree comes from the French *pied de grue*, which literally means crane's foot. Like the branched footprint of a bird, a pedigree represents the branching process by which genes are transmitted from one generation to the next.

Autosomal diseases should occur in equal frequency in both sexes, if the phenotype is neither sex-specific nor sex-influenced. More important, however, is that autosomal traits or disorders should be transmitted independently of the sex of parent and offspring. Some general guidelines for recognizing autosomal dominant disorders from pedigree data are as follows:

1. All affected individuals should have at least one affected parent. Therefore, affected individuals are usually found in every generation.
2. Both males and females are affected in approximately equal numbers.
3. Both males and females transmit the trait to both sexes of offspring.
4. Matings of a heterozygous affected × normal produce approximately a 1:1 ratio of affected:normal offspring. This is, of course, a function of sibship size.
5. The trait or disorder does not appear in descendants of two normal persons, unless there is *incomplete penetrance* or recurrent mutations. This means that some branches of a pedigree can be completely free of the trait.

Autosomal recessive disorders must display the same general patterns of transmission, that is, transmission must be independent of the sex of the

Table 2-1. General features of disease distribution in families and populations under the four major forms of Mendelian inheritance.

	Autosomal dominant	Autosomal recessive	X-linked dominant	X-linked recessive
Both males and females affected in equal frequency in population	Yes	Yes	No For rare diseases, approximately 2/3 of affecteds will be female	No For rare diseases, female frequency equals square of male frequency
Transmission by both sexes	Yes	Yes	No Father-son transmission not possible	No Father-son transmission not possible
Status of parents of an affected child	At least 1 parent of affected child must be affected	For rare disorders, typically, both parents normal; consanguinity more common than in general population	At least 1 parent affected; affected males must have affected mothers (except for new mutations)	Usually both parents normal, although maternal male relatives frequently affected
Most common at-risk mating type (for a rare disorder)	$Aa \times aa$ Affected × normal	$Aa \times Aa$ Normal × normal	$XY \times XX^-$ Normal × affected heterozygote	$XY \times XX^-$ Normal × normal heterozygote

Segregation ratio in offspring (normal: affected) from most common mating type	1:1 from mating of affected × normal; no risk to children of 2 normals, barring incomplete penetrance and new mutation	3:1 segregation	1:1 for both sons and daughters	1:1 in males only; all daughters phenotypically normal, but 50% are carriers
Other prominent mating types to be considered	$Aa \times Aa$ Affected × affected	$aa \times AA$ Affected × normal	X–$Y \times XX$ Affected male × normal female	X–$Y \times XX$ Affected male × normal female
Segregation ratio	3:1 affected to normals; frequently homozygous individuals are more severely affected	All offspring normal, but all are carriers	All daughters affected, no sons affected	No affected offspring, all daughters carriers
Variations on pattern	Late onset; incomplete penetrance; variable expressivity	Complementation between genetically distinct forms of disease; incomplete penetrance	Variable expression in heterozygous females, possibly mimicking incomplete penetrance; more severe in males	Heterozygous females may show decreased levels of gene product, but with substantial variation

Each model assumes the disease is caused by a single Mendelian locus with two alleles (one disease allele and one normal).

parent and child. Differences arise in the expression of the phenotype: heterozygous carriers do not differ from homozygous normal individuals in their phenotype. General guidelines for identifying rare autosomal recessive disorders in pedigrees are as follows:

1. Most affected individuals have two normal parents. Thus, the trait will appear to skip generations.
2. The trait is expressed and transmitted by both sexes.
3. Mating between heterozygotes who are phenotypically normal yield both normal and affected offspring in approximately a 3:1 ratio. Again, this is a function of sibship size.
4. When dealing with rare traits, the normal heterozygous parents of affected individuals are more frequently related to one another compared to the general population. Sometimes, however, the relationship may not be recognized or reported.
5. Matings of affected × normal yield phenotypically normal offspring who are carriers.
6. Regardless of the population frequency, when both parents are affected, all of their children will be affected. However, there may be *complementation* among genetically distinct forms of the same disease where the children are phenotypically normal because their parents were homozygous for the disease-producing allele at two different loci.

The X-linked recessive pattern of inheritance is so striking that several X-linked diseases were recognized well before anything was understood about Mendelian genetics. The uniqueness of this X-linked pattern of transmission of diseases and traits partially accounts for the large number of recognized X-linked recessive diseases. Some general guidelines for identifying X-linked recessive traits are as follows:

1. If it is a rare trait, many more males than females will be affected. The frequency of affected females is approximately the square of that among males. For extremely rare disorders, affected females are virtually unknown.
2. Father to son transmission is impossible. By virtue of being male, sons obviously must have received the Y chromosome from their father and not the X.
3. Among sons of carrier mothers, approximately 50% will be affected and 50% will be normal.
4. All daughters of carrier females × normal males will be phenotypically normal, but approximately half will be carriers.
5. All daughters of affected male × normal female matings will be heterozygous, while all sons of such matings will be normal.

It is more difficult to identify XD transmission because it is easily confused with autosomal transmission. Segregation of the 2 X chromosomes in heterozygous females is no different from that of the other 22 autosomes. Only the male shows differences in transmission, so matings involving an affected male will be most informative. For rare XD diseases, approximately two-thirds of affected individuals in the population are female and only one-third male, so it is the rarer case that will provide sufficient information to distinguish between autosomal and X-linked dominant traits. Some general guidelines for identifying XD transmission are as follows:

1. No father-son transmission is possible. This can be best identified in affected male × normal female matings.
2. All daughters of affected males are affected. The phenotypic expression in heterozygous females is more variable, however, due to the random inactivation of all but one X chromosome in somatic cell lines. This *random X inactivation* process occurs early in development and is irreversible, but which X chromosome is inactivated in a given embryonic cell is randomly determined. Therefore, heterozygous females may, by chance alone, have a majority of cell lines with the normal allele active.
3. For rare traits or disorders, children of affected females × normal males have an equal probability of being affected and normal. Therefore, children of affected females have the same risk as expected under an AD mechanism.
4. If the trait is rare, there are approximately twice as many affected females as affected males.

While Y-linked or *holandric* transmission is possible and must exist at least for the testes determining factor, it has proved difficult to document for other traits. For Y-linked transmission to exist, the phenotype must be strictly limited to males, and transmission must be exclusively from father to son. Except possibly for hairy pinnae (hair on the outer rim of the ears), very few phenotypes in humans have been found to be transmitted on the Y chromosome. *Sex-limited* traits, where only males express the phenotype, can easily be confused with holandric traits. The key difference is that daughters of affected males can neither express *nor* transmit the trait in question. Clearly, since fully half the species must function without the product of any holandric gene, genes for vital functions must be shared by both sexes.

2.4.3. Factors Affecting Patterns of Single Gene Transmission

There are many factors that create exceptions to these general rules and guidelines for identifying patterns of Mendelian transmission. These factors usually do not affect probabilities of allele transmission, but are related to the phenotypic expression of genes. Since inferences about the presence of genetic mechanisms must be drawn by examining the distribution of the trait (or disease) in families, such factors do have to be considered in the analysis of pedigree data.

Sex-Influenced and Sex-Limited Traits

Beyond the differences directly due to genes on the sex chromosome, there are both *sex-limited* and *sex-influenced* phenotypes. Sex-limited traits are those expressed exclusively in one sex and not the other, while sex-influenced traits are those whose expression differs in the two sexes. Any gene affecting the primary or secondary sex characteristics will be sex-limited, although the analogous organ or tissue in the other gender might also be detectably different. One example of a sex-limited disorder is hydrometrocolpos, an anomaly of the vagina, which is inherited as an autosomal recessive in the Old Order Amish (catalog #23670, McKusick, 1990). An example of a sex-influenced trait is pattern baldness, a common autosomal trait with more pronounced expression of the genotype in males (Stern, 1973). Both males and females transmit the trait to their offspring with equal probability, however. Another example would be a mutant gene leading to increased risk for breast cancer which would largely be limited to expression in females, but some cases of the exceedingly rare male breast cancer also occur in such families (Newman et al., 1988).

Penetrance and Expressivity

Two concepts often arise in discussions of the exceptions to Mendelian patterns of inheritance: *incomplete penetrance* and *variable expressivity*. These concepts are often confused and understandably so. Incomplete penetrance is a statistical concept to reflect the observation that not everyone who has the genotype of interest will manifest the phenotype of interest (be it a trait or disease). Retinoblastoma illustrates the concept of incomplete penetrance, since unaffected individuals with both an affected parent and an affected child have been reported. Such individuals must obviously carry the mutant allele; however, they may have passed through some critical developmental stage for this embryonic tumor and escaped the disease. Penetrance of the retinoblastoma gene has been estimated as 90%, that is, any one heterozygote has a 90% chance of being affected (Sutton, 1988). Many Mendelian disorders have documented instances of incomplete penetrance where individuals known to have the at-risk genotype fail to develop the disorder.

Variable expressivity, on the other hand, refers to the range of phenotypic expression possible among affected individuals. This concept of a phenotypic range is illustrated by polydactyly, an autosomal dominant malformation, where an affected individual may have one or more extra fingers or toes (and occasionally both). In addition, however, polydactyly often displays incomplete penetrance, since there are reports of normal offspring of affected parents passing the trait onto their own children. A complicating factor in this particular phenotype arises in that there are several forms of polydactyly where the pattern of transmission in families is not clearly Mendelian.

Another example of the difficulties created by variable expressivity is found with Marfan's syndrome, a connective tissue disorder inherited in an autosomal dominant fashion and characterized by long fingers (arachnodactyly), eye abnormalities (lens dislocation and visual impairment), and cardiac disease (aortic dilatation with high risk of aneurysm). The range of phenotypic manifestations in this disease is quite impressive. Some affected individuals have multiple and severe organ system involvement, while others have only mild manifestations, and some obligate carriers of the Marfan allele have no apparent clinical manifestation. Any time the phenotype of interest is a syndrome, that is, a collection of clinical abnormalities that may or may not be present in any one patient, the lower limit of variable expressivity is incomplete penetrance.

Variable Age of Onset

Another complicating factor frequently seen in autosomal dominant traits is variable age of onset. For example, Huntington disease (HD) has been recognized as an autosomal dominant disease for almost 90 years, and, typically, onset of clinical symptoms is late in life (between ages 35 and 50). For uniformly progressive and degenerative diseases, such as Huntington disease, late onset is not generally interpreted in terms of incomplete penetrance but more in terms of censorship of the observations in a family, and sometimes due to death from another cause. It would not be considered incomplete penetrance. This disease is considered to have complete lifetime penetrance, that is, any heterozygote will eventually develop the disease if he or she lives long enough. Variation in age of onset complicates genetic analysis considerably, however, primarily because younger individuals below the age of risk provide little information. Sometimes this situation is referred to as *covariate dependent penetrance*, with age serving as the covariate.

Etiologic Heterogeneity

Another factor that may distort observed patterns of transmission in pedigrees is etiologic heterogeneity: the situation where a particular phenotype, usually a disease, can be produced by several causes, both genetic and environmental. Traditionally, affected individuals with the normal genotype are called *phenocopies*; these are nongenetic cases in which the disease is caused by environmental factors. Of course, it is frequently impossible to discriminate genetic from nongenetic cases without extensive family history information. Furthermore, the presence of several distinct genetic forms of the same disease in different pedigrees can also obscure the overall pattern of transmission if all pedigrees are pooled as part of a formal genetic analysis. Retinitis pigmentosa is an excellent example of etiologic heterogeneity with autosomal recessive, two or more autosomal dominant, and at least two X-linked recessive forms of the disease, already well documented (Humphries et al., 1992). In addition, a large number of cases with no apparent family history (*simplex cases*) have been observed, suggesting there may be nongenetic factors that can cause this disease (Boughman et al., 1980).

Genetic Interaction

Although experimental genetics has clearly established that effects of Mendelian traits can depend on the presence of other genetic factors, human examples of genetic interaction remain ill-defined. The vague concept of a "genetic background" effect is often mentioned but rarely explored. In experimental settings, it is possible to show that the manifestation of a single-gene trait can be affected by other genetic loci. The term *epistasis* refers to the suppression or alteration of expression of one gene by another locus, that is, nonallelic interaction between different genes. In humans, the complex interaction among the ABO, secretor, and Lewis loci offers one example of a complex epistatic system, where the phenotype of the Lewis antigen system is jointly determined by gene products of the Lewis and secretor loci (Levitan, 1988). It is important to note, however, that gene interaction can also occur between alleles at the same locus (e.g., the S and C alleles at the β-globin locus interact to produce a phenotypically milder anemia in heterozygotes compared to SS homozygotes), in addition to that between genes at different loci. Predicted patterns of these two types of interaction are distinct and can be exploited to separate these components. In general, however, it is difficult to document genetic interaction solely from observational studies in humans.

Environmental Interaction

The phenotypic manifestation of a single gene may depend on the presence of environmental triggers or exposures, and this phenomenon is central to genetic epidemiology. At this point, it suffices to state that if the manifestation of a single-gene trait requires the presence of some unmeasured environmental factor, the patterns of Mendelian segregation may be so distorted that the single gene can no longer be identified. Specialized analytic methods and sampling strategies are needed to document such interaction between genes and environmental factors (see Chapters 5 and 6).

2.4.4. Genetic Linkage

Genetic linkage represents departures from Mendel's second law, the independent assortment of genes, and is a reflection of the cosegregation of alleles at loci physically located near one another on the same chromosome. While gametes produced by two independently segregating genes contain the four combinations of alleles in equal proportion, gametes arising from two linked loci will have a predominance of alleles paired in the same combinations seen in their parents. Due to *crossing over* or *recombination* during meiosis, however, linked genes are not always transmitted together. The amount of recombination depends on the physical distance between linked genes along the chromosome. The longer the distance, the more the opportunity for meiotic crossing over, resulting in observable genetic recombination. Conversely, the shorter the physical distance, the less recombination will occur and the tighter the linkage.

In the population as a whole, genetic linkage creates only minor imbalances in the possible combinations of genotypes, and overall there may be no discrepancy in the expected proportion of the various combinations of alleles at two linked loci (i.e., certain *haplotypes* or combinations of alleles at linked loci). At equilibrium, the frequencies of pairs of alleles at different loci (i.e., haplotypes) is simply the product of their respective allele frequencies (Weir, 1990). When there is an excess/deficiency of certain haplotypes, however, the loci are said to be in *linkage disequilibrium*. Linkage disequilibrium will decay with time, but this is a function of the recombination between loci. The rate of decay can be quite slow for tightly linked loci, and may span scores of generations. Observed disequilibrium in a population may merely reflect a transition point on the way to true multilocus equilibrium, or it may be due to recent merging of two or more subpopulations with different gametic frequencies. Random fluctuation in haplotype frequencies due to small population sizes, or possibly selection for certain multilocus combinations, should also be considered (Hartl and Clark, 1989).

Although extreme linkage disequilibrium between a marker locus and a disease locus can result in a statistical association between a marker allele and the disease when population samples are examined, it is important not to confuse the effects of linkage with a more general association between a marker allele and a disease. Association can occur between an allele at a marker locus and a disease due to a number of complex biologic interactions, including any in which the marker allele plays a direct or indirect role in the pathogenesis of the disease (see Chapter 5). For example, the association between the *PiZ* null allele and emphysema may be due to the lack of functional α_1-antitrypsin in homozygotes, while the association between the allele *B27* of the *HLA-B* locus and the disease ankylosing spondylitis may involve cross-reactivity of this antigen and a pathogen. Linkage, however, is a property of the relative position of loci, not their alleles, and the observed cosegregation within a given family can involve any allele at the marker locus.

The demonstration of genetic linkage in humans and the localization of genes on specific chromosomes can be accomplished by both statistical and experimental methods. Statistical methods involve linkage analysis of two or more genetic traits (i.e., two markers or a marker and a disease locus), using pedigree data, as described in more detail in Chapter 9. On the other hand, experimental methods to map a locus to a chromosome include rodent-human somatic cell hybridization techniques, in situ hybridization, chromosome sorting techniques, as well as other techniques (McKusick, 1988).

2.4.5. Patterns of Multiple Locus Transmission

While the patterns of multiple locus transmission are straightforward and can be worked out for any number of loci, there are many different types of interactions possible. If the observed phenotype is binary (e.g., affected versus nonaffected), it can be very difficult to distinguish among distinct genetic mechanisms involving two or more loci. The phenomenon of epistasis described above, even when strictly recessive or dominant, leads to patterns of familial aggregation and recurrence risk that are quite different from those expected under single-locus mechanisms. In general, recurrence risks under two locus models are functions of the allele frequencies at the individual loci and the amount of information on affected relatives (e.g., if normal parents are involved, if any normal sibs exist). Expected risks to a sib of an affected individual can be calculated under Mendelian principles, but these can range from very low to very high, often reflecting the effects of one segregating mating type (Beaty et al., 1988a). Consider the two-locus model represented in Table 2–2: If only the genotype *aabb* manifests the disease, then the probability of an affected child from a *AaBb* × *AaBb* mating is 1/16. The term *emergenesis* has been proposed when multiple loci are involved and only one multiple homozygote is affected (Li, 1987). Such traits, although

Table 2–2. Distribution of genotypes among progeny of $AaBb \times AaBb$ mating under a Mendelian two-locus model

Genotype	Genotype frequency	"Phenotypic score" on an additive scale	Frequency with A or B alleles*
$AABB$	1/16	4	1
$AABb$	2/16 ⎱	3	
$AaBB$	2/16 ⎰		4(2 + 2)
$AAbb$	1/16 ⎱		
$AaBb$	4/16 ⎬	2	6(1 + 4 + 1)
$aaBB$	1/16 ⎭		
$Aabb$	2/16 ⎱		
$aaBb$	2/16 ⎰	1	4(2 + 2)
$aabb$	1/16	0	0

*Under the two-locus model used by Li (1987), only doubly homozygous genotypes are at risk. Termed *emergenesis*, this can also be thought of as a recessive disease masked by a dominant allele at an epistatic locus.

strictly Mendelian, show very little familial aggregation (see column 3 of Table 2–2).

While the terms "multilocus," "multifactorial," and "polygenic" are often used synonymously in the literature, certain distinctions among these terms should be kept in mind. Multilocus refers to the situation where more than one distinct genetic locus influences a single phenotype, possibly with pre-defined patterns of epistatic interaction. Skin pigmentation in humans likely qualifies as a multilocus trait, since it is estimated that four distinct loci contribute to skin pigmentation in a simple additive manner (Cavalli-Sforza and Bodmer, 1971).

The term *multifactorial* should be reserved for situations where the phenotype is determined by both genetic and environmental factors, frequently without specifying the number of genetic loci involved (one, few, or many). Many common diseases serve as examples of multifactorial inheritance, for example, heart disease and diabetes.

The term *polygenic* should be reserved for situations where an unspecified large number of independently segregating loci contribute in a simple additive fashion to the phenotype. This latter concept of polygenic inheritance derives from R. A. Fisher's concept of equal and additive effects across many independent loci. This polygenic concept served as a bridge between Mendelian genes (which are intrinsically discrete) and continuous or quantitative phenotypes. Dermatoglyphic traits serve as an example of a continuous phenotype apparently under polygenic control. In the example with a two-locus model above, if one assumes that alleles A and B each contribute 1 unit to the phenotype (height, weight, etc.), then the genotype $AABB$ would have a phenotypic value of 4 units, while the genotype $aabb$ will have a phenotypic value of 0 units. As shown in Table 2–2, the mating $AaBb \times AaBb$ will lead to a distribution of progeny with 0, 1, 2, 3, and 4 phenotypic units with relative frequencies of 1, 4, 6, 4, and 1, respectively (see column 2 of Table 2–2). If a still larger number of polygenic loci were involved, then the shape of the distribution of the phenotypes in these progeny would better approximate a normal distribution.

2.4.6. Quantitative Genetics

The polygenic model of inheritance bridged the gap between Mendelian genetics, which traditionally involved the study of discrete traits (most frequently diseases) and biometric or quantitative genetics, which traditionally involved the study of continuous traits. Quantitative genetics developed along with and served as a catalyst for much of statistics. Many of those who developed the early principles of statistics (Galton, Pearson, Fisher) were motivated by questions of familial resemblance and human genetics. Several common statistical techniques (correlation, regression, analysis of variance) were first developed to measure genetic factors underlying continuously varying traits. These traits showed obvious familial aggregation, but were quite intractable under the principles of simple Mendelian genetics.

In domestic organisms such as plants, it is possible to modify Mendel's original experimental design to study quantitative traits. When a quantitative trait (e.g., flower length) showed effectively nonoverlapping distributions in purebred lines, crosses between two parental lines and among the resulting progeny lines could be done. Crossing a purebred line having a short flower length with a line having a long flower length gave offspring with an intermediate flower length, although all three groups showed substantial variation in flower length (East, 1916). Although the phenotypic means differed considerably for the two parental and the offspring lines, their variances were quite similar. This variance is all nongenetic or residual variation because all three groups are genetically homogeneous (i.e., the two parental lines are homozygous at all loci affecting flower length, and all offspring plants are heterozygous). When the progeny individuals were selfed, however, the observed variance among their offspring (where one would expect Mendelian segregation to occur) was much larger than for the two prior generations. Using this increased variance in the third generation, as well as the difference in phenotypic means for the two parental lines, it is possible to estimate the number of independent loci influencing a quantitative trait (Bulmer, 1985). While truly purebred lines of humans are never available, it is possible to take advantage of certain experiments of nature. This type of analysis has been used to estimate, for example, that skin pigmentation in humans is under the control of only about four loci, which appear to act strictly additively, that is, the alleles controlling the amount of pigment are codominant (Cavalli-Sforza and Bodmer, 1971).

In human populations, it is more difficult to use the techniques of statistical genetics to extrapolate to biologic mechanisms, and the earliest work in quantitative genetics was aimed at simply measuring the degree of familial resemblance. For example, Galton's early work on the inheritance of height in humans helped him develop the concept of regression and correlation. Because he had no knowledge of Mendelian principles, Galton attempted to relate the observed "regression to the population mean" seen in children's height to the then-accepted blending model of inheritance. Later workers showed that such regression to the mean could easily result if the observed phenotype (here height) were influenced by both genetic and environmental forces acting independently. Since parents with high phenotypic values can transmit only the genetic component to their offspring, their offspring would be expected to be closer to the population mean, that is, they will be, on average, shorter than their tall parents. If the genetic component to height is the result of many independent genes each contributing in an additive fashion (i.e., polygenes), such a regression of the child's phenotype on the midparent value will serve as an estimator of the proportion of phenotypic variance which is attributable to genetic differences, a quantity known as *heritability* (the ratio of genetic variance to the total variance) as discussed in detail in Chapter 7. In 1918, R. A. Fisher showed that if there were no dominance for a large number of independently segregating loci, it is possible to express the observed correlation between types of relatives as a linear function of the phenotypic variation directly attributable to genetic differences and that attributable to nongenetic differences. Effects of these independent polygenes are summarized by *genetic components of variance* (Mather, 1949).

2.4.7. Mitochondrial Inheritance

Mitochondria are cytoplasmic organelles whose most important cellular function is the synthesis of adenosine triphosphate (ATP) via the process of oxidative phosphorylation. Each mitochondrion contains several circular chromosomes, and most of its DNA serves some coding function. Until recently, mitochondrial inheritance was rarely mentioned as a source of genetic disease; however, several disorders are now attributed to defects in mitochondrial genes. The cardinal feature of mitochondrial inheritance is that transmission occurs only through the mother, and all her children should receive her mitochondrial genes regardless of their own genomic makeup. This maternal transmission occurs because maternal mitochondria are passed with the cytoplasm of the ova, while paternal mitochondria from the sperm are not donated to the zygote—only the nucleus of the sperm participates in fertilization. Incomplete penetrance of mitochondrial traits should be expected because there is an element of randomness in the transmission of mitochondria from mother to offspring, on top of the random distribution of mitochondria in cell lines among different tissues in the offspring.

2.5. THE GENETIC MATERIAL IN HUMAN POPULATIONS

In this section, the principles underlying the behavior of genes in populations are reviewed. For more comprehensive discussions, the reader is referred to several textbooks on population genetics (Cavalli-Sforza and Bodmer, 1971; Crow, 1986; Hartl and Clark, 1989; Weir, 1990).

2.5.1. The Hardy-Weinberg Principle

The cornerstone of population genetics is summarized in the Hardy-Weinberg principle, which was independently derived by G. H. Hardy and W. Weinberg in 1908. This principle offered a simple explanation for how genetic diversity for Mendelian traits can be maintained in a population. The Hardy-Weinberg law also defined the simple relationship between the frequency of genes in a population and the frequency of genotypes (i.e., individuals), and is therefore useful for estimating allele frequencies from the prevalence of Mendelian disease.

Since at any one autosomal locus, an individual carries two alleles (one paternal and one maternal), the population's pool of all alleles at a single autosomal locus can also be represented by the familiar Punnett square. For example, if A and a are alleles at a single locus, and if the relative frequency of A is denoted p, with the relative frequency of a denoted q (where $p + q = 1$), then the genotypes of a random-mating population can be presented as in the top half of Figure 2–5. Once these proportions of genotypes are established, working out the expected frequencies of genotypes among off-spring in the next generation shows that an equilibrium exists. Specifically, the frequencies of the three genotypes (AA, Aa, and aa) will be the same in all subsequent generations, that is, p^2, $2pq$, q^2 (see Table 2–3). Thus, these genotype frequencies represent the *Hardy-Weinberg equilibrium*. The derivation is somewhat different for X-linked genes, but the logic is identical.

UNDER RANDOM MATING

		gametes with **A**	gametes with **a**	
gametes with **A**	p	p^2	pq	$p^2 + pq = p(p + q) = p$
gametes with **a**	q	pq	q^2	$q^2 + pq = q(p + q) = q$
		p	q	1.0

UNDER INBREEDING

		gametes with **A** p	gametes with **a** q	
gametes with **A**	p	$p^2(1 - F) + pF$	$pq(1 - F)$	p
gametes with **a**	q	$pq(1 - F)$	$q^2(1 - F) + qF$	q
		p	q	1.0

Figure 2–5. Punnett square showing genotypes possible for a single Mendelian locus with two alleles in a randomly mating population, where the frequency of A is p, and the frequency of a is q ($= 1 - p$).

Table 2–3. Maintenance of Hardy-Weinberg equilibrium in a population.

Given a population in initial Hardy-Weinberg equilibrium, with

Genotype AA Aa aa
Frequency p^2 $2pq$ q^2

At equilibrium		Genotypic probability in offspring			Genotypic frequency in next generation		
Mating type	Frequency	AA	Aa	aa	AA	Aa	aa
$AA \times AA$	p^4	1	0	0	p^4	0	0
$AA \times Aa$	$2p^3q$	1/2	1/2	0	p^3q	p^3q	0
$AA \times aa$	p^2q^2	0	1	0	0	p^2q^2	0
$Aa \times AA$	$2p^3q$	1/2	1/2	0	p^3q	p^3q	0
$Aa \times Aa$	$4p^2q^2$	1/4	1/2	1/4	p^2q^2	$2p^2q^2$	p^2q^2
$Aa \times aa$	$2pq^3$	0	1/2	1/2	0	pq^3	pq^3
$aa \times AA$	p^2q^2	0	1	0	0	p^2q^2	0
$aa \times Aa$	$2pq^3$	0	1/2	1/2	0	pq^3	pq^3
$aa \times aa$	q^4	0	0	1	0	0	q^4

Total frequency of
$$AA = p^4 + 2p^3q + p^2q^2 = p^2(p^2 + 2pq + q^2) = p^2$$
$$Aa = 2p^3q + 4p^2q^2 + 2pq^3 = 2pq(p^2 + 2pq + q^2) = 2pq$$
$$aa = q^4 + 2pq^3 + p^2q^2 = q^2(p^2 + 2pq + q^2) = q$$

Similarly, Hardy-Weinberg equilibria can be worked out for multiple alleles and multiple loci.

An assumption here is that mating is random with respect to the locus in question. The conditions necessary to maintain the Hardy-Weinberg equilibrium can be summarized as follows: random mating, no migration into or out of the population, no inbreeding, no selective survivorship among genotypes, large population sizes (to avoid loss of alleles due to sampling errors), no mutation, and absence of any other force that would alter the allele frequencies. If these conditions are met, the allele frequencies can be directly estimated from observed genotypic or phenotypic frequencies in the population.

Ideally, one would always estimate allele frequencies by methods of gene counting, but this can work only for codominant traits where homozygotes can be distinguished from heterozygotes. When dominance exists, it is not possible to count alleles directly. In such situations, by assuming a Hardy-Weinberg equilibrium, one can estimate allele frequencies and from that the proportion of gene carriers. For example, if a recessive disease has a frequency of 1/10,000 in the population (i.e., $q^2 = .0001$), the allele frequency expected under Hardy-Weinberg equilibrium is .01 (i.e., the estimated allele frequency is the square root of the observed prevalence). From this, the frequency of heterozygous carriers is computed as .0198 or almost 2% of the population.

2.5.2. Factors Affecting Gene and Genotype Frequencies

Numerous factors affect the frequency of genes and genotypes at any particular locus and thus will perturb Hardy-Weinberg equilibrium. This, in turn, will affect the genetic structure of a population over time. Human populations never truly meet the conditions necessary for Hardy-Weinberg equilibrium, since there is always some mutation, selection, migration, nonrandom mating; in addition, small population sizes are common (which lead to genetic drift). It becomes important to appreciate which forces may be important in determining the genetic structure of human populations.

Mutation and Selection

The equilibrium frequency of a mutant allele in a population depends on a balance between the mutation rate (which introduces new copies) and the effect of selection (which removes copies of the mutant allele from the population). Selection is broadly defined in terms of genetic fitness or the ability of an individual to contribute genes to the next generation. Two factors affect fitness: viability and fertility. Many mutations are harmful to the extent that they reduce the life span of the affected individual (e.g., Mendelian diseases generally reduce the life span), while others reduce the ability of the person to reproduce (i.e., causing sterility), and some interfere with both. Thus, a new mutation with deleterious effects on the phenotype tend to be selected against and will be eliminated from the population with time.

Mutations that have some advantage over the original wild-type allele can persist and spread through human populations, of course. However, it is difficult to document examples of positive selective pressure in human populations because obtaining adequate data on genotype-specific fertility and mortality is difficult even in existing populations. Obtaining such estimates for environments experienced by previous generations is impossible. The best example of selection for a mutant allele in humans is the case for a selective advantage to heterozygotes carrying the sickle cell allele at the β-globin locus. Homozygotes for this allele tend to have a severe anemia that leads to substantial morbidity and early death, while the heterozygotes appear to have a selective advantage over the homozygous wild-type individuals in areas with endemic falciparum malaria. This heterozygote advantage is the likely explanation for high frequency of the sickle cell allele in many West African populations, but it is difficult to document increased fitness in the heterozygote directly (Cavalli-Sforza and Bodmer, 1971). Moreover, recent molecular genetic studies of DNA polymorphisms in the region of the β-globin locus raise the possibility that more that one mutational event gave rise to this single allele in different populations, complicating the process of estimating genetic fitness.

Chance Fluctuations: Founder Effect/Genetic Drift

The sampling process by which gametes are selected from a gene pool to form the individuals of the next generation is subject to random variation. When large numbers of gametes are formed (i.e., when the population itself is large), these "sampling errors" will be small and there will be little change in gene frequencies across generations. However, for small populations the sampling errors can be substantial, and furthermore they are cumulative in their effect, since the next generation must be sampled from the current generation. Thus, the smaller the gene pool in the current generation, the greater the chance that allele frequencies will differ in the next. Cumulative changes in gene frequency due to sampling variation is termed *genetic drift*.

The history of the human species is dominated by life in small, relatively isolated populations, and is filled with episodes of smaller groups of related individuals splitting off from existing populations. Simple geographic constraints often place limits on mate selection. Even in relatively large populations, mating structures are influenced by social, ethnic, and religious forces that act to stratify the general community into smaller subpopulations. Subdivision of any large population into smaller units, each of which may internally maintain a random mating structure, will also lead to deviation from an overall Hardy-Weinberg equilibrium due to genetic drift because each subpopulation is subject to the random effects of minor changes in gene frequencies and will constantly diverge from the mean of the overall population (Hartl and Clark, 1989). Genetic migration or admixture among subgroups can only partially counter this divergence.

When a new population is founded by a small group of individuals (a small sample of the original gene pool) there may also be substantial differences in gene frequencies. The smaller the group of original founders, the greater the probability that their genes are not representative of the general population, and therefore the allele frequencies in descendants may be quite different from the original group. This is known as *founder effect*, and it will be compounded by genetic drift over many generations, if the descendant populations remain small. Both founder effect and genetic drift result from a random sampling of genes into gametes, and both act to increase the genetic diversity among populations. The cumulative effects of these random fluctuations in allele frequencies over many generations is to increase the probability of fixation of allele frequencies, where some alleles are completely lost from some populations.

A notable consequence of founder effect (and genetic drift) is that frequently rare diseases become hallmarks of certain populations. For example, the Ellis-van Creveld syndrome is an autosomal recessive form of dwarfism that reaches unusually high frequencies in the Lancaster County, Pennsylvania Amish population, but is essentially unknown in other populations. Genealogic data from this reproductive isolate has traced all cases of the disorder to a single migrant couple who came to North America from Europe in the 1700s. Inbreeding in this closed population has also acted to increase the frequency of affected individuals.

Nonrandom Mating: Inbreeding

Inbreeding results from *consanguineous matings* where the two parents have one or more ancestors in common. Offspring of a consanguineous mating are *inbred*, and have some nonzero probability of receiving two copies of any autosomal allele, which are merely exact copies of a single allele carried by a common ancestor. All homozygous individuals have two copies of a single allele that are *identical by state* (*ibs*), but only inbred individuals may have alleles that are *identical by descent* (*ibd*). Inbreeding is measured by the *inbreeding coefficient*, F, which is the probability that the individual receives two alleles (at any autosomal locus) that are identical by descent. Obviously, the inbreeding coefficient is a relative measure based on the pedigree structure over the last several generations only, since generally the founding ancestors are not assumed to be inbred.

At the population level, inbreeding alone alters the genotypic frequencies at all loci, but does not affect their allele frequencies. This can be demonstrated by noting that inbreeding creates a correlation among uniting gametes, which modifies the familiar Punnett square as shown in the bottom half of Figure 2–5. In essence, inbreeding increases the probability of homozygosity at a locus, and conversely decreases the probability of heterozygosity, but without altering allele frequencies.

One consequence of inbreeding is to bring about a decrease in the overall fitness of the population when high rates of homozygosity increase the prevalence of recessive genetic diseases. The decrease in fitness due to suboptimal genotypes has been termed "genetic load" (Morton, 1982).

Nonrandom Mating: Assortative Mating

Selection of mates is rarely random. Individuals may preferentially select one another because of physical and behavioral characteristics, many of which are influenced by genetic factors. While assortative mating can, in theory, be either positive or negative (i.e., individuals may prefer similar mates or purposefully select for phenotypic differences), positive assortative mating is better documented in humans. While most traits thought to be influenced by assortative mating are *not* controlled by single loci but by many loci, the end result of positive assortative mating is also to create a correlation among uniting gametes in the population, as seen with inbreeding. One difference is that the effects of assortative mating are limited to those loci influencing the trait in question (and possibly those tightly linked with them). In general, positive assortative mating increases the proportion of homozygotes and decrease that of heterozygotes, although the effect of assortative mating is substantially less than that of inbreeding (Hartl, 1980). Assortative mating, on the other hand, will increase the variance from genes affecting quantitative traits more than will inbreeding (Crow, 1986).

It is important to note that the effects of inbreeding, positive assortative mating, and genetic drift among subpopulations are identical. Each creates a correlation between uniting gametes in the overall population that reduces heterozygosity below what is expected under a simple Hardy-Weinberg equilibrium.

2.6. CONCLUDING REMARKS

It is not the purpose of this chapter to provide a comprehensive treatment of human genetics, but briefly to summarize key principles as they relate to genetic epidemiology. Readers are referred to other sources for further details (Vogel and Motulsky, 1986; Levitan, 1988; Sutton, 1988; Mange and Mange, 1990). The larger field of human genetics is rapidly evolving and further knowledge is being acquired at an exponential rate. The challenge to genetic epidemiology is to incorporate new molecular and biochemical discoveries into a systematic investigation of disease at the level of family and population studies. The fundamentals of genetics still hold, although the molecular structure of the gene is now recognized as more complex and demands expansion of models to describe the genetic structure of human populations.

Fundamental Epidemiologic Concepts and Approaches

3.1. OBJECTIVES AND STRATEGIES OF EPIDEMIOLOGY

"Epidemiology is concerned with the patterns of disease occurrence in human populations and of the factors that influence these patterns" (Lilienfeld and Lilienfeld, 1980). In genetic epidemiology, genetic factors are explicitly considered along with environmental factors in the search for determinants of disease occurrence in populations. This search necessitates combining traditional epidemiologic methods with those of genetic analysis, and incorporating genetic and other biologic markers into epidemiologic studies. This chapter presents a brief overview of basic epidemiologic concepts and approaches, specifically relating these concepts to the study of genetic factors in disease. As this overview of epidemiology is far from comprehensive, the reader is referred to other textbooks for further details (e.g., Lilienfeld and Lilienfeld, 1980; Mausner and Kramer, 1985; Kelsey et al., 1986; Rothman, 1986; Kahn and Sempos, 1989).

The following list indicates the epidemiologic strategy for the study of disease and the relevant discussions in this chapter:

1. *Defining the disease, trait, or phenotype under study*. In sections 3.2 and 3.3, epidemiologic views of disease and disease causation are reviewed. In particular, the understanding of disease heterogeneity and natural history is emphasized. Then, traditional epidemiologic views are applied to genetic factors. It can be shown that many epidemiologic concepts and terms in the area of infectious agents have counterparts in human genetics (section 3.4).

2. *Assembling and analyzing data on the occurrence of disease in populations (or families)*. This leads to the formation of hypotheses concerning the role of etiologic factors. The basic tools for measuring disease frequency are outlined (section 3.5).

3. *Testing for associations between diseases and suspected risk factors.* The types of epidemiologic studies and various approaches to measuring associations between disease and risk factors are reviewed (sections 3.6 and 3.7).
4. *Searching for mechanisms of disease and natural history.* Once associations are found, the next step is to assess biologic mechanisms of causation and pathogenesis. The sources of bias in epidemiologic studies and approaches to the evaluation of associations are reviewed (section 3.8).
5. *Applying knowledge of etiology, pathophysiology, and natural history of disease to intervention and prevention strategies.* This topic is further discussed in Chapter 10.

3.2. EPIDEMIOLOGIC CONCEPTS OF DISEASE

In this section, epidemiologic concepts of disease classification and natural history are briefly reviewed.

3.2.1. Disease Classification

An essential prerequisite to any epidemiologic study is the "case definition." Similarly, an essential prerequisite to a genetic investigation is the definition of the "phenotype." Classification of disease usually proceeds from the general to the specific, from a phenotypic classification (based on the presence of clinical or pathologic manifestations) to a pathogenetic classification (based on the underlying pathophysiologic processes) and eventually to an etiologic classification (based on the underlying causal mechanisms). A phenotypic classification can range from pure clinical criteria (such as constellations of signs and symptoms, often used in psychiatric disorders) to the reliance on laboratory tests, such as radiologic examinations and physiologic measures, and genotypic classification. Frequently, the final phenotypic classification is nonspecific and causally heterogeneous. For example, pneumonias include a wide range of underlying infectious agents, including viruses, bacteria, and fungi, and noninfectious mechanisms such as allergic and inflammatory processes.

The goal of epidemiologic investigations is to help elucidate the role of etiologic mechanisms underlying such clinical phenotypes. This can be achieved by combining epidemiologic tools with clinical information and laboratory tests. Advances in biomedical research have identified extensive heterogeneity within many disorders where several biologically distinct entities with different etiology, pathophysiology, and clinical manifestations had been lumped together previously, for example, peptic ulcer and diabetes mellitus (Rotter, 1983; Rotter and Rimoin, 1983; Orchard et al., 1986).

In Figure 3–1, the problem of clinical and etiologic heterogeneity is illustrated for Down syndrome. With improvements in clinical and laboratory techniques, the definition of this syndrome has evolved from descriptive,

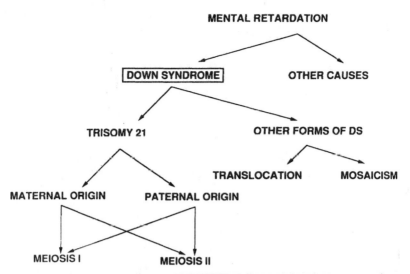

Figure 3–1.   Refinement of disease classification illustrated with Down syndrome.

symptomatic states (such as mental retardation with peculiar facial appearance) to more refined pathogenetic classifications (such as trisomy 21 derived from nondisjunction versus a Down's phenotype based on a translocation). The further refinement of trisomy 21 cases by parental origin of the nondisjunction event may be important in the identification of different parental factors affecting the ultimate risk of occurrence of trisomy 21 (Hassold and Jacobs, 1984). Heterogeneity of disease is important not only in the clinical setting where it can influence the diagnosis, management, and prognosis of individual patients, but also in epidemiologic analyses where it implies pathogenetic and etiologic variability among affected individuals. In both genetic and epidemiologic studies of disease, lumping heterogeneous conditions under one phenotype can result in overlooking important etiologic factors if these factors are critical in only one subgroup of the disease (Weiss and Liff, 1983; Adams et al., 1989). In the example of Down syndrome, if advanced paternal age increases the risk of paternally derived trisomy 21, this effect may not be readily appreciated if a study cannot separate trisomy 21 cases by parental origin of the nondisjunction event. Most cases of Down syndrome appear to be due to maternal nondisjunction that is strongly influenced by maternal age. Importantly, Down syndrome cases due to chromosome translocation are likely to have no parental age association, a point that can be totally missed if such cases (which constitute less than 5% of all Down's syndrome cases) are not distinguished in an epidemiologic study.

3.2.2. Natural History of Disease

The definition of the disease or phenotype used in any epidemiologic study is also inevitably connected with the stage of disease natural history. As shown in Figure 3–2, the spectrum of disease can be viewed as ranging from the

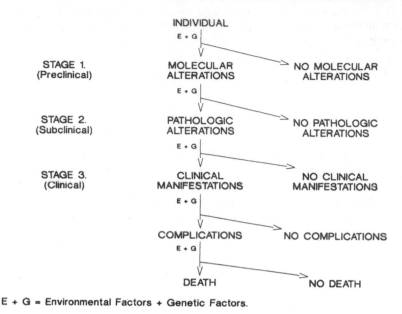

E + G = Environmental Factors + Genetic Factors.

Figure 3–2. Spectrum of disease and natural history in relation to genetic and environmental factors. E + G, environmental factors + genetic factors.

preclinical to the clinical levels (Mausner and Kramer, 1985; Evans, 1987). The first stage can be considered predisease status and resides in the molecular alterations at the subcellular level (e.g., carrying the gene for familial hypercholesterolemia, an autosomal dominant genetic condition). The next stage of disease represents subclinical illness, which involves the biochemical, cellular or physiologic changes that may be detectable with laboratory methods (e.g., a lipoprotein profile showing high blood cholesterol levels) in the absence of clinical signs and symptoms. The clinical stage begins with onset of signs and symptoms that leads to diagnosis of the disease entity (e.g., angina pectoris). The next stage refers to complications of the disease in different organ systems (e.g., stroke, peripheral vascular disease). Death may or may not be the ultimate outcome. Different diseases vary in pattern and speed of progression from one stage to another. For certain conditions, this progression occurs quickly (such as with some acute infectious diseases), while for others, it may take years or decades to occur (such as with some slow virus infections). For some diseases, progression from subclinical to clinical illness occurs in only a few affected individuals, while for others, this progression occurs in the majority of persons.

The splitting of disease into stages by natural history not only is of academic or theoretical interest, but also can provide insight into the pathogenetic mechanisms of disease and factors affecting the progression of the disease from one stage to another. Ultimately, these pathogenetic mechanisms can influence the development of effective preventive and intervention strategies. In infectious diseases, the identification of subclinical infection is crucial in understanding the transmission of disease in the population (Last, 1986). In chronic diseases, the observation that often only a small proportion of individuals with disease show overt clinical manifestations (i.e., clinically affected individuals represent only the tip of the iceberg) led Lilienfeld and Lilienfeld (1980) to state: "One of the major deterrents in elucidating the epidemiology of diseases of unknown etiology is the absence of methods to detect the subclinical state—the bottom of the iceberg."

3.3. EPIDEMIOLOGIC CONCEPTS OF CAUSATION

Traditionally, epidemiologists have thought of disease causation as an interaction among agent, host, and environment, "the epidemiologic triangle" (Mausner and Kramer, 1985), or as a web of causes ranging from external exposures to internal pathogenetic mechanisms (MacMahon and Pugh, 1970). The challenge to epidemiology is to disentangle this web and measure the relative impact of the various component parts. Therefore, epidemiologists routinely examine a large number of candidate "risk factors" and test for possible associations with disease.

3.3.1. Disease Risk Factors

Factors that influence the risk or occurrence of a disease are generally labeled *risk factors*, and these encompass a wide range of variables, including demographics (race, sex, age, and socioeconomic status), physical and biologic agents (chemical exposures, drugs, infectious agents, etc.), and behavioral factors (smoking, alcohol consumption, and life-style), as well as numerous others. Frequently, however, epidemiologic studies make no distinction among initiating factors (e.g., infectious agents), factors affecting the risk of exposure to such initiating factors, or the pathogenesis and the natural history of the disease following exposure (Evans, 1987). For example, malnutrition, alcoholism, and steroid therapy have all been shown to be risk factors in the development of tuberculosis (Stehbens, 1985). Although these factors contribute to the development of clinical illness, they cannot, combined or separately, produce tuberculosis in the absence of exposure to tubercle bacilli (Stehbens, 1985).

While the example of tuberculosis represents a clear-cut infectious disease, the situation is much more complicated for most chronic diseases in which multiple initiating factors can lead to clinical disease, along with multiple factors affecting pathogenesis and natural history. The distinction among initiating factors, pathogenetic factors, and interacting factors may not always be apparent. Moreover, knowledge of the initiating factor may not always be adequate to prevent the occurrence of disease. For example, in an epidemic of food poisoning, knowledge of the cause (e.g., *Salmonella*) does not automatically identify the source of the outbreak. An epidemiologic investigation may implicate a specific food item as a risk factor for the disease and thereby identify the source of the contamination. Implicating specific persons who handled these food items as risk factors may also lead to the source of the infectious agent and help control of the epidemic. Likewise, in the case of sickle cell anemia, knowledge of the etiology (in this situation, a point mutation in the β-globin gene) does not automatically provide an insight into the pathogenesis of the disease, why sickle cell crises occur, how and when anemia occurs, and why certain complications occur in some individuals but not others. Also, for cigarette smoking and lung cancer, the fact that cigarette smoking has been associated with lung cancer does not automatically explain the pathogenesis of lung cancer, nor does it pinpoint the presence of other components in disease progression. Although undoubtedly, smoking is an important cause of lung cancer (Fielding, 1986), not all smokers develop lung cancer (Mattson et al., 1987), a fact that indicates the presence of other interacting, genetic and environmental factors that contribute to the development of lung cancer (Rothman, 1986; Caporaso, 1991). Moreover, because lung cancer can develop in nonsmokers (albeit at a much lower risk than smokers), it is clear that lung cancer is etiologically heterogeneous.

Clearly, in order for epidemiologic risk factors to have biologic significance, they need to be examined in the context of the natural history and pathogenesis of the disease. Laboratory methods could be used to identify the initiation of the general pathologic process following exposure to an etiologic agent, and this must be combined with a search for factors that lead to clinical disease in some individuals and to mild or subclinical illness in other individuals (Evans, 1987). Figure 3–2 shows that at each stage of the disease process from the subclinical through the clinical levels, a combination of genetic and environmental factors, broadly defined, can alter the natural history of disease.

If disease is viewed as the result of a dynamic interaction between environmental and genetic factors, then risk factors can be classified into several conceptually distinct groups, shown in Table 3–1 (Evans, 1987).

Thus, epidemiologists have begun to address questions such as the following: "Why do certain heavy smokers develop lung cancer while others do not?" (Rothman, 1986). "Why do certain carriers of hepatitis B antigen develop hepatocellular carcinoma while others do not?" (Evans, 1987). "Why do certain individuals develop islet cell antibodies of the pancreas?" (Lipton and LaPorte, 1989). Also, "Why do only some of these individuals go on to develop insulin-dependent diabetes mellitus?" (Krolewski et al., 1987). And finally, "Why do certain patients with insulin-dependent diabetes mellitus develop complications such as diabetic nephropathy while others do not?" (Seaquist et al., 1989).

3.3.2. Necessary and Sufficient Causes

Because the onset of disease is rarely due to a single event even in the case of purely mendelian or purely infectious diseases, a useful epidemiologic concept is that of necessary and sufficient causes. This concept is illustrated here with a few examples of single genetic factors (Table 3–2). Some diseases have been attributed to single causes that are both necessary and sufficient. One example is Tay-Sachs disease, an autosomal recessive condition that

Table 3–1. Types and examples of epidemiologic risk factors

Type	Examples
Factors affecting risk of exposure to initiating factors	Intravenous drug use and HIV infection
Initiating factors	Bacteria, viruses, radiation, drugs, chemicals
Factors affecting pathologic course of disease	
Environmental factors	Steroid use, nutritional status, and tuberculosis
Genetic factors	Hemochromatosis gene and iron intake Acetylator phenotype and aryl compounds in bladder cancer
Factors affecting inheritance of genetic factors	Consanguinity, founder effect, and inheritance of susceptibility genotypes
Pathogenetic mechanisms (cellular, biochemical)	Hypercholesterolemia, elevated low-density lipoprotein in the genesis of coronary heart disease
Factors affecting clinical course of disease	Stress, type A personality in myocardial infarction

Modified from Evans (1987).

involves accumulation of G_{M2} gangliosides in the central nervous system because of an enzyme deficiency (hexosaminidase A) and manifests clinically with degenerative neurologic signs leading to death in early childhood (Sandhoff et al., 1989). Inheritance of the Tay-Sachs genotype is both a necessary and sufficient cause for this disease. On the other hand, if the broader definition of disease is infantile G_{M2} gangliosidosis, the Tay-Sachs genotype can be viewed as a sufficient but not necessary cause, since other genetic disorders, such as Sandhoff disease, have similar clinical manifestations. Sandhoff disease, like Tay-Sachs disease is an autosomal recessive disease, but it can be distinguished from Tay-Sachs disease because it is characterized by deficiency of both hexosaminidase A and B enzymes (Sandhoff et al., 1989). Thus, different mutations leading to similar clinical manifestations reflect genetic heterogeneity in the disease.

An example of a disease with a necessary but not sufficient cause is phenylketonuria (PKU), an autosomal recessive disease that manifests with mental retardation and hypopigmentation due to the deficiency of the enzyme phenylalanine hydroxylase (Scriver et al., 1989). In this situation, phenylalanine (present in a normal diet) is crucial for manifestation of the disease among homozygous carriers of the deficiency allele and also provides the basis for secondary prevention of the mental retardation. Removing phenylalanine from the diet and supplementing with tyrosine, an environmental intervention, offers an effective therapy for this disease.

Perhaps the largest group of risk factors are those that are neither necessary nor sufficient for the development of disease. These reflect both underlying etiologic heterogeneity and the presence of genetic-environmental in-

Table 3–2. Examples of necessary and sufficient causes applied to genetic factors in disease

Disease	Genetic factor	Necessary	Sufficient	Comment
Tay-Sachs	Hexosaminidase A deficiency (homozygous genotype)	Yes	Yes	Genetic disorder with complete penetrance
G_{M2} gangliosidosis	Hexosaminidase A deficiency (homozygous genotype)	No	Yes	Genetic heterogeneity in G_{M2} gangliosidoses (Sandhoff's disease and Tay-Sachs disease)
Phenylketonuria	Phenylalanine hydroxylase deficiency (homozygous genotype)	Yes	No	Gene-environment interaction required (phenylalanine)
Ankylosing spondylitis	*HLA-B27* allele	No	No	Etiologic heterogeneity and gene-environment interaction

teractions. Examples here include *HLA-B27* and ankylosing spondylitis (Ahearn and Hochberg, 1988), α_1-antitrypsin deficiency, and emphysema (Kueppers, 1978).

3.3.3. The Sufficient Cause Model

The sufficient cause model summarized by Rothman (1986) provides a useful approach for studying the interrelation of several "risk factors" or circumstances that lead to the onset of disease in any one individual. Under this model, a *sufficient cause* may be defined as "a set of minimal conditions and events that inevitably produce disease. . . . In disease etiology, the completion of a sufficient cause may be considered equivalent to the onset of disease" (Rothman, 1986). The component factors of a sufficient cause are the combination of genetic and environmental factors that participate in the initiation and the pathogenesis of the disease and are rarely totally identified.

In diseases with etiologic heterogeneity, more than one sufficient cause is involved in disease occurrence. Two sufficient causes for a hypothetical disease are presented in Figure 3–3. Component factors for each individual sufficient cause are a mixture of genetic (G) and environmental factors (E), and these may overlap for the various sufficient causes. This scheme could easily apply to the example of smoking and lung cancer. Because not all smokers develop lung cancer, only a proportion of smokers must possess the other component factors in a sufficient cause needed for the development of lung cancer. Such component factors, in addition to smoking, can be genetic and/or environmental (e.g., genetically determined enzyme systems such as the debrisoquine oxidation phenotypes [Caporaso et al., 1989a, 1989b] as well as other risk factors [Sarucci, 1987]). Moreover, because lung cancer occurs in nonsmokers, at least one additional sufficient cause exists for lung cancer, that does not include smoking as a component cause.

As another simple representation of the model, let us consider phenylketonuria (PKU) where only one sufficient cause is involved, comprising one genetic factor (phenylalanine hydroxylase deficiency) and one environmental factor (phenylalanine in the diet). Clinical disease will ensue if, and only if, the genetic and the environmental factors are both present, and thus their

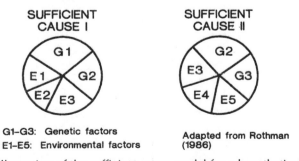

G1–G3: Genetic factors
E1–E5: Environmental factors

Adapted from Rothman (1986)

Figure 3–3. Illustration of the sufficient cause model for a hypothetical disease. G1–G3: genetic factors; E1–E5: environmental factors. [Adapted from Rothman (1986).]

combined presence is a sufficient cause for the development of disease. Each of the component causes is necessary but not sufficient to the development of disease. The sufficient cause model can be used to estimate the proportion of individuals who are susceptible to a risk factor (Khoury and Flanders, 1989; Khoury et al., 1989c). Susceptible individuals are those who have (or will have) all the other components of a sufficient cause and will thus develop disease if exposed to the risk factor of interest. The usefulness of the sufficient cause model lies in interpreting the apparent "strength" of a risk factor-disease association, and in assessing "interaction" among component factors (Rothman, 1986). Under this scheme, one can estimate the proportion of persons who are susceptible to each component cause. In the case of PKU, the proportion of susceptibles to phenylalanine is simply the frequency of the PKU genotype in the population. On the other hand, the proportion of susceptibles to the genetic factor (i.e., phenylalanine hydroxylase deficiency) is simply the proportion of individuals exposed to phenylalanine, which is 100% as exposure is universal.

3.4. EPIDEMIOLOGIC CONCEPTS APPLIED TO GENETIC FACTORS

Many concepts and terms applicable to genes have striking counterparts in the epidemiologic study of infectious agents. Some of these concepts, summarized in Table 3–3, have long been used by geneticists in the context of well-defined Mendelian disorders (Khoury and Cohen, 1988).

3.4.1. The Incubation Period

An important epidemiologic characteristic of disease is the incubation period (or latent period)—the interval between the time of contact with the agent to the time of onset of clinical disease. The incubation period is a classical concept for infectious agents, but has been applied as well to noninfectious diseases and is a biologic attribute of any agent (Lilienfeld and Lilienfeld, 1980; Armenian and Lilienfeld, 1983). In single-gene disorders with onset after birth, the age at onset defines the equivalent of the incubation period (Armenian and Khoury, 1981), since the time of exposure to the agent occurs at conception (actually, the incubation period of the gene is the period from the time of conception to the age at onset). Even for single-gene diseases, there is wide variation in the age at onset (Childs and Scriver, 1986). Although most recessive disorders frequently have onset during infancy and childhood, more dominant disorders have onset later in life (Costa et al., 1985).

The usefulness of the comparison between age at onset and incubation period can be appreciated by examining the shape of its distribution. In common-source outbreaks of infectious diseases, the incubation period is lognormally distributed and is skewed to the right (Lilienfeld and Lilienfeld, 1980). Likewise, for many single-gene, especially recessive, disorders with a defined biochemical defect, the age at onset also follows a lognormal distri-

Table 3–3. Some similarities in concepts and terms between genetic epidemiology and infectious disease epidemiology

	Genetic epidemiology	Infectious disease epidemiology
Agent	Genes	Viruses, bacteria, etc.
Latency	Age at onset	Incubation period
Subclinical disease	Penetrance Carrier state	Pathogenicity Case-infection ratio Carrier state
Clinical disease	Expressivity	Virulence, case fatality
Mode of transmission	Person-to-person (parent to offspring)	Person-to-person Common vehicle
Occurrence in populations		
Measures	Gene, genotype, and phenotype frequencies	Incidence, prevalence
Clusters	Ethnic, geographic clusters, founder effect	Epidemics
Mathematical modeling	Population genetics	Epidemic modeling
Familial clustering		
First case	Proband	Primary or index case
Measure	Recurrence risk	Secondary attack rate
Pattern	Vertical (or horizontal)	Horizontal (or vertical)
Time	Clustering by age at onset	Clustering by calendar time
Statistical issues	Lack of independence	Lack of independence

Adapted from Khoury and Cohen (1988).

bution (Armenian and Khoury, 1981), indicating that expression of disease likely depends solely on the exposure at conception (i.e., the genetic defect), as expected. On the other hand, other single-gene disorders do not follow a lognormal distribution in their age at onset, suggesting factors other than the genetic defect itself (such as environmental triggers) may be important in the manifestation of the disease.

3.4.2. Clinical and Subclinical Disease

Both for infectious agents and genetic disorders, there exists a gradient of disease ranging from the subclinical to the clinical stages. The observation that not all individuals infected with a specific microorganism develop illness can be measured by the case-infection ratio. A similar concept in genetics is penetrance, a measure that refers to the probability that an individual who carries a specific genotype will manifest clinically the expected phenotype. These parallel concepts are important in understanding the natural history of disease, disease pathogenesis, and disease transmission in populations. For example, for both genes and infectious agents, a "carrier state" exists—

referring to individuals with the infection (e.g., individuals carrying hepatitis B surface antigen) or the gene (e.g., heterozygotes for α_1-antitrypsin deficiency gene) who may or may not develop clinical manifestations of disease but can transmit the factor to other individuals.

Furthermore, depending on the virulence of the agent, individuals affected with infectious diseases may show a variety of clinical manifestations ranging from mild to severe disease, complications, and death (Lilienfeld and Lilienfeld, 1980; Mausner and Kramer, 1985). Terms such as "case-fatality ratio" are widely used. Similarly, many genetic disorders are known to show variation in clinical expression from mild to severe disease—a concept known as *variable expressivity*. Also, in genetics the term *pleiotropy* is used to denote the multiple indirect effects of a single gene on different organs or organ systems.

3.4.3. Disease Transmission in Populations and Families

Despite obvious differences in mechanisms of transmission between genes and infectious agents, some common concepts and approaches emerge. Infectious agents are transmitted either indirectly (common source, airborne, etc.) or directly (person-to-person spread). The mode of transmission leads to characteristic patterns of occurrence of the disease in populations and families (Lilienfeld and Lilienfeld, 1980; Last 1986). The spread of an infection in populations has been studied extensively, both empirically in outbreak investigations (Mausner and Kramer, 1985) and theoretically, using mathematical models (Bailey, 1975; Rvachev and Longini, 1985).

Likewise, genes are transmitted as a special type of person-to-person spread following Mendel's laws of inheritance. Such transmission leads to characteristic patterns of occurrence in families. In populations, the behavior of genes typically follows the predictions of the Hardy-Weinberg principle as well as other factors affecting the distribution of genes and genotypes in populations over time and space. The actual distribution of genes in populations can also be studied by using empirical methods of population surveys. A combination of observational and theoretical approaches leads to the measurement of genes in populations in terms of genotype and gene frequencies. Conversely, the occurrence of infectious diseases is measured by using the standard epidemiologic tools of prevalence and incidence. The occurrence of "epidemics" of infectious diseases depends on a combination of factors, such as exposure, incubation period, generation time, and herd immunity. On the other hand, "epidemics" of genetic traits in populations depend on factors such as founder effect, genetic drift, assortative mating, migration, selection, and exposure to mutagens. An example of an "epidemic" of a genetic condition is the exceptionally high frequency of Ellis-van Creveld syndrome (an autosomal recessive type of dwarfism) in the Old Order Amish of Lancaster County, Pennsylvania. Such an "epidemic" has been attributed to the combination of genetic drift and founder effect in this isolated population (McKusick, 1978).

In addition, both genes and infectious agents are known to cluster in families. In infectious diseases, the individual who introduces the disease to the family is the primary case (or index case). In genetics, the first affected person ascertained in a family is called the proband (or index case). Epidemiologists refer to secondary attack rates in describing disease transmission in families (Mausner and Kramer, 1985), whereas geneticists refer to recurrence risks, although conceptually the terms are identical. The pattern of familial spread of infectious agents is primarily horizontal (affecting the same generation), although vertical transmission does occur. Examples of vertical transmission include transplacental transmission of hepatitis B virus (Blumberg et al., 1966), and kuru, an infectious disease long mistaken for a genetic entity (Bennett et al., 1959). On the other hand, although genes are always transmitted vertically in families, horizontal clustering of phenotypes can be observed, especially with rare autosomal recessive conditions, where multiple siblings may be affected, but parents rarely. For infectious agents, there may be a tendency for familial clustering by calendar time, whereas for genes there may be greater clustering by age at onset (Susser and Susser, 1987a, 1987b), and this may be a useful distinction when examining patterns of familial aggregation. For both genes and infectious agents, familial clustering leads to the statistical problems of dependence between observations that necessitate special statistical approaches in data analysis (Bonney, 1986).

3.5. MEASURES OF DISEASE FREQUENCY

In order to characterize diseases in populations and families and to compare their occurrence among different subgroups of the population, epidemiologists have traditionally used several measures describing disease frequency. The three main measures (incidence, cumulative incidence, and prevalence) are briefly summarized in Table 3–4.

3.5.1. Incidence

The *incidence rate* measures the instantaneous force of disease occurrence (Rothman, 1986). Referred to as incidence density, or force of morbidity or mortality, the incidence rate is equal to the number of new (or incident) cases of disease divided by the sum of the time period for all individuals at risk in the population. Technically, a person may be counted more than once as an incident case if he or she has multiple new occurrences of disease. The denominator of incidence rate is a measure of persons at risk in a defined time period, that is, person-time. The underlying assumption of the incidence rate is that one unit of person-time is considered equivalent to and independent of another unit of person-time. Thus, if one case of a disease occurs in a population of 100 persons, each followed for 1 year, or in a population of 50 persons each followed for 2 years, the incidence rate of the disease in both cases is 1 in 100 person-years. Incidence rates are used in follow-up epidemiologic studies and for several vital statistics indices (such as birth, death, and marriage rates).

Table 3—4. Summary of basic epidemiologic measures of disease frequency

	Incidence	Cumulative incidence	Prevalence
Numerator	No. of new disease onsets	No. of new cases in a period of time	No. of cases at a point in time
Denominator	Sum of time periods of all individuals, person-time	Size of population at the start of observation	Size of the population at same point or period of time
Dimension	1/time	None	None
Other terms	Incidence density, force	Disease risk, probability of of morbidity or mortality	Proportion or fraction with disease
Examples	Birth, death rates	Attack rate, lifetime risk, penetrance	Allele and genotype frequencies
Comments	Useful in etiologic studies	Useful in etiologic studies	Not as useful in etiologic studies
		Time element is crucial	Function of incidence times duration
		Frequently approximated with the odds of disease	

3.5.2. Cumulative Incidence

Cumulative incidence (Table 3–4) is a measure of the risk or probability of acquiring disease. Basically, it is the number of new cases of disease in a specified period of time divided by the number of individuals at the beginning of the observation period. Technically, cumulative incidence is not a rate but a proportion, although the terms "rates" and "proportions" continue to be used interchangeably in the literature. Two examples of cumulative incidence are as follows:

1. *Attack rate*: For instance, in an acute outbreak of vomiting and diarrhea, if 2 cases occur in a specified period of time (say 3 days) following a luncheon attended by 100 people, the attack rate (or cumulative incidence) is 2%. This can be contrasted with the incidence rate, which is 2 per 300 person-days, if information is available on all 100 people for 3 days.
2. *Penetrance of a gene*: The term "penetrance" is traditionally used in genetics to denote the proportion of persons known to carry a genotype, who will manifest clinical disease during their lifetime (Khoury et al., 1988c).

Although often not explicitly stated, the time element is crucial in interpreting cumulative incidence measures. For late-onset diseases, it can be difficult to measure accurately the true cumulative incidence without considering competing causes of death.

Cumulative incidence is a useful measure in etiologic studies of disease where subgroups of the population are compared. Also, it is important to derive a measure of risk or probability of disease in counseling situations. Frequently, in epidemiologic analyses, disease risk is replaced by disease odds, which is the ratio of disease risk over one minus disease risk. In the case of rare conditions, these odds closely approximate risk and often may be more conveniently used for statistical analyses.

3.5.3. Prevalence

Prevalence measures the proportion of individuals who have disease at a specific point (or period) of time. Prevalence does not differentiate between new and old cases and can be shown to be a function of the product of incidence rate and the mean duration of illness. Therefore, at any point in time, prevalence is usually skewed for diseases that have a chronic clinical course (such as arthritis, diabetes, and chronic obstructive pulmonary disease). The prevalence of a condition is influenced by factors affecting (1) the incidence of the disease and (2) factors affecting the course of the illness, including treatment, survival, and cure. Because of this, comparisons of prevalence between subgroups of the population are generally less useful for etiologic studies of disease than comparing incidence rates or cumulative incidence. While prevalence proportions are easily obtained in cross-sectional surveys of the population and are frequently the only information available, they must be interpreted cautiously.

It is important to understand that genotype and allele frequencies constitute prevalence measures. For example, in the case of the ABO blood groups, the proportion of individuals with blood group AB at a point in time is the prevalence of AB phenotype in the population. Also, because the Hardy-Weinberg principle allows us to estimate gene (= allele) frequencies from phenotypes, the frequency of the *A* allele is the prevalence of this allele in a population of gametes at any one point in time. In the face of selection, the prevalence of a genotype or a gene may change with age and across generations.

The frequency of birth defects offers another example of prevalence data (Hook, 1982; Schulman et al., 1988). Although often treated as an incidence measure, the proportion of births affected with malformations is more appropriately considered a measure of prevalence because it depends not only on the incidence of defects at conception or during embryogenesis but also on the prenatal survival of affected fetuses. For many types of malformations, there is a great deal of selective prenatal loss of affected fetuses during pregnancy. From that perspective, risk factors affecting the prevalence of a specific defect at birth need to be carefully interpreted in terms of their implications regarding incidence, prenatal survival, or both. For example, an apparent risk factor associated with an increase in a specific birth defect may be merely acting to improve prenatal survival of fetuses who would otherwise not survive to birth.

3.6. TYPES OF EPIDEMIOLOGIC STUDIES

As discussed earlier, the term "risk factor" is used to denote any factor that increases the risk of disease, including demographic factors, environmental exposures, genetically determined traits, and biochemical characteristics. The fundamental epidemiologic approach to the study of disease is to compare two or more subgroups of a population with regard to disease occurrence and risk-factor characteristics. This approach can be carried out either in an experimental setting where investigators assign individuals to different groups or in an observational setting where researchers simply observe disease outcomes in different subgroups or observe the history of the presence of risk factors among individuals with and without disease. Clearly, most epidemiologic data are derived from observational studies, as experimental studies in humans are quite limited. However, the field of experimental epidemiology has recently burgeoned, with increasing interest in controlled clinical trials (Meinert, 1986).

Conceptually, there are four types of epidemiologic studies: ecologic, cross-sectional, case-control, and cohort studies. The cohort approach applies to both experimental and observational studies, although no further distinction will made between them in this discussion. The four types of studies are summarized in Table 3–5. For more in-depth discussion of the design, con-

Table 3–5. Types of epidemiologic studies

Type of study	Characteristics	Measures of disease frequency	Measures of association
Cohort	Follow-up of groups of people that differ with respect to risk factor characteristics	Incidence, cumulative incidence rates	Relative risk, difference in incidence, odds ratio
Case-control	Persons with and without disease studied for past risk factors	None	Odds ratio
Cross-sectional	Persons ascertained for disease and risk factors simultaneously	Prevalence rate	Relative prevalence, difference in prevalences
Ecologic	Cohort or cross-sectional studies, where risk factor characteristics are not known for each person but only for the total group	Same as cohort and cross-sectional studies	Same as cohort and cross-sectional studies

duct, analysis, and interpretation of the various types of epidemiologic studies, readers are referred to other texts on these subjects (Lilienfeld and Lilienfeld, 1980; Schlesselman, 1982; Mausner and Kramer, 1985; Kelsey et al., 1986; Rothman, 1986).

3.6.1. Ecologic Studies

Ecologic studies provide preliminary evidence for the role of specific risk factors in disease. Generally, ecologic studies involve the comparison of disease frequency (incidence or prevalence) between populations that are different with respect to one or more risk factors of interest. A distinctive feature of an ecologic study is that the risk-factor information is not known for individual subjects but rather as a total population characteristic. For example, the inverse association between gastric cancer risk and socioeconomic status led to the hypothesis that a high carbohydrate diet may increase the risk of gastric cancer (Howson et al., 1986). To test this hypothesis, an ecologic study was conducted to correlate gastric cancer mortality levels in different countries with different per capita consumption of cereals such as flour. A high degree of correlation was found in the 16 countries examined (Hakama and Saxen, 1967). Because carbohydrate consumption was not measured on individual subjects, it may well be that such an association can be explained on the basis of other factors (e.g., confounding; see section 3.8). In fact, further testing of the relationship between gastric cancer and consumption of rice, cereals, and starches, using case-control studies, has yielded equivocal or negative findings (Howson et al., 1986).

Nevertheless, ecologic studies often provide initial clues for further epidemiologic research that can be applied in the context of the study of the distribution of genetic traits in populations (Chapter 4) and the evaluation of the role of genetic factors in disease, using migrant studies (Chapter 5). In the absence of risk factor data on individuals, however, associations obtained from ecologic studies can occasionally be spurious. The term *ecologic fallacy* is frequently used to refer to such spurious associations obtained from ecologic studies (Morgenstern, 1982). More discussion on ecologic studies is available elsewhere (Kelsey et al., 1986).

3.6.2. Cross-Sectional Studies

In cross-sectional studies, a set of individuals (either total populations or subgroups of populations) is studied at a single point in time (or over a defined period of time) for the prevalence of disease. Individuals with different risk-factor characteristics are compared with respect to the prevalence of the condition. In cross-sectional studies, both risk factors and disease status are ascertained at the same time. The main disadvantages of cross-sectional studies are as follows:

1. Cross-sectional studies are not suitable for rare diseases or for diseases that have a short duration or poor survival rate.

2. Cross-sectional studies do not readily distinguish between factors affecting disease risk (incidence) and factors affecting the natural history of disease, particularly its duration.
3. Risk-factor characteristics ascertained simultaneously with disease may or may not be relevant to the etiology of the disease, especially for conditions with long latency periods, or the risk factor may have been modified or caused by the presence of the illness itself.

On the other hand, the advantages of cross-sectional studies are as follows:

1. Cross-sectional studies are relatively quick and inexpensive.
2. Cross-sectional studies may provide clues for further etiologic research, using cohort or case-control studies.

3.6.3. Case-Control Studies

Case-control studies have emerged as a powerful tool in epidemiologic research with numerous refinements in approaches, design, and analytic techniques (Schlesselman, 1982). The characteristics of a case-control study are as follows:

1. There is preferential sampling of the numerator over the denominator of an incidence rate. In a case-control study, all cases with disease are sampled, but controls represent only a sample of the person-time experience of the underlying population.
2. Ascertainment of risk factors for the disease occurs retrospectively for both cases and controls, and the measure of disease–risk factor association is based on the direct comparison of past exposure rates between cases and controls, rather than on the comparison of disease frequency.

It is important to keep in mind that cases and controls selected for study must be drawn from the same underlying population. The appropriateness of control groups in case-control studies is a critical issue much discussed in the epidemiologic literature (Cole, 1979; MacLaughlin et al., 1985; Schlesselman, 1985; Poole, 1986). The lack of appropriate ascertainment procedures may introduce various biases and prevent proper interpretation of results (see section 3.8). The main advantages of case-control studies, which have made them increasingly popular in epidemiologic research, are the same disadvantages of the cohort approach, namely:

1. Completion time is relatively short.
2. Multiple risk factors can be examined.
3. Case-control studies are usually not expensive.
4. Case-control studies are suitable for rare diseases.

On the other hand, the main disadvantages of case-controlled studies are as follows:

1. Case-control studies are not suitable for rare exposures.

2. Direct information about disease risk is not provided; only an estimate of relative risk is available (see section 3.7).
3. Risk factors are ascertained retrospectively and may be subject to potential recall bias.

3.6.4. Cohort Studies

Cohort studies are follow-up studies in which two or more groups of individuals with different risk-factor characteristics are followed and compared for morbidity or mortality outcomes. Cohort studies can be either prospective (if the cohorts are followed for future outcomes), or nonconcurrent prospective (if the outcomes of interest occurred in the past), or a mixture of both. Appropriate measures of disease frequency are incidence and cumulative incidence rates. The main advantages of cohort studies are as follows:

1. The natural history of disease from the preclinical through the clinical stages can be studied.
2. Cohort studies are suitable for rare exposures.
3. Multiple disease outcomes can be studied.
4. Risk factors can be ascertained before the onset of disease.

The main disadvantages of cohort studies are as follows:

1. Cohort studies are usually expensive.
2. A long time is usually required to complete the study, depending on the disease frequency and its latency period following the exposure of interest.
3. Cohort studies are usually limited to one or a few exposures of interest.
4. Cohort studies are ill-suited to rare outcomes.

Although cohort studies are often viewed as the ideal epidemiologic study design, they are not totally free from some of the biases that plague other types of studies, namely, selection and confounding (section 3.8). In contrast to the experimental setting of clinical trials where subjects are randomized to one treatment group or another, for observational cohort studies individuals are selected with respect to their risk factor characteristics. For example, despite the overwhelming evidence of deleterious health effects of cigarette smoking (Fielding, 1986), some have suggested that the higher mortality of smokers compared with nonsmokers may be due to unrecognized life-style factors (such as stress) that could be different for smokers compared with nonsmokers (Gantt and Lincoln, 1988). Although confounding can never be completely ruled out in observational studies, the application of indirect methods to search for potential confounding highlights the implausibility that other factors, such as stress, can account for the strong association between smoking and lung cancer (Flanders and Khoury, 1990). Further discussions and illustrations of these types of epidemiologic studies are given in the context of population studies of genetic traits (Chapter 4) and the study of the role of genetic factors in disease occurrence (Chapter 5).

3.7. MEASURES OF ASSOCIATION

In comparing measures of disease frequency between groups with different risk-factor characteristics, traditional epidemiologic analysis is based on the cross-classification of disease outcomes and different risk factors in multiway contingency tables. In its simplest form, when a risk factor is either present or absent, and the disease is either present or absent, the basic building block of standard epidemiologic analysis becomes the 2 × 2 table. Such 2 × 2 tables are appropriate for the basic analysis of cohort, cross-sectional, and case-control studies, with modifications to suit the sampling scheme (e.g., matched versus unmatched design) and the measures of disease frequency for each type of study (Table 3–6). The goal of the analysis is always to test for association between the disease outcome and the risk factor. Also, the basic arrangement can be modified to accommodate risk factors or outcomes that have multiple levels (polychotomous), and those that are inherently continuous in nature (such as measures of height, weight, and blood pressure).

3.7.1. Strength of Association

An association between a disease and a risk factor may represent a cause-effect relationship and still span a broad range of numerical values. Two types of measures for such an association are available: measures of differences in

Table 3–6. Measures of association: the 2 × 2 table

Disease	Risk factor		
	Present	*Absent*	*Total*
Present	a	b	$a + b$
Absent	c	d	$c + d$
Total	$a + c$	$b + d$	$a + b + c + d$

E = probability of disease among people with risk factor exposed = $a/(a + c)$.
U = probability of disease among people without risk factor unexposed = $b/(b + d)$.

Difference measure
Difference in incidence, cumulative incidence, or prevalence:

$$E - U = \frac{a}{a + c} - \frac{b}{b + d}$$

Ratio measures
Relative risk (or prevalence):

$$\frac{E}{U} = \frac{a/(a + c)}{b/(b + d)}$$

Odds ratio:

$$\frac{E/(1 - E)}{U/(1 - U)} = \frac{ad}{bc}$$

For incidence, the denominators are measures of person-time for both absolute and relative effects.

risk, and ratios of risks or probabilities. The most appropriate measure for an association depends in part on the true role of the risk factor, and Table 3–7 lists the expected values for measures of effect difference and ratios of risk when the necessary and sufficient nature of a causal risk factor is considered.

A *difference measure* of a risk factor denotes the excess of disease incidence rate, cumulative incidence rate, or prevalence associated with exposure to the risk factor. As shown in Table 3–7, the difference in the measure of disease frequency between persons with the risk factor and persons without the risk factor quantitates the association between disease and risk factor. As such, this cannot be obtained directly from the case-control design. Other terms used to describe measures of difference are "attributable rate" and "attributable risk."

On the other hand, the ratio of a measure of disease frequency among persons with the risk factor over that among persons without the risk factor also quantitates the association between a disease and a risk factor. If the disease frequencies are incidence rates, cumulative incidence rates, and prevalence, then the relative effects are the *rate ratio*, *risk ratio*, and *prevalence ratio*, respectively. These terms have been collectively known as measures of relative risk, although they may have different interpretations. If the measure of disease frequency is the odds of disease, then the relative effect is the ratio of the odds of disease among persons with the risk factor over the odds of disease among persons without the risk factor, that is, the odds ratio. The importance of the odds ratio as a measure of association lies in the fact that in case-control studies, where direct measures of relative risk cannot be obtained because of the sampling design, the ratio of the odds of exposure to the risk factor among cases over the odds of exposure to the risk factor among controls, that is, the odds ratio of exposure, is identical to the odds ratio of disease in follow-up studies. The use of the odds ratios has become increasingly popular for measuring effects of risk factors in epidemiologic studies for several reasons:

1. The odds ratio is a good approximation of the relative risk for rare diseases.

Table 3–7. Measures of strengths of association of risk factors, in the context of necessary and sufficient causes

| | | Disease risk | | Measure of association | |
| | | With factor (exposed) | Without factor (unexposed) | Difference | Ratio |
Necessary	Sufficient				
Yes	Yes	1	0	1	∞
No	Yes	1	U	$1 - U$	$1/U$
Yes	No	E	0	E	∞
No	No	E	U	$E - U$	E/U

E = probability of disease in exposed persons (individuals with risk factor).
U = probability of disease in unexposed persons (individuals without risk factor).

2. The odds ratio can be obtained from cohort, case-control, and cross-sectional studies.
3. The odds ratio is amenable to statistical techniques of adjustment, using both stratified and multivariate analyses (Schlesselman, 1982; Rothman, 1986; Kahn and Sempos, 1989).

Despite the increasing use of risk-ratio measures (especially the odds ratio) in the analysis and presentation of epidemiologic studies, such measures have some disadvantages that demand caution in making inferences (Greenland, 1987a). First, the magnitude of a relative risk estimate greatly depends on the background risk of disease and is not due solely to the factor of interest. As shown in Table 3–7, if the risk factor is not sufficient (i.e., there is etiologic heterogeneity in the disease), the relative risk measure is inversely related to the magnitude of disease risk among persons without the risk factor. Thus, the higher the background risk not due to a given factor, the lower the relative effects of the factor (Rothman, 1986; Adams et al., 1989). For example, suppose one is interested in quantitating the relative impact of untreated phenylketonuria on the frequency of mental retardation. The risk of mental retardation in untreated persons with the PKU homozygous genotype is effectively 100%, while the risk of mental retardation among children without PKU is about 4% (due to numerous factors and disorders other than PKU). Thus the risk ratio would be close to 25 in this instance. A smaller risk ratio would be seen if the PKU genotype were incompletely penetrant, or if the incidence of mental retardation in the population were more than 4%.

The artificial nature of measures of relative risk can also be seen in Table 3–7 for factors that are necessary for the occurrence of disease, whether they are sufficient or not. In this instance, the relative-risk measure becomes infinitely large because no individual without the risk factor will develop the disease. In the example of PKU, one can see that manipulating the definition of the disease outcome also has marked effects on the magnitude of the relative risk. Since mental retardation is a nonspecific and etiologically heterogeneous disease endpoint, one could define the disease outcome as mental retardation associated with a mousy urine odor and fair skin—cardinal clinical manifestations of untreated PKU. In this situation, the risk of this particular clinical outcome is negligible among persons without the PKU genotype, and the relative risk becomes infinitely large.

A second disadvantage is that a relative risk measure does not readily convey the magnitude of risk to the individual who has a specific risk factor, and thus has to be interpreted in the context of the magnitude of the background disease risk in the population. Consider, for example, two risk factors for two separate diseases (with risks in individuals without the factor of 1/1,000,000 and 1/1,000, respectively) both having a relative risk of 100. These identical relative risks have different interpretations in terms of disease risk for any one individual. The same relative risk could translate into a higher risk of disease for persons with the risk factor. In the example above, the disease risks for persons with the factor are 1/10,000 and 1/10, respectively.

The third disadvantage of a relative risk measure is that it does not convey the importance of the risk factor in the etiology of disease in the population, and it always must be interpreted in conjunction with the frequency of the risk factor itself in the population. For example, the risk ratio associating cigarette smoking with lung cancer is about 20, that is, there is a 20-fold increase in risk among smokers compared to nonsmokers. Likewise, the risk ratio associating the α_1-antitrypsin deficiency homozygous genotype with chronic obstructive pulmonary disease is also 20. It turns out, however, that, although these two risk ratios are virtually identical, cigarette smoking accounts for more than 90% of cases of lung cancer in the population, while α_1-antitrypsin deficiency accounts for only about 1% of COPD in the population. This is a function of the very low prevalence of α_1-antitrypsin deficiency genotype (1/2000) compared with the prevalence of smoking (30%) in the general population.

3.7.2. Attributable Fraction

As discussed above, measures of relative risk and risk difference do not convey automatically the overall contribution of a risk factor to a disease in a particular population. The concept of attributable fraction is useful to address this issue and has grown in importance in the epidemiology literature (Leviton, 1973; Rothman, 1986; Greenland and Robbins, 1988; Adams et al., 1989; Browner and Newman, 1989). This measure is important in quantitating the role of a specific factor in disease etiology and in terms of the public health impact of a risk factor. The public health relevance of this measure lies in estimating the proportion of cases of disease in the population that could be prevented if the exposure of interest were absent.

Although there are still some conceptual problems in its definition and interpretation measures of attributable fraction (Greenland and Robbins, 1988), the term "attributable fraction" is used primarily to refer to the excess fraction of cases of a disease in a population that would have not occurred within a certain time period had the risk factor or the exposure been absent. Several formulas for computing attributable fraction (or excess case load) are available (summarized in Table 3–8). These formulas usually give similar results in the absence of confounding, but only insofar as the odds ratios obtained from case-control studies approximate ratios of cumulative incidences in cohort studies (Greenland and Robbins, 1988). These formulas can be used to calculate the attributable fraction of disease due to simple genetic traits with known allele frequencies and relationship to disease in terms of relative risk (or odds ratios). For example, as discussed earlier, using Levin's formula, one can estimate that the attributable fraction of *PiZ* homozygous genotype in the occurrence of COPD is about 1% (see Table 3–9).

Within the framework of a sufficient cause model, one can theoretically calculate the attributable fraction for each sufficient cause in the occurrence of disease. In the example given in Figure 3–3, suppose that sufficient cause I accounts for 70 percent of the disease and sufficient cause II accounts for 30 percent of the disease. In other words, the removal of a sufficient cause I would result in a 70 percent decline in disease risk in the population. The

Table 3–8. Measurement of attributable fraction (AF) in epidemiologic studies

1. Using overall disease risk in the population (Kelsey et al., 1986)

$$AF = \frac{p - p_0}{p}$$

where p is the probability of disease risk in the total population and p_0 is the probability of disease in individuals without the risk factor

2. Using the frequency of the risk factor in the population (Levin, 1953)

$$AF = \frac{f(R - 1)}{1 + f(R - 1)}$$

where f is the frequency of the risk factor in the population and R is the measure of relative risk (or odds ratio for rare diseases)

3. Using the frequency of the risk factor among cases (Miettinen, 1974)

$$AF = \frac{f_c(R - 1)}{R}$$

where f_c is the fraction of cases with the risk factor and R is the measure of relative risk (or odds ratio for rare diseases)

removal of a sufficient cause can be accomplished by interrupting at least one of the component factors underlying that sufficient cause. Thus, each component factor in a single sufficient cause will have the same value of attributable fraction as the other components (unless individual factors are part of more than one sufficient cause). In the example of PKU discussed earlier, only one sufficient cause is involved with two component factors: that is, PKU homozygous genotype and dietary phenylalanine. Therefore, each of these

Table 3–9. Measures of absolute and relative risks, risk difference and attributable fraction for selected genetic traits that have been associated with certain diseases

	Disease		
	Ankylosing spondylitis	Chronic obstructive pulmonary disease	Lung cancer
Disease risk	0.002	0.05	0.058
Genetic trait	HLA-B27	α_1-antitrypsin deficiency (PiZ homozygote)	High aryl hydrocarbon hydroxylase inducibility
Type of trait	Autosomal dominant	Autosomal recessive	Autosomal dominant
Allele frequency	0.036	0.02	0.324
Genotype relative risk	100	20	20
Risk difference (%)	2.48	94.3	9.74
Penetrance (%)	2.50	99.2	10.20
Attributable fraction (%)	88	0.8	91

From Khoury and Flanders (1989).

component causes accounts for 100% of the disease in the population. Thus 100% of PKU in the population could be prevented by one of two ways: either by removing the susceptible genotype from the population, or by removal of phenylalanine from the diet. This leads to the concept that values of attributable fraction for individual factors that contribute to a single sufficient cause in disease can sum to more than 100%.

This somewhat paradoxical notion has important implications in the study of the role of genetic factors in disease etiology and in interpreting risk factor-disease associations in the context of biologic interactions (see Chapter 5). For complex diseases with multiple sufficient causes, a mixture of genetic and environmental factors likely operates in each of these sufficient causes. Thus, as commented by Rothman (1986), "it is easy to show that 100 percent of any disease is environmentally caused, and 100 percent is inherited as well." Because genotypes are not easily modifiable, the prevention of disease occurrence will likely depend on the manipulation and interruption of the environmental factors that interact with genetic susceptibility. In the example of PKU used here, it is obvious that instead of removing phenylalanine from the diet of all individuals in the population (thereby risking possible harmful nutritional effects), the best prevention strategy is the removal of phenylalanine from the diet only for persons who have inherited the homozygous genotype. These individuals can be identified through newborn screening. The topic of disease prevention in the context of genetic-environmental interaction is discussed further in Chapter 10. Finally, the concept of attributable fraction can be used in the design of epidemiologic studies of genetic factors in disease (Adams et al., 1989; Browner and Newman, 1989). See Chapter 5 for further discussion of this issue.

3.8 CAUSAL INFERENCE IN EPIDEMIOLOGY

When an association is found between a disease and a suspected risk factor in an epidemiologic study, the next step is to attempt to interpret such an association in the context of disease natural history and mechanisms of pathogenesis. However, many associations can arise artifactually because of circumstances connected with study design, selection of subjects, collection of data, and methods of analysis. Observational studies are particularly vulnerable to biased associations.

3.8.1 Sources of Bias in Epidemiologic Studies

Some common types of bias that occur in epidemiologic studies are summarized in Table 3–10. Chapters 4 through 6 provide further details and illustrations of the kinds of bias with particular emphasis on confounding that arise both in population and family studies in genetic epidemiology, as well as available approaches to minimize these biases by appropriate study design and/or analytic strategies.

Table 3–10. Common types of bias in epidemiologic studies

Type of bias	Comments
Selection	Can occur when there are differential selection rates of subjects by disease and/or risk factor characteristics; e.g., bias related to hospital-based studies (Berkson, 1946)
Detection	Can occur when persons with a risk factor are more likely to have disease detected because of more intense medical follow-up, e.g., issue of endometrial cancer and estrogen use (Hulka et al., 1978)
Information	Can occur when interviewers who are aware of the identity of subjects or factors of interest (e.g., case or control) and collect information unevenly between subjects
Recall	Can occur in retrospective studies when persons with disease tend to report past events and exposures differently from persons without disease
Misclassification	Can occur when there is error in classifying subjects by disease or risk factor that tends to distort associations between disease and risk factors (Flegal et al., 1986)
Confounding	Can occur when an association between a risk factor and disease can be explained by a factor associated with both disease and risk factor (Miettinen and Cook, 1981)
Type I errors	Can occur due to chance associations between disease and a risk factor, especially when numerous associations are examined, e.g., hypothesis-generating case-control studies

3.8.2 Assessment of Epidemiologic Associations

In addition to the evaluation of possible biases that could account for an epidemiologic association, several guidelines have been proposed for various aspects of associations and their interpretation from a biologic and pathogenetic perspective (Hill, 1965). They include (1) the strength of the association, (2) possible dose-response effects, (3) consistency of the association, (4) temporality, and (5) biologic plausibility and coherence (Table 3–11).

Table 3–11. Some guidelines used in the assessment of the causal role of epidemiologic associations

Guideline	Comments
Strength of association	The larger the relative effect of a factor, the more likely the causal role of the factor.
Dose-response	If the risk of disease increases with increasing dose of exposure to the risk factor, the likelihood of a causal relation is strengthened; e.g., amount of cigarettes smoked and lung cancer risk.
Consistency	If a similar association can be found in different studies and different populations, the likelihood of a causal role is increased.
Temporality	Risk factors and exposure must precede disease if a causal role is to be implicated.
Coherence	Associations need to be biologically plausible and/or consistent with existing knowledge.

These guidelines have been debated extensively in the literature (Rothman, 1986) and may or may not apply in all situations. For example, as discussed earlier, an association as measured by relative risk may not be strong, but yet the factor involved may actually have an important role in the development of disease, if it is common in the population. On the other hand, the higher the relative risks, the more unlikely that the association is simply the result of hidden biases and the more likely the association is real. Also, dose-response effects may not always apply. The absence of a dose-response effect may reflect some threshold phenomenon; and its presence could still occur with confounding. These points should not be considered as absolute criteria for causal inference but rather viewpoints that may be helpful in the evaluation of empirical observations (Rothman, 1986; Susser, 1991).

3.9. CONCLUDING REMARKS

In summary, epidemiology approaches the study of disease by assessing and comparing the frequency of disease in different groups of the population. Epidemiology seeks to identify "risk factors" for the occurrence of disease. Risk factors can be thought of broadly as factors or circumstances that contribute to the development of disease; and the measurement of associations between risk factors and disease should be viewed as the first step toward unraveling the etiology, pathogenesis, and natural history of disease, with the ultimate goal of prevention (Wynder, 1985). Careful consideration must be given to guard against biases in the design, conduct, and analysis of etiologic studies. The epidemiologic approach to disease and risk factors should not be reduced to a "black box" approach where statistical associations are generated and examined without appropriate evaluation or interpretation. Rather, the approach should be based on a sound biologic foundation in which associations are carefully assessed in terms of disease progression and mechanisms of action for each risk factor, considering the spectrum of natural history.

To accomplish its goals, epidemiology must synthesize information obtained from the various fields of biomedical sciences, such as immunology, microbiology, and biochemistry, in order to provide a meaningful basis for the associations derived from observational studies. Such a synthesis is particularly important in genetic epidemiology where the epidemiologic approach to measuring disease and risk factors complements the molecular, biochemical, cytogenetic, clinical, and statistical tools available in human genetics to provide a better understanding of disease mechanisms.

4

Study of Genetic Traits

4.1. INTRODUCTION

This chapter focuses on epidemiologic concepts and methods for studying genetic traits as outcomes. Here, "genetic traits" are broadly defined to include any variation in the human genome that can be detected at the molecular, biochemical, or clinical levels. These comprise classical Mendelian disorders and traits, structural or numerical chromosomal abnormalities, and genetic polymorphisms regardless of their association with clinical disease. A genetic trait may represent a genotype at a single locus but often is not so limited. This chapter presents (section 4.2) an overview of methods of ascertaining and measuring genetic traits, methods for quantifying the distribution of genetic traits in populations (section 4.3), and approaches for identifying factors that influence the occurrence of new genetic mutations (section 4.4). Finally, section 4.5 deals with approaches to studying determinants of the genetic structure of populations.

4.2. ASCERTAINMENT AND MEASUREMENT OF GENETIC TRAITS

Genetic variation can be studied at different levels. Molecular alterations in a single gene, when observable, provide the ultimate endpoints for study (Cooper and Schmidtke, 1991). The numerous genetic mutations that have been described in the thalassemias and other hemoglobinopathies constitute an appropriate example (McKusick, 1988). As a group these disorders have contributed tremendously to our evolving knowledge of molecular genetics and have served as a model for studying the varieties of mutations that can occur in human populations (Antonarakis et al., 1985). Molecular consequences of mutations may involve single nucleotide substitutions, as well as deletions, and duplications ranging from small pieces of DNA to whole chromosomes (Sutton, 1988). The biochemical consequences of mutations range from no effect to the complete absence of the gene product and its precursor. Other effects include alterations in the structure of the gene product and its function.

4.2.1. Genetic Traits as Outcomes

Selected examples of the classification of genetic traits by level of identification are given in Table 4–1. As shown by the example of Down syndrome discussed in Chapter 3, the outcome used in population studies must depend on the level of current knowledge about the genetic trait. Traditional strategies for identifying genes began with the study of a clinical phenotype. Study of the patterns of familial occurrence can often point to the presence of a distinct genetic mechanism. The next step of inquiry is often the identification of physiologic or pathologic characteristics that could serve as a more precise endpoint for further study, instead of merely a clinical definition. Eventually, further genetic studies may identify a protein or enzyme system underlying a physiologic abnormality. The last step usually is the identification of the actual gene(s) involved to delineate the particular mutation(s) leading to the abnormality. An alternative approach, termed "reverse genetics" or "positional cloning," relies on molecular mapping techniques to locate a gene on a specific chromosome within the genome and then identify its structure function.

The gradual improvement in classification of a disease associated with a simple genetic trait can be exemplified by phenylketonuria (PKU) (McKusick, 1988; Scriver et al., 1989; Konecki and Lichter-Konecki, 1991). As shown in

Table 4–1. Classification of genetic traits by level of identification: Examples and disease associations

Levels of identification	Examples	Disease/phenotype associations
Molecular	A → T at 6th codon leads to Glu-Val substitution in β-globin	Sickle cell anemia/trait
Chromosomal, numerical	Meiotic nondisjunction of chromosome 21	Trisomy 21 (Down) syndrome
Chromosomal, structural	Deletion in 15q11	Prader-Willi syndrome
Biochemical	Phenylalanine hydroxylase deficiency	Phenylketonuria
Physiologic or pathologic	Abnormal sweat chloride	Cystic fibrosis
Clinical	Penetrant lethal dominant mutations diagnosed early in life	"Sentinel" phenotypes

Table 4–2, PKU was first identified clinically as an autosomal recessive form of mental retardation associated with hypopigmentation and peculiar mousy odor to the urine. The physiologic abnormality associated with the disease is hyperphenylalaninemia. The next step was the identification of the deficiency of the gene product, the enzyme phenylalanine hydroxylase. Finally, molecular efforts have identified the actual location of the gene on chromosome 12 (DiLella et al., 1986), and several distinct gene mutations have been identified (Guttler and Woo, 1986). Phenylketonuria also illustrates the increasing diagnostic specificity and resolution of disease heterogeneity at each step. For example, if investigators study the epidemiology of PKU at the clinical level, other disorders that manifest with mental retardation may be inadvertently lumped with PKU, and this could distort inferences concerning the geographic and ethnic distribution of this disease. If one seeks to study PKU at the physiologic level (i.e., a study of hyperphenylalaninemia), causes of hyperphenylalaninemia other than PKU (both genetic and nongenetic) would be lumped with the condition. The study of PKU at the enzyme level has indicated that, in addition to phenylalanine hydroxylase deficiency, PKU can be caused by the deficiency of other enzymes, such as dihydropteridine reductase and dihydrobiopterin synthetase (Sutton, 1988).

The traditional progression from phenotypes (be they clinical or physiologic) to genotypes has been altered by advances in molecular biology (Orkin, 1986). In this process investigators seek to identify the role of genes using DNA probes or DNA polymorphisms (e.g., restriction fragment length polymorphisms [RFLP] or variable number tandem repeats [VNTR]), in patients and their relatives affected with certain diseases before the specific gene products underlying the disease are known. This process can be illustrated by Duchenne muscular dystrophy, an X-linked Mendelian disease, in which the gene was mapped and cloned before the discovery of the protein gene product (dystrophin) deficient in this disease (Ray et al., 1985; Kunkel, 1986). This molecular approach is gaining popularity in investigations of complex disorders where genes are thought to play a role but cannot explain all occurrence of disease (National Research Council, 1988). A number of recent studies have started to test candidate genes for their possible role in the etiology of relatively common disorders, such as oral clefts (Ardinger et al.,

Table 4–2. Levels of analysis of a genetic trait illustrated with phenylketonuria

Level	Endpoint
Clinical	Phenotype of mental retardation, hypopigmentation, and mousy odor to urine
Physiologic	Hyperphenylalaninemia
Biochemical	Phenylalanine hydroxylase deficiency
Molecular	G to A donor splice mutation, intron 12, PKU gene, on chromosome 12, band q24.1. (Other mutations exist)

1988) and insulin-dependent diabetes mellitus (Field, 1988; Morel et al., 1988).

The expansion of molecular techniques is also leading to the gradual erosion of the barrier between the concept of a genetic locus and a chromosome abnormality (Emanuel, 1988). The distinction between chromosomal and single-gene pathologies is becoming blurred with the realization that many conditions previously classified as Mendelian disorders are in fact due to small chromosomal deletions not detectable by regular cytogenetic techniques. With advances in high-resolution banding, several disorders have been shown to exhibit subtle chromosomal pathology, possibly related to the loss of one or more genes, the so-called contiguous gene syndromes (Schmikel, 1986). Some examples include abnormalities of 15q11 in the Prader-Willi syndrome (Mattei et al., 1985), deletions of 17p13 in the Miller-Dieker syndrome (Schwartz, 1988), and deletions of 22q11 in the DiGeorge syndrome (Greenberg et al., 1988). The variability in size of these deletions may contribute to the phenotypic variability seen in the clinical syndromes involved.

Despite the current enthusiasm for molecular techniques, one should not overlook the importance of measuring genetic traits at the biochemical level. After all, the final function of a gene is determined by the protein product it encodes, and advances in biochemical genetics continue to occur in the "inborn errors of metabolism" (Valle and Mitchell, 1988). For example, some enzyme deficiency has been demonstrated for about a third of all autosomal recessive traits listed in McKusick's catalog. Also, deficiencies in structural proteins are being increasingly described, especially for autosomal dominant traits (McKusick, 1988). Electrophoretic techniques have long been used to examine variants in proteins to monitor mutational events in human populations (Neel et al., 1983, 1988a, 1988b). Improvements in this technology, together with the increasing utility of isoelectric focusing, immunologic methods, and two-dimensional electrophoresis have enhanced the ability to detect and measure genetic variation at the protein level (Skolnick and Neel, 1986; Neel et al., 1986). Naturally, the kinds of genetic mutation that can be detected by electrophoretic methods are those that result in substitutions of differently charged amino acids (Neel et al., 1988b). While not all genetic mutations can be detected using such methodology, this problem can be surmounted by molecular approaches to detect mutations at the DNA level (Delehanty et al., 1986; Mendelsohn, 1987; Jeffreys et al., 1988; Kovacs et al., 1989).

Meanwhile the identification of genetic traits continues at the phenotype level. McKusick's updated catalogs represent a synthesis of the growing number of single-gene mutations that have been identified. Because the presence of a Mendelian phenotype in an individual can be due to either inheritance from prior generations or a new mutation, investigators continue to look for those Mendelian disorders that can serve as markers for new mutations, the so-called "sentinel phenotypes" (Holmes et al., 1981; Mulvihill and Czeizel, 1983; Nelson and Holmes, 1989). In brief, Mulvihill and Czeizel (1983) observed that a sentinel mutation is a disorder that

> (i) occurs sporadically as a consequence of a single, highly penetrant, mutant gene,

(ii) is a dominant or X-linked trait of considerable frequency and low fitness, and

(iii) is uniformly expressed and accurately diagnosable with minimal effort, at or near birth.

Examples of such sentinel phenotypes include achondroplasia, Crouzon craniofacial dysostosis, and incontinentia pigmenti (Mulvihill and Czeizel, 1983). Sentinel phenotypes have been proposed as monitoring tools to detect environmental mutagens. Despite the large number of dominant phenotypes recognized clinically, only a few can be considered as candidate sentinel phenotypes, and these are individually quite rare (Mulvihill and Czeizel, 1983). It is anticipated that with improved identification of molecular mechanisms underlying these sentinel phenotypes, the measurement of new mutations will become more accurate, although the discovery of further heterogeneity must also be expected. For example, most cases of osteogenesis imperfecta type II have been shown to be due to new mutations affecting the various collagen genes (Tsipouras and Ramirez, 1987).

4.2.2. Methods of Ascertainment of Individuals with Genetic Traits

How are individuals with specific genetic traits ascertained in epidemiologic studies? Aside from the sentinel phenotypes that can be diagnosed clinically only, the ascertainment of genetic traits usually requires laboratory testing (biochemical, molecular, cytogenetic, etc.) with or without clinical evaluation. For example, the phenotyping of HLA antigens, serum proteins, and blood groups requires laboratory testing of each individual. Sometimes the ascertainment of a genetic trait in an individual requires also testing family members. With HLA antigens, establishing an individual's HLA haplotype at the separate loci of the HLA complex generally requires testing both parents.

When the genetic trait is associated with a clinical phenotype, ascertainment is usually done in a sequential fashion. For example, in the case of autosomal trisomies, such as trisomies 13 and 18, affected individuals manifest patterns of multiple malformations at birth that may suggest the diagnosis to a clinician. The clinical suspicion of a chromosomal syndrome would lead to appropriate cytogenetic testing for confirmation. However, some cytogenetic disorders may not be associated with a recognized phenotype until later in life. For example, clinical recognition of the sex chromosome aneuploidies XYY or XXX at birth may be difficult (Jones, 1988). It is usually much later that the phenotypic features associated with these conditions appear, and there is substantial variability in their expression. Some genetic traits may be phenotypically silent but can lead to disease in the progeny of the individual, such as balanced chromosome translocations that are not associated with clinical manifestations in carriers but produce abnormalities in offspring who inherit the abnormal chromosome in an unbalanced combination.

Thus, because of reliance on laboratory methods to detect genetic traits, the study of genetic traits in populations is complicated by problems of both ascertainment and measurement. Some methods used to ascertain genetic traits in populations are shown in Table 4–3. If all individuals in a defined population were systematically tested for the presence or absence of a specific genetic trait, this would permit complete characterization of its distribution in that population. Also, if other types of information were collected on all individuals, such as race, age, inbreeding, and sociodemographic and personal variables, this would permit direct investigation into factors affecting the distribution of the genetic trait in this population and its relationship to disease. Such an endeavor is rarely possible, except in situations where total populations have been followed over time. A notable example of this approach are studies of genetic effects on survivors of the atomic bomb in Japan (Neel et al., 1988b). Under most conditions, however, these investigations are prohibitively expensive.

A second approach is that of screening programs targeted to select groups, for example, those programs designed to detect individuals who are heterozygotes for certain recessive disorders. This approach is usually applied to subgroups of the population that are at high risk for lethal or devastating disorders (e.g., Tay-Sachs disease carrier screening among Ashkenazi Jews). Advantages, uses, and limitations of programs for heterozygote screening have been discussed elsewhere (Kaback, 1983).

A third method used to ascertain individuals with genetic traits in populations relies on general newborn genetic screening programs. These programs can be used to compute the frequency of selected genetic disorders, usually rare autosomal recessive diseases associated with inborn errors of metabolism (e.g., PKU or galactosemia), as well as to identify conditions requiring early therapeutic intervention.

A fourth method relies on birth defects surveillance systems and registries of chromosomal abnormalities. Birth defects surveillance systems have rapidly

Table 4–3. Some methods used in the ascertainment of genetic traits in human populations

Method	Comments
Total population studies (e.g. atomic bomb survivors)	Can evaluate frequency and determinants of a wide variety of genetic endpoints; very expensive.
Heterozygote screening	Ascertains carriers of selected genetic disorders in high-risk groups
Newborn screening	Ascertains frequency of selected genetic disorders in entire birth cohort
Cytogenetic registries and surveillance systems	Ascertain frequency and determinants of chromosomal anomalies that are clinically detectable at or shortly after birth
Genetic clinics/hospitals	Could be used in etiologic studies but complex patterns of referral and selection could make them unsuitable for evaluating frequency of genetic traits

proliferated in many countries around the world as response to the thalidomide tragedy. The primary objective of these systems is to serve as an early
warning signal to detect new teratogens in the environment; and they usually
rely on multiple sources of ascertainment. Such surveillance systems can also
detect genetic traits associated with chromosomal abnormalities and any structural birth defects apparent at or shortly after birth. Surveillance systems such
as the New York chromosome registry (Hook and Porter, 1981), and the
Metropolitan Atlanta Congenital Defects Program (Edmonds et al., 1981)
have been used extensively in epidemiologic studies of chromosomal abnormalities and other birth defects.

Finally, ascertainment of most genetic traits is usually made as part of
special studies in teaching hospital settings and/or referral centers with separate genetics clinics. Due to problems in referral patterns and other factors
influencing selection of individuals or families, however, it may not be possible
to identify any underlying reference population. Therefore, it becomes difficult to make valid inferences about the population frequency of the genetic
trait. However, with careful consideration of such limitations due to sampling,
such settings can still be used in epidemiologic studies of genetic traits (see
section 4.4).

4.2.3. Measurement Errors in Genetic Traits

The choice of a particular outcome for study influences the design and interpretation of any epidemiologic study. To assess the distribution and determinants of genetic traits in populations, one must always be aware of the
potential for measurement errors. If the genetic trait of interest is measured
directly at the DNA level, or is a simple codominant Mendelian trait, where
the observed phenotype corresponds directly to a single genotype, then only
routine problems of laboratory or labeling misclassification need be considered. In all other settings, however, more careful consideration should be
given to problems of misclassifying the genetic traits in individuals. Physiologic, biochemical, or clinical tests used to identify genetic traits in individuals
are often accompanied by measurement errors. Two types of errors need to
be considered: (1) errors associated with accuracy and (2) errors associated
with reproducibility.

Accuracy of Measurement

The concepts of sensitivity, specificity, and predictive value can shed some
light on the utility of a particular laboratory method for identifying genetic
traits. For a thorough review of these concepts and their relevance to general
epidemiologic studies, readers are referred elsewhere (Fletcher et al., 1982;
Kelsey et al., 1986). In the context of a genetic-epidemiologic study, one is
interested in identifying individuals with and without a genetic trait. A simple
classification of the presence and absence of the genetic trait according to
some laboratory test is presented in Table 4–4. Here, *sensitivity* refers to the
fraction of people with the genetic trait who are correctly classified by the

Table 4–4. Parameters of accuracy in the measurement of a genetic trait

Test	Truth		
	Genotype+	*Genotype−*	*Total*
Genotype+	$se \times g$	$(1 - sp) \times (1 - g)$	g'
Genotype-	$(1 - se) \times g$	$sp \times (1 - g)$	$1 - g'$
Total	g	$1 - g$	1

Genotype +: present; genotype −; absent.

g is the frequency of the genotype in the population; g' is the frequency of the positive test in the population.

$$\text{Sensitivity } (se) = P(\text{test} + \mid \text{genotype} +)$$

$$\text{Specificity } (sp) = P(\text{test} - \mid \text{genotype} -)$$

$$\text{Positive predictive value } (PPV) = P(\text{genotype} + \mid \text{test} +)$$

$$= \frac{se \times g}{se \times g + (1 - sp)(1 - g)}$$

$$\text{Negative predictive value } (NPV) = P(\text{genotype} - \mid \text{test} -)$$

$$= \frac{sp \times (1 - g)}{(1 - se) \times g + sp \times (1 - g)}$$

test. *Specificity* refers to the fraction of people without the genetic trait who are correctly classified as such by the test.

The concepts of sensitivity and specificity can also be applied to various methods of ascertainment of genetic traits. For example, in trying to ascertain whether an individual has the PKU genotype using the conventional newborn screening test for phenylalanine blood concentration, it has been shown that, among infants subsequently shown to have PKU, phenylalanine levels rise with age (in days). Therefore, depending on the particular cutoff used to define elevated phenylalanine level and the timing of the test, some affected individuals may be missed. Thus, the screening test may not have 100 percent sensitivity. Maximal rates of missed cases (false negatives) have been estimated as 16%, 2% and 0.3% for screening done on days 1, 2, and 3, respectively (Scriver et al., 1989). Moreover, the simple biochemical test most frequently used for newborn screening is not specific for phenylalanine hydroxylase deficiency because it picks up other causes of hyperphenylalaninemia.

Another important concept is the predictive value of a test. The *positive predictive value* (PPV) refers to the fraction of persons classified as having the genetic trait who actually do have the trait. The *negative predictive value* (NPV) refers to the fraction of persons classified as not having the genetic trait who actually do not have the trait. PPV and NPV are functions of sensitivity, specificity, and the frequency of the underlying trait in the population tested (Table 4–4). The rarer the genetic trait in the tested population, the lower the PPV will be for any given levels of sensitivity and specificity. In the example of PKU, because PKU is very rare (about 1 per 10,000 newborns), PPV is extremely small, even for a test that is 100% sensitive (Fletcher et al., 1982). Unless the test used is both 100% sensitive and 100% specific, there will always be some misclassification.

Misclassification of genetic traits in epidemiologic studies can affect the estimated frequency of a genetic trait in a population and, perhaps more importantly, can lead to either spurious differences between the groups or to a dilution of real differences between the groups when the frequency of the genetic trait is compared among subgroups of the population stratified by exposures or other risk factors (see section 4.4).

Reproducibility of Measurement

As with any other type of test, potential problems in measuring genetic traits can come from lack of reproducibility. These difficulties can be due to random errors alone or to more systematic ones affected by external factors. Complex enzyme assays may be difficult to reproduce across laboratories or over time within a single laboratory. One example is the relatively complex lymphocyte enzyme assay to measure aryl hydrocarbon hydroxylase inducibility. This enzyme system was originally reported by Kellerman and colleagues (1973) to be strongly associated with lung cancer risk, but it was difficult to replicate this association in other laboratories. When genotype assignment is based on a cutoff point (e.g., enzyme activity less than a certain level, or substrate level more than a certain level), repeated measurements on the same or different blood samples from the same person, tested by the same or different laboratory personnel, can lead to fluctuations of measured levels and quite possibly to different assignments of genotypes. Quality control measures must be established to assess reproducibility in any laboratory measurement. Measures of reproducibility involve computing correlations between repeated observations for continuous variables. When the outcome is binary, one can calculate the proportion of agreement, and the kappa index for the assignment of genotypes should be computed, using repeated tests based on a single specimen or on separate specimens from the same individual. For example, the assignment of an apparent genotype from two measurements (test 1 and test 2) leads again to a 2 × 2 table from which the percent agreement can be calculated (Table 4–5). To correct for chance agreement that can occur, especially if one class is rare, the kappa index can be computed as shown in Table 4–5 (Fleiss, 1981). According to Fleiss, values of kappa > 75% can be taken as excellent agreement (beyond chance alone), while kappas < 40% indicate poor agreement. Similar measures of agreement can also be computed

Table 4–5. Parameters of agreement in the measurement of a genetic trait

Test 1	Test 2		
	Genotype +	Genotype −	Total
Genotype +	a	b	p_1
Genotype −	c	d	q_1
Total	p_2	q_2	1

Genotype +, present; genotype −, absent.

Proportion of agreement = $a + d$

Kappa index = $\dfrac{2(ad - bc)}{(p_1 q_2 + p_2 q_1)}$

when dealing with polychotomous outcomes such as assignment of homozygosity and heterozygosity at a single locus (Fleiss, 1981).

It must be understood that reproducibility is not the same as accuracy. Accuracy can be measured only when the true genotypic status of the individual is known by using some "gold standard." On the other hand, reproducibility can always be measured by comparing the performance of two or more tests in the assignment of an apparent genotype, even if the true status of the individual remains unknown. It is entirely possible that a laboratory test can be highly reproducible but always gives the wrong assignment of genetic trait (inaccurate) due to systematic errors (Kelsey et al., 1986). On the other hand, poor reproducibility of a test is almost always an indicator of poor accuracy. This type of measurement error in epidemiologic studies of genetic traits can be critical to issues of random and/or differential misclassification of the endpoints (sec sections 4.4 and 4.5).

4.3. DESCRIPTIVE STUDIES: DISTRIBUTION OF GENETIC TRAITS IN POPULATIONS

This section reviews genetic and epidemiologic approaches to characterizing the distribution of genetic traits in populations. At any given point in time, the distribution of genetic traits in populations is a function of the combination of (1) occurrence of mutation and (2) forces that can alter allelic and genotypic frequencies, such as migration, selection, and drift due to population size. Thus, when measuring genetic traits in populations, it is necessary to distinguish at the outset whether one wishes to focus on the study of de novo mutations or on the study of all genetic traits (both "new" allelic variants and those inherited from previous generations). When considering the available tools for measuring genetic traits in populations, several apparent differences between classic genetic and epidemiologic approaches are noted.

4.3.1. Genetic and Epidemiologic Approaches

Geneticists traditionally have sought to measure the distribution of not only phenotypes in populations, but also of the underlying alleles and genotypes. For example, using carefully conducted epidemiologic surveys, one can measure the frequency of PKU at birth as 1 per 10,000 live births. Epidemiologic principles alone, however, cannot relate this measure of disease prevalence to the frequency of the PKU allele as 1%, but this is done by assuming Hardy-Weinberg equilibrium in the population.

Differences in the nomenclature and terminology used by geneticists and epidemiologists in describing disease and genetic trait frequencies often create unnecessary confusion. Although both geneticists and epidemiologists can arrive at 1 per 10,000 livebirths as the estimate of frequency of PKU at birth, different terms (such as incidence, prevalence, frequency, or rate) may be used in the literature. As discussed in Chapter 3, even among epidemiologists there is disagreement on the definitions and the usage of basic terms, such as "rates" (Elandt-Johnson, 1975; Schulman, 1988). This different nomenclature can be reconciled by applying unified principles to express estimates of frequency (Elandt-Johnson, 1975; Rothman, 1986). (See Chapter 3.)

Another major area of differing orientation between the two fields is the emphasis epidemiologists place upon identifying the strengths and weaknesses of the sources of data used to derive measures of frequency. For example, blood donors have long been used in population genetics to estimate allele frequencies for genetic systems such as HLA, various blood group antigens, and other genetic traits (such as hemochromatosis; Edwards et al., 1988). Another example is a study of genetic polymorphisms of human serum ribonuclease I (RNase), in which laboratory workers, students, and other convenient volunteer families were used to estimate frequencies of the two common alleles RNASE*1 and RNASE1*2 (Yasuda et al., 1988). Epidemiologists would question the representativeness of such samples of convenience. Specifically, it is likely that volunteer samples are different from the underlying population with respect to factors such as ethnic background, socioeconomic status, consanguinity, and other factors that may or may not be related to the frequency of the genetic traits of interest. These concerns about study populations, collection of data, completeness of ascertainment, selection factors, methods of detection of genetic traits and phenotypes, confounding factors, sample size, and statistical power are rooted in the epidemiologic approach. These concerns apply to studies that seek to compare frequencies of various genetic traits between groups, or that aim to examine the role of specific genetic traits in the etiology of disease (Chapter 5).

4.3.2. Prevalence Measures of Genetic Traits

The measures of disease frequency reviewed in Chapter 3 can also be applied to genetic traits and, in many circumstances, to alleles in populations. A prevalence measure denotes the proportion of individuals with a specific genetic trait in the population at a given point or time period. It is not a measure of risk. Prevalence is often confused with incidence in the literature (Hook, 1982), just as a proportion is often confused with a rate (Elandt-Johnson, 1975). For example, the frequencies of various chromosomal abnormalities detected in liveborn surveys are prevalence and not incidence measures (Schulman, 1988). Prevalence is most appropriate here because a large fraction of fetuses with chromosomal anomalies are lost early in pregnancy.

Prevalence measures can be applied to phenotypes as well as to genotypes and alleles. For both phenotypes and genotypes, the denominators used in the calculation are individuals, whereas for alleles, the denominator is the number of genes in the population (for autosomal traits this is twice the number of individuals; for X-linked traits this is twice the number of females plus the number of males). To illustrate issues and problems related to the measurement of the prevalence of a genetic trait, consider the following example. In a survey of 11,065 healthy blood donors, Edwards et al. (1988) examined the prevalence of hemochromatosis genotype, an autosomal recessive disorder characterized by excessive absorption of iron through the gastrointestinal tract and progressive accumulation of iron in parenchymal organs, frequently leading to liver cirrhosis, cardiac myopathy, skin pigmentation, and endocrine problems. The disease locus is tightly linked with the HLA locus on chromosome 6 (Kravitz et al., 1979). Previous studies of this disease had given conflicting information regarding its prevalence and, thus, the allele frequency in the population. In part, these problems arose because of the lack of established diagnostic criteria for this condition. One phenotypic marker for the disease is the laboratory measurement of transferrin saturation. A value of 62% saturation or more, previously determined to predict homozygosity accurately in 92% of the cases (Dadone et al., 1982), was used in Edwards' (1988) study as an initial screening test. Individuals who had this value of ferritin saturation (or greater) were further evaluated for liver biopsy, pedigree analysis, and HLA studies. In this study, the prevalence of the high ferritin saturation phenotype was .008 in men and .003 in women. However, further workup of the "positive" group based on transferrin assay revealed a prevalence proportion of the homozygous genotype of .0045 in men. Assuming Hardy-Weinberg equilibrium, this corresponds to an allele frequency of .067 $[- (.0045)^{1/2}]$. Information on the "positive" transferrin phenotype in women could not be used directly because it identified only half as many female homozygotes as predicted by this allele frequency under Hardy-Weinberg equilibrium (which predicts the allele and genotype frequencies would be similar in both sexes). This example illustrates not only the use of prevalence data to estimate allele frequencies, but also points out problems inherent in case definition and classification related to sex-specific sensitivity and -specificity of both screening and diagnostic tests.

4.3.3. Incidence Measures of Genetic Traits

Measurement of the frequency of new mutations has long been of interest to population geneticists and is particularly relevant to quantitating the impact of environmental agents such as radiation and chemicals on the human genome (Vogel and Rathenberg, 1975; Hook and Porter, 1981; Vogel and Motulsky, 1986). However, when one applies incidence measures to genetic traits, some problems arise. Theoretically, when measuring disease incidence in a defined population, individuals free of disease are followed over time and new cases of disease counted, permitting investigators to compute incidence rates directly (per unit of person-time) as well as cumulative incidence proportions up to any given time. In this context, the term "mutation rate" has been used to refer to "the probability with which a particular mutational event takes place in a fertilized germ cell per generation" (Vogel and Motulsky, 1986). This measure should rightly be considered a proportion and carries the implication of cumulative incidence, that is, risk of genetic change per generation. The measure also refers to fertilized germ cells only, since the measurement of mutation in unfertilized gametes has so far been difficult and is of dubious consequence. Because of this, one is limited to measuring the frequency of mutations either in recognized spontaneous abortions, at birth, or later in life. Thus, in practice, measurement of mutation rates is usually not an incidence measure per se but rather a prevalence measure (Hook, 1982). In spite of this drawback, the term "mutation rates" will be used throughout this chapter for consistency with the literature.

Direct Method

As a hypothetical example, assume that the methodology existed to measure a mutational event at birth. In a newborn survey, suppose that, of 100,000 newborns, 10 are found to manifest a given genetic trait. In order to calculate the mutation rate at this specific locus, first, one has to determine how many of these 10 cases represent "new" mutations (i.e., the trait was not present in either parent). Second, if one makes the assumption that the mutational event does not interfere with fertilization and does not affect prenatal survival, then, the proportion of individuals at birth with the new mutation can be used to compute mutation rates directly. In this example, assuming that all 10 cases are "new" mutations, one can estimate that the mutation rate at this hypothetical locus is $10/2 \times 10^{-5}$, or 5 per 10^{-5} per gamete per generation. The division by 2 is necessary because the number of gametes is double the number of individuals. Furthermore, if one can determine the parental origin of the mutation (which is becoming increasingly possible using molecular techniques, Chandley, 1991), one can measure the mutation rate in fertilized ova versus that in sperm. In the example above, if one assumes that of the 10 cases, 8 occurred in the mother and 2 in the father, the mutation rates at this locus would be 8 per 10^{-5} per fertilized ova, and 2 per 10^{-5} fertilized sperm.

This method for measuring mutation rates is known in population genetics as the *direct method* (Vogel and Motulsky, 1986) and has been used to study mutations in chromosome number (e.g., trisomy 21), chromosome structure (such as deletions), as well as dominant single-locus mutations. This method, however, cannot be applied to autosomal recessive disorders, as new mutations cannot be readily distinguished from those transmitted from prior generations (Morton, 1981).

An illustration of the direct approach to measuring mutation rates for a chromosomal abnormality is provided by the example of Down syndrome. The frequency at birth of trisomy 21 is about 1 per 1000 livebirths. Thus, the mutation rate for trisomy 21 can be estimated as 5 per 10^{-4} fertilized germ cells per generation. This estimate is, of course, not correct, since a large proportion (75% to 80%) of trisomy 21 fetuses are lost during gestation. Moreover, this estimated mortality may be conservative because many trisomy 21 zygotes may be lost before the pregnancy is recognized clinically. Also, there is the possibility of differential fertilization between germ cells containing a normal chromosomal complement and those that have an extra chromosome 21 as a result of nondisjunction, although confirmation of this hypothesis would be extremely difficult. Because of recent advances in cytogenetic and molecular techniques, it is now frequently possible to separate nondisjunction events as to their parental origin and meiotic stage. If one assumes that about 20% of trisomy 21 cases have a paternal origin (Magenis,

1988), one can estimate a mutation rate of paternal trisomy 21 as 2 per 10^{-4} fertilized sperm cell per generation. On the other hand, about 80% of trisomy cases have a maternal origin, and most of those arise in meiosis I. Similar estimates for the mutation rate of maternal nondisjunction events per fertilized ovum per generation are approximately 8 per 10^{-4} fertilized ova per generation. Based on molecular studies, recent data suggest, however, that only about 5% of trisomy 21 cases are due to paternal errors in meiosis (Antonarakis et al., 1990; Sherman et al., 1990).

In measuring mutations for dominant traits, the direct method can be applied to specific molecular or biochemical endpoints. This approach has also been used to estimate mutation rates based on the so-called "sentinel" phenotypes as discussed in section 4.2.1. Problems in this direct method for measuring mutation rates have been previously reviewed by Vogel and Motulsky (1986) and can be briefly summarized as follows:

1. *Study population:* Ideally, estimates of mutation rates should be made from population-based newborn surveys or registries, or follow-up investigations of entire populations, or at least well-defined subgroups.

2. *Ascertainment of genetic traits*: The accuracy and completeness of ascertainment of the genetic trait under study are important. For example, if one is measuring the frequency of trisomy 21 in a population of newborns, unless all newborns in the population are screened for chromosomal abnormalities, the number detected depends on the completeness of recognition of the trisomy 21 clinical phenotype by pediatricians or medical practitioners, karyotype examination, and reporting. Underascertainment of affected individuals leads to underestimates of mutation rates. This issue becomes more crucial for disorders with incomplete penetrance, where the characteristic phenotype or disease may not be expressed at all in some individuals carrying the mutation. Such disorders should not be used as "sentinel" phenotypes. For Mendelian phenotypes that are not apparent at, or shortly after, birth, mutation rates can still be calculated within the context of an epidemiologic study in which a cohort of births is followed and the genetic trait of interest is ascertained at various ages. Cumulative incidence proportions in this situation, but not the prevalence of the trait, will provide estimates for mutation rates. Prevalence measures in a cross section of the population depend, of course, on both incidence and survival of affected individuals (i.e., the duration of this "disorder"). Thus, in a population survey, the prevalence of a genetic trait associated with shortened survival will underestimate the cumulative incidence, and will produce estimates of mutation rates that are biased downward. Reduced survival and death due to competing causes complicate the interpretation of cumulative incidence measures.

3. *Ascertainment of "new" genotypes*: To calculate a mutation rate, one has to know the proportion of individuals with a given genetic trait whose parents did not transmit the genetic trait. These are commonly known as sporadic cases. For autosomal dominant traits, ascertainment of "new" mutations can be done only after evaluation of the family history and the verification that the trait was not present in either parent (Nelson and Holmes, 1989). This can be a particular problem in the event of nonpaternity, where

the father of record is not the biologic father. In the case of aneuploidies (such as trisomy 21) where all affected individuals are usually "new," assignment of the parental origin of the extra chromosome still requires direct examination of parents of affected individuals, using multiple chromosome polymorphisms and/or DNA markers.

Another problem related to the ascertainment of "new" mutations in offspring is the possibility of germ-line mosaicism in otherwise normal parents (Hall, 1988b; Edwards, 1989). For several dominant disorders and some X-linked recessive diseases, there are reports of more than one affected offspring from parents that are phenotypically normal by all known methods of testing. These findings have suggested that "phenotypically normal individuals may transmit several gametes that are clonal descendants of a single progenitor germ cell in which a de novo mutation occurred during the development of the parent" (Hall, 1988b). Identification of germ-line mosaicism in males may become possible in the near future with the further development of molecular techniques for examining sperm (Hecht, 1987). The same applies to other forms of mutations, such as cytogenetic changes, which are becoming more amenable to study in semen samples, for example, fusion with hamster oocytes (Evans, 1988). On the other hand, mosaicism (and other types of mutations) in female germ cells are far more difficult to study because of the relative inaccessibility of these cell lines. Recently, however, women enrolled in in vitro fertilization programs or embryo transfer have been used to study chromosomal anomalies in oocytes (Wramsby et al., 1987). It should be noted that for some of the examples cited in the literature, alternative explanations to germ-line mosaicism may also be involved, such as etiologic heterogeneity and genetic interaction (Hall, 1988b).

4. *Etiologic heterogeneity:* When genetic traits are studied at the phenotypic level, the existence of multiple etiologic mechanisms associated with a single phenotype interferes with estimation of mutation rates. Nongenetic cases of a phenotype (known as "phenocopies"), where the etiology is presumably environmental, may be misclassified as a new mutation leading to an overestimation of mutation rates. Likewise, for many single-gene traits, the existence of several patterns of inheritance in different pedigrees (autosomal dominant, autosomal recessive, and X-linked) may also affect the calculation of mutation rates unless the various phenotypic forms can be clearly distinguished by clinical or laboratory methods. In particular, if an X-linked recessive form of a genetic disease exists, there will be a greater frequency of affected males that might inflate the apparent maternal mutation rate.

Indirect Method

Indirect approaches to estimating mutation rates have been proposed in population genetics (Vogel and Rathenberg, 1975; Vogel and Motulsky, 1986). Haldane's original indirect method is based on the concept of an equilibrium between mutation and selection in human populations. To illustrate this concept, consider the autosomal dominant sentinel phenotypes. One of the components of the definition of a sentinel phenotype is low fitness, meaning reduced ability to reproduce. Under this scheme, all new cases are eliminated by natural selection as they arise. Thus, any cases in a particular generation must be de novo mutations, that is, none of the parents has the same trait. Thus, the mutation rate is simply the proportion of births affected with the trait (divided by 2 as for the direct method). More generally, if the relative fertility of individuals with the trait is f, with $f = 1$ implying fertility levels equivalent to that of the general population and $f = 0$ implying affected individuals are completely sterile, the indirect estimate of a mutation rate for an autosomal dominant trait is

$$\mu = \frac{1}{2}(1 - f)p, \tag{4-1}$$

where p is the birth prevalence of individuals with the trait, or cumulative incidence in a cohort of births. When the trait is a genetic lethal (i.e., f is 0), μ is simply $p/2$. Under this condition, the direct method gives the same result, since all individuals with the trait must be new mutations. Formulas for indirect estimation of mutation rates have been derived for autosomal recessive, X-linked, and Y-linked genetic traits (Vogel and Rathenberg, 1975) and are shown in Table 4–6.

While the indirect method has the advantage over the direct method, in that it is not affected by problems of nonpaternity, its main disadvantage (in addition to the ones listed for the direct method) is that accurate estimates of relative fertility (f) are rarely available. Another problem arises from improved medical care that now permits individuals with some genetic traits traditionally associated with poor fitness to live longer and to reproduce. This violates the assumption of equilibrium between mutation and selection, and leads to distorted estimates of mutation rates. Thus, the indirect method can give only approximate values of mutation rates and can rarely be used to study determinants of mutations in humans.

Table 4–6. Indirect method for estimating mutation rates of single-gene traits, with various modes of inheritance

Mode of inheritance	Mutation rate
Autosomal dominant	$\frac{1}{2}(1 - f)p$
Autosomal recessive	$(1 - f)p$
X-linked recessive	$\frac{1}{3}(1 - f)p_{males}$
X-linked dominant	$\frac{2}{3}(1 - f)p$
Y-linked	$(1 - f)p_{males}$

Adapted from Vogel and Rathenberg (1975).

f = relative fertility of persons with the genetic trait, where $f = 1$ implies no impairment in fertility relative to the general population, $f = 0$ corresponds to complete infertility.

p = prevalence proportion of the trait in a cohort of births.

p_{males} = proportion among males only.

4.4. ANALYTIC STUDIES: DETERMINANTS OF MUTATIONS IN POPULATIONS

As has been indicated, the determinants of genetic traits can be divided conceptually into those that are associated with the formation of de novo mutations in populations, and those that are associated with the genetic structure of an existing population at a given point in time. Approaches to the first group of determinants are all too familiar to epidemiologists and largely involve the evaluation of environmental risk factors (mutagens), while approaches to the second group of determinants are more familiar to population geneticists. As emphasized by Roberts (1983), it is the second group of determinants that gives genetic epidemiology its uniqueness. In this section, approaches to studying determinants of new genetic traits in terms of study design, ascertainment of risk factors, and analytic issues are discussed.

4.4.1. Study Design

Factors affecting the occurrence of mutations in populations may be environmental (such as radiation and chemicals) or genetic in nature (e.g., genes that possibly affect the rate of autosomal nondisjunction [Alfi et al., 1980]). To assess these factors, genetic outcomes (discussed in section 4.2) can be studied with classical epidemiologic methods, despite all the limitations and difficulties in identifying such outcomes. Two epidemiologic study designs are discussed in this section: cohort and case-control designs. Table 4–7 summarizes the main characteristics of these two types of studies, their relative advantages and possible limitations.

Cohort Approach

The cohort design involves the comparison of the frequency of occurrence of specific new mutations among subgroups of the population identified on the basis of characteristics of interest (such as groups exposed or nonexposed to radiation). As discussed in Chapter 3, cohort studies are difficult, lengthy, and costly. This is particularly relevant in the area of mutation epidemiology, where the outcomes are extremely rare, relatively complex to measure, and tend to occur many years after putative exposures (Miller, 1983).

Examples of available cohort-type studies in this area have been rather opportunistic, relying on cohorts formed by either man-made or natural disasters (e.g., atomic bomb studies, studies in the Sevesco population). Other international collaborative studies involve the assessment of mutation rates in humans by studying the offspring of cancer patients who have survived and reproduced after having had chemotherapy and radiotherapy (Lyon, 1985). Another example is the Collaborative Perinatal Project, a large multicenter prospective study of more than 50,000 women ascertained during pregnancy and followed prospectively for pregnancy outcomes, morbidity, and mortality in their children through age 7 years. In this study, a variety of prenatal exposures and events were studied in relation to outcomes of pregnancy

Table 4–7. Comparison between the main characteristics of cohort and case-control studies of mutations

Characteristic	Cohort	Case-control
Ascertainment basis	Exposure-driven	Outcome-driven
Examples	Studies of atomic bomb survivors in Japan	Case-control studies of Down syndrome examining the effects of parental ages and exposure to radiation
Study population	Entire populations, exposed individuals	Individuals with specific genetic outcomes
Comparison group	Unexposed individuals	Individuals without specific outcomes (controls)
Risk factor ascertainment	Prospective (or retrospective)	Retrospective
	Usually one main exposure	May be multiple exposures
Genetic condition or outcomes	Multiple genetic and non-genetic outcomes studied	Specific genetic outcome studied
Measures of association	Absolute and relative measures	Relative measures only
Estimation of mutation rates	More direct	Less direct
Sample size and statistical power		
Risk factor	Better for rare exposures	Better for common exposures
Mutation	Better for common outcomes	Better for rare mutations
Limitations and possible biases	Selection bias, confounding	Recall bias, confounding
Relative cost	More costly	Less costly

including chromosomal abnormalities and other birth defects (Niswander and Gordon, 1972; Heinonen et al., 1977).

Another example of cohort studies involves the use of population-based registries of chromosomal abnormalities, such as trisomy 21. These registries, used primarily for surveillance purposes, ascertain infants born with chromosomal abnormalities and other structural defects among birth cohorts in well-defined populations. In the example of trisomy 21, this method, used to study the relationship between parental ages and the birth prevalence of trisomy 21, is feasible because parental ages are usually recorded in vital records (birth certificates) and thus available for both trisomy 21 cases and the population at large without conducting separate interview studies. Such data have been used to compare the prevalence of trisomy 21 at birth among mothers of different age groups. The well-known increased frequency of trisomy 21 among offspring of older mothers has been documented, using this type of surveillance system (e.g., Adams et al., 1981).

One limitation to keep in mind is the problem of prenatal loss discussed earlier. Studies based on birth prevalence of genetic traits should be more correctly thought of as cross-sectional in nature rather than cohort (since ascertainment is at birth and not at the time of conception). However, as discussed above, problems with estimation of mutation rates essentially make all studies of reproductive outcomes based on birth cohorts cross-sectional in nature. Although the distinction is acknowledged, nevertheless, these types of studies are used to derive estimates of mutation frequencies and to evaluate their associations with risk factors. On the other hand, the usual cross-sectional studies based on population samples of different age groups can be used only to derive prevalence estimates of genetic traits. Differences in the prevalence of specific genetic traits between subgroups of the population (e.g., on the basis of age, race, or exposures) may be due to factors also affecting mutation rates, and/or those related to population dynamics (e.g., fertility, migration, selection). Thus, cross-sectional studies are always limited to some extent when measuring mutation rates and the effects of potential risk factors on the occurrence of new genetic traits.

Case-Control Approach

As already noted in Chapter 3, case-control studies are being utilized increasingly in epidemiologic studies of disease (Schlesselman, 1982; Kelsey et al., 1986; Rothman, 1986). A comparison of the major features of case-control design with those of the cohort approach is shown in Table 4–7. Case-control studies have a particular appeal in the study of mutations in humans for several reasons: First, they are less costly than cohort studies, especially when one considers that laboratory testing is required for only a sample of unaffected individuals (controls) rather than the total population. Second, because the outcomes of interest are rare (1 per 10,000 or less), most cohort studies would require very large and often unattainable sample sizes. Finally, the theoretical base and methodology of case-control studies is well developed, so that inferences regarding measures of effects obtained from this type of design, when properly conducted, can be valid and applicable in the context of cohort studies as well (Rothman, 1986).

The idea that controls are a sample of the population-time experience from which cases are derived is important to keep in mind when designing any case-control study of genetic mutations. Frequently this population base is difficult to conceptualize, and therefore an appropriate control group may not be readily apparent. A nearly ideal situation exists when a case-control study of a specific genetic trait (e.g., trisomy 21) is designed where cases are drawn from population-based birth defect surveillance systems. In this situation, an appropriate control group can be derived from the total population of births from which the cases are drawn. The situation becomes more difficult when dealing with clinic- or hospital-based studies. Here, the population base from which cases are selected is usually ill defined; therefore, care must be exercised in the choice of a control group.

For example, consider the Prader-Willi syndrome, a dysmorphic syndrome where the majority of cases are associated with a deletion in chromosome 15.

The origin of this deletion is frequently in paternal germ cells (Ledbetter and Cassidy, 1988; Magenis, 1988). Recent reports suggested that paternal occupational lead exposure may be a risk factor for this disorder (Strabowski and Butler, 1987; Cassidy et al., 1989). To test this hypothesis, a case-control study would be more cost-effective than a cohort study because of the extreme rarity of this genetic disorder. Given that the diagnosis of Prader-Willi syndrome is usually made only in selected genetic centers, a problem arises in choosing an appropriate control group for a series of cases ascertained through one or more genetic clinics. Because the diagnosis may or may not be done at birth, another problem arises from having a series of cases of different age groups (prevalent versus incident cases). Ideally, only incident or new cases ascertained at birth or in a more or less delineated cohort of births should be used as the case group. Incident cases are preferable over prevalent cases because the primary interest is in factors causally related to the occurrence of the mutation. Prevalent cases are also affected by factors related to the prognosis and natural history of the disorder. An ideal control group should derive from the same cohort of births, but in a clinic or referral center situation, this often is not feasible. To test specific hypotheses (e.g., occupational exposures), it is important to choose a control group that is comparable to the case group with respect to sociodemographic, educational, and ethnic backgrounds because any one or more of these factors may act as confounding variables in the interpretation of any positive association that may be observed (see the subsection entitled "Confounding" later in this chapter).

The choice of appropriate controls is a difficult and controversial area in epidemiology (Schlesselman, 1982; Kelsey et al., 1986). When total populations are under disease surveillance or medical follow-up, controls can be readily drawn from the same population. In fact, studies of cohorts of individuals or populations can generate their own case-control studies (so-called nested case-control design). However, the example of Prader-Willi syndrome is typical of situations in the study of mutations, where ascertainment of the outcomes is usually done in a tertiary care center (sometimes collaboratively among several such centers). Thus, it is often impossible to determine the underlying population from which cases have been derived. For this reason, a variety of control groups have been used in epidemiologic studies. One control group consists of individuals ascertained at the same medical facility as the cases (hospital controls). These persons may be healthy or have other conditions unrelated to the exposure(s) or risk factor(s) under study. Another control group consists of neighbors of the cases, a sample selected from the same community from which cases are derived (community controls). A third control group may involve friends and other acquaintances of families of cases. Each type of control group has its advantages and limitations, as discussed elsewhere (e.g., Lilienfeld and Lilienfeld, 1980; Schlesselman, 1982; Kelsey et al., 1985). Many investigators choose multiple control groups to test a particular hypothesis, especially because the different comparison series are not likely to involve the same limitations. It is comforting to find that a particular association between a suspected exposure and an outcome holds when different types of controls are used (e.g., Cohen, 1980).

4.4.2. Ascertainment of Risk Factors

To study determinants of new mutations, it is necessary to compare the frequency of such traits in different subgroups of the population for risk factors of interest. Risk factors can range from environmental variables, such as pollutants and radiation exposures, to personal exposure via occupations and life-styles, and other demographic factors, such as parental age. Risk factors may also include genetic and other host variables, such as consanguinity, and the presence or absence of certain genetic markers.

One of the most studied genetic mutations is trisomy 21, which accounts for 95% of Down syndrome. This may be due in part to the prevalence of this mutation as a recognizable cause of mental retardation, the relative ease of phenotypic recognition, and the availability of prenatal diagnosis. Several factors have been identified to be associated with excess risk of Down syndrome. The best known, of course, is advanced maternal age. Other suggested risk factors include parental radiation exposures, maternal autoimmune disease, viral infections, advanced paternal age, familial tendency, consanguinity, cigarette smoking, certain genetic markers (*dNOR* variants) (Hassold and Jacobs, 1984; Jackson-Cook et al., 1985; Janerich and Bracken, 1986).

There are multiple methods for ascertainment of risk factors. As shown in Table 4–8, different sources are available. For example, parental ages are readily available on vital records (birth certificates) and recorded with reasonable accuracy. Where population-based registries of Down syndrome exist, vital records can thus be used to derive maternal and paternal age-specific birth prevalences. Other kinds of risk factors may be readily available from review of hospital medical records. For example, information on maternal chronic conditions, such as diabetes mellitus, are usually obtainable from medical records. Other types of data, such as life-style and personal habits (e.g., cigarette smoking and alcohol intake), are not consistently available in medical records, however, and questionnaires are usually used to obtain such information. Available environmental data are occasionally used to estimate personal exposures. For example, in studies of survivors of the atomic bombs

Table 4–8. Sources of data regarding risk factors in epidemiologic studies of genetic traits: some examples

Source of data	Risk factor
Vital records	Maternal age, paternal age, parity
Hospital medical records	Maternal chronic diseases (e.g., diabetes, thyroid disorders)
Questionnaires	Smoking, alcohol, occupational history, family history
Environmental data	Radiation exposure, pesticides, chemical pollutants
Laboratory measures Exposures	Dioxin levels, smoking + serology for certain viral diseases
Genetic markers	dNOR variants, HLA haplotypes

in Japan, gonadal radiation exposure was assessed, using an elaborate scheme that involved computing distance from the epicenter in addition to other variables (Radiation Effects Research Foundation, 1987).

Finally, biologic markers of exposures and genetic susceptibility are increasingly useful in epidemiologic studies of mutations (National Research Council, 1987). The use of such laboratory tests to refine exposure classification can result in improved validity of exposure classification obtained from questionnaires (Stein and Hatch, 1987; Hogue and Brewster, 1988). Markers are becoming increasingly available for a variety of exposures, such as smoking, alcohol, cocaine, many prescription drugs, and certain environmental contaminants.

In some instances, laboratory markers of susceptibility have been used directly as risk factors for mutations. For example, in the case of trisomy 21, staining variants of nucleolar organizer region (NOR) in parents have been thought to play an etiologic role in the process of nondisjunction that leads to trisomy 21 (Jackson-Cook et al., 1985). More recent studies have not confirmed this original observation, however (Hassold et al., 1987; Schwartz et al., 1989; Spinner et al., 1989).

4.4.3. Analytic Issues

Analytic issues in epidemiologic studies of genetic traits and mutations include decisions regarding the choice of appropriate measures of effect to be used with different study designs, the effect of misclassification on inferences, and the ways in which confounding between risk factors and genetic traits can influence inferences.

Measures of Association

Measures used to evaluate the association between the specific risk factors and the occurrence of new mutations are similar to those used in general epidemiology. Cohort studies provide the opportunity to measure risk ratios (relative risks), odds ratios, absolute risks, and risk difference, while case-control studies can yield measures of odds ratios that are, for practical purposes, equivalent to risk ratios, as mutation events are generally rare. In the event that a case-control study is nested within a cohort study and/or conducted in a defined population with known frequency of the outcomes measured, such a study can indirectly yield measures of both absolute risks and risk difference. Furthermore, both types of studies yield measures of attributable fraction (Chapter 3).

For example, the best-known risk factor in the occurrence of trisomy 21 is advanced maternal age. Numerous epidemiologic studies (both cohort and case-control studies) have shown an increasing risk of Down syndrome with increasing maternal age (Lilienfeld, 1969; Janerich, 1986). An illustration of the magnitude of the association is shown in Table 4–9, based on results published by Adams and coworkers (1981) on the prevalence of Down syndrome diagnosed within the first year of life, using the Metropolitan Atlanta population-based birth defects registry. With this cohort approach, it is easy

Table 4–9. Association between maternal age and the prevalence of Down syndrome in the first year of life based on data from the Metropolitan Atlanta Congenital Defects Program

Maternal age (years)	Prevalence per 1000 livebirths	Difference in prevalence	Relative effect
15–19	0.66	0.05	1.08
20–24	0.61	Reference	Reference
25–29	0.78	0.17	1.28
30–34	1.54	0.93	2.52
35–39	2.63	2.02	4.31
40–44	14.29	13.68	23.4
45+	34.19	33.58	56.1

Adapted from Adams et al. (1981).

to compute absolute and relative effects of different maternal ages on the occurrence of Down syndrome. More than 50-fold excess risk is seen for women 45 years or older at the time of delivery. In addition, for these women, there is an excess of 3.36% over the prevalence in women between 20 and 24 years (prevalence difference). Absolute risk and risk difference measures are helpful in assessing the magnitude of the biologic effect of advanced age in terms of the proportion of women who are at risk for a trisomy 21 conception (Khoury et al., 1989c). Of course, any inference about risk from a prevalence study at birth is only approximate because of the effects of prenatal loss in trisomic concepti (which cannot be measured accurately but may well vary by maternal age; Khoury et al., 1989b). Another issue to be kept in mind is that, due to the advent of prenatal diagnosis and elective abortion, the prevalence of Down syndrome at birth is likely lower than during mid-pregnancy (Kallen and Knudsen, 1989). The impact doubtless varies for different maternal ages, since prenatal diagnosis is mainly done for women 35 or older. Finally, analysis of effects of maternal age grouped by five-year intervals may mask differences in yearly maternal age-specific rates, especially at the upper extreme of maternal age, as shown by Hook and Lamson (1980).

In addition to the above measures of effects of advanced maternal age on trisomy 21, it is important to estimate the magnitude of the attributable fraction associated with age. In a well-defined population, what proportion of Down syndrome cases can be attributed to advanced maternal age (say 35 years or older)? Although this analysis has been done in many studies, data presented by Goldberg and coworkers (1979) are used to illustrate the application of the concept of attributable fraction. Based on the Metropolitan Atlanta Registry, Goldberg and associates (1979) found that the rate of all chromosomal anomalies (most of which were trisomy 21 cases) was 1 per thousand births for women under 35 years old and 5.8 per 1000 births for those 35 or older (relative risk of 5.8). To compute attributable fraction, the prevalence of the risk factor (maternal age 35+) must be known. In this population, 4.5% of deliveries occurred to women 35 or older. The proportion of infants with all chromosomal anomalies attributed to maternal age 35+

can then be calculated as $.045(5.8 - 1)/[1 + .045(5.8 - 1)] = 18\%$. Thus, the vast majority of Down syndrome cases (and other chromosomal abnormalities) cannot be attributed to advanced maternal age, despite the strong relative and absolute effects of advanced maternal age on the prevalence of Down syndrome. This phenomenon has to be considered both for public health prevention and intervention strategies, as well for etiologic research into trisomy 21.

To illustrate measures of association in case-control studies, consider the study of Olshan and colleagues (1989), a case-control study of Down syndrome that explored paternal occupation as a risk factor. Cases included 1008 liveborn Down syndrome infants ascertained by the British Columbia Health Surveillance Registry between 1952 and 1973. Two liveborn controls were matched for each case by hospital and date of birth. The fathers' job titles were obtained from the birth certificate. Fifty-nine job categories were grouped and compared between cases and controls. Several job categories were significantly associated with having a Down syndrome offspring (Table 4–10). Note that, since the study was designed as a matched case-control study, a matched odds ratio was calculated. Attributable fractions were computed for these job titles using Miettinen's formula (Miettinen, 1979). Overall, none of these job categories accounted for more than 3% of all Down syndrome cases in the population. This finding is not unexpected, since the vast majority of Down syndrome cases appear to be related to maternal rather than paternal nondisjunction events.

Thus far, risk factors have been treated as either dichotomous (present/absent) or polychotomous (several categories). However, many risk factors represent continuously distributed measures of exposure dose. For example, one can define cigarette smoking not only by type (filter/no filter, low tar, etc.), but also by number of cigarettes smoked per day, or cumulative dose (such as number of pack-years). Likewise, alcohol consumption can be quan-

Table 4–10. Association between paternal occupation and the risk of Down syndrome, British Columbia Case-Control Study

Paternal occupation	No. of cases*	No. of controls*	Odds ratio	95% Confidence interval	Attributable fraction (%)
Janitor	12	7	3.26	1.02–10.4	0.8
Mechanics	26	22	3.27	1.57–6.80	1.8
Farm managers/ workers	59	56	2.03	1.25–3.03	3.0

Data from Olshan et al. (1989).
Attributable fraction (AF) based on Miettinen formula:

$$AF = f_c \frac{(RR - 1)}{RR}$$

where f_c is the proportion of cases with risk factor and RR is the relative risk of Down syndrome associated with exposure to risk factor.
*1008 Down syndrome cases and 2016 matched controls.

titated by type (beer, wine, etc.) and the amount drunk daily, in binges, or cumulatively over time. Usually dose-response relationships have been evaluated, using nonparametric methods such as the Mantel trend test (Mantel, 1963). Increasingly, however, parametric methods (e.g., linear and logistic functions) are being used in epidemiologic analyses.

Similarly, maternal age can be treated as a continuous variable (single years) when predicting the rate of trisomy 21. Dose-response relationships can be defined using a linear model:

$$y = ax + b, \tag{4-2}$$

where y is the probability of trisomy 21, and x is maternal age, a and b are parameters to be estimated. Of course, this is not an ideal example, since it is known that the relationship between the rate of Down syndrome and age is not linear but seems to be more or less flat until the age of 30, with a marked increase after age 35. Alternatively, one could use the logistic regression model, where the relationship between age and probability of Down syndrome is linear on a logit scale:

$$y = \frac{\exp(a + bx)}{1 + \exp(a + bx)}. \tag{4-3}$$

Another variation of this logistic function was recently suggested by Morton and colleagues (1988) in modeling the effect of maternal age on the rate of trisomy

$$y = \frac{d + \exp(a + bx + cx^2)}{1 + \exp(a + bx + cx^2)} \tag{4-4}$$

where d is an age-independent component and cx^2 is a quadratic component.

Although any parametric model that characterizes a specific mathematical relationship between the exposure and the rate of genetic mutation can improve statistical power over the more general polychotomous analyses of maternal age (such as the ones presented in Table 4–9), such modeling should be based on biologic theory, an accurate assessment of a meaningful measure of exposure, and large enough numbers of individuals with various levels of exposure. Unfortunately, these requirements have been rarely attainable in epidemiologic analyses of genetic mutations and in most diseases in general. This is one of the main reasons why epidemiologists have often resorted to nonparametric models for analysis, and tend to dichotomize or polychotomize variables which are inherently continuous in nature.

For example, in the studies of the effects of radiation from the atomic bombs on genetic mutations in offspring of survivors, parental gonadal radiation exposure was estimated using several methods, including distance from epicenter, and the effects of various kinds of intervening shielding (Radiation Effects Research Foundation, 1987). Since actual gonadal radiation exposure was never directly assessed, such methods provide only approximate estimates for the total amount of radiation incurred. In the final report on genetic mutations altering protein charge and/or function in offspring of atomic bomb survivors, simple dichotomous categories were used for the cohort identification: proximally exposed parents versus distally exposed parents (Neel et al., 1988b).

Misclassification

The difficulties inherent in the measurement of both genetic traits and exposures in human populations have already been discussed. With regard to exposures, epidemiologic approaches to their measurement can be as crude as relying on ecologic data only (e.g., residence in proximity to a toxic waste site) or quite refined, such as obtaining biologic specimens from each individual. The range of refinement is listed in Table 4–11 with some selected examples. Any proxy measure of exposure, such as ecologic data and reported exposures, always creates problems of misclassification of exposure (accuracy and reliability), just as it does for genetic traits. Thus, parameters of sensitivity and specificity (Table 4–4) for these proxy measures, as well as those of agreement (Table 4–5), can be applied as in the case of specific outcomes.

What then are the potential effects of misclassification on measuring determinants of genetic traits in epidemiologic studies? The problem of misclassification has recently received much attention in the epidemiologic literature (Shy et al., 1978; Kelsey et al., 1986; Flegal et al., 1986; Khoury et al., 1988d). Two types of misclassification have been recognized: nondifferential and differential, both of which can modify measures of effect in any epidemiologic study.

Nondifferential misclassification exists if the magnitude of the measurement error for one variable does not depend on the value of other variables (Kelsey et al., 1986). Specifically, consider a binary exposure (present/absent). Measurement error is nondifferential if values of sensitivity and

Table 4–11. Examples of levels of refinement of exposure classification

Level	Examples
1. Proxy for exposure	Occupation title, residence data
2. Reported exposure	Reported patterns of cigarette smoking, alcohol intake, and drug ingestion, perceived exposures to pesticides, Agent Orange, occupational chemicals
3. Biologic exposure	Documented exposure as measured in blood or tissue systems, e.g., dioxin levels, alcohol levels, smoking measures
4. Relevant biologic exposure	Documented gonadal exposure at the pertinent time prior to or at conception; issues of dose, timing, and actual molecular or biochemical processes (usually unattainable)

specificity are constant over other variables, including those for disease or outcome status. For example, in a hypothetical case-control study of Down syndrome and radiation exposure, nondifferential misclassification exists if the ability of mothers to report accurately any radiation exposure (e.g., during the five years prior to conception) does not differ for cases and controls (i.e., their sensitivity and specificity are identical). The impact of this type of misclassification will be generally but not always (Kristensen, 1992) to dilute all measures of effects such as odds and risk ratios toward unity. An example is given in Table 4–12, where radiation exposure is assumed to have a true relative effect of 10 (odds ratio), and the prevalence of exposure is 50%. Assuming that recall of radiation exposure has various levels of sensitivity and specificity (60%, 90%, and 99%), Table 4–12 shows how lower sensitivity and specificity of maternal recall results in a lower expected odds ratio. If sensitivity and specificity are 60%, then the observed odds ratio is 1.4, barely elevated over the null hypothesis value of 1. The amount of dilution also depends on the prevalence of exposure or risk factor. Greater dilution is obtained at very high and very low prevalences of exposures (Kelsey et al., 1986).

Differential misclassification exists if the magnitude of the measurement error for a given variable varies according to the value or category of one or more of the other variables (Kelsey et al., 1986). A notable example is the problem of recall bias often discussed in case-control studies (Schlesselman, 1982; Kelsey et al., 1986). Again, consider the problem of maternal radiation exposure in a case-control study of Down syndrome. Pertinent exposures could have occurred throughout the childhood or adulthood of mothers. The opportunity therefore exists for both recall loss of true events and memory distortion. Such recall problems may occur differentially for mothers of Down syndrome cases as compared with mothers of control subjects. One explanation might be that mothers of children with Down syndrome might be more motivated to look for a cause of their infants' problem. Under these conditions, there is a distortion in the magnitude of the observed association (odds ratio) between the exposure and the outcome. The distortion can go in either direction. It could inflate the magnitude of the association (i.e., result in higher odds ratios). This could result in a spurious association, when in fact none exists, if mothers of Down syndrome cases have higher sensitivity and/ or lower specificity of recall than mothers of control subjects. On the other

Table 4–12. Effects of random (nondifferential) misclassification of a binary exposure on the observed odds ratio in an epidemiologic study

	Sensitivity		
Specificity	*60%*	*90%*	*99%*
60%	1.4	3.2	6.5
90%	2.3	4.8	8.4
99%	2.7	5.4	9.1

The true odds ratio is assumed to be 10 and the prevalence of exposure is 50%.
Adapted from Kelsey (1986).

hand, it could also dilute a truly elevated odds ratio toward unity (or even below 1) if the reverse occurs (lower sensitivity and/or higher specificity in mothers of cases).

The problem of bias in reporting past exposures, pregnancy-related events, and drug intake has been a major source of concern in case-control studies of birth defects and other pregnancy outcomes (Klemetti and Saxen, 1967; Bracken, 1984). In fact, the types of questions asked in an interview instrument have been shown to affect the reporting of drug intake during pregnancy (Mitchell et al., 1986). Also, when interviews are compared with medical records, disagreements in reporting conditions are frequently found (Klemetti and Saxen, 1967; Hewson and Bennett, 1987; Bryant et al., 1989). Granted that data collected through interviews are not likely to be perfect, the issue is whether such imperfections affect the inferences regarding the associations between exposures and pregnancy outcomes. More recent investigations of this problem, however, do not provide evidence of widespread differential reporting of past exposures (MacKenzie and Lippman, 1989; Mulinare et al., 1989). Nevertheless, in view of the potential impact of exposure misclassification problems inherent in observational studies relying only on interview data, the use of accurate and reproducible laboratory markers of exposure is preferable whenever possible (Stein and Hatch, 1987; Hogue and Brewster, 1988).

Confounding

In analyzing the relationship between a risk factor and a genetic trait, the issue of confounding has to be considered and addressed either in the study design and/or in the analysis. Consider, for example, the question as to whether advanced paternal age may be an additional risk factor for the occurrence of nondisjunction of chromosome 21. Any study examining this question has to take into account the possible powerful confounding effect of advanced maternal age. Advanced maternal age is a confounder because it meets the following criteria: (1) it is causally related to the outcome and (2) it is associated with the risk factor of interest—advanced paternal age (Gordis, 1988a). Thus, if the effects of maternal age are not accounted for, an indirect (noncausal) association might be expected between advanced paternal age and trisomy 21.

Confounding can be handled in the design of the study, in the analysis, or in both. In designing a case-control study of trisomy, this can be minimized by choosing a control group matched by maternal age to the trisomy group. Matching can be done 1 to 1 (e.g., Cohen et al., 1963; Sigler et al., 1965) or on a frequency basis (Schlesselman, 1982). Matching by maternal age is reasonable when the investigators are assessing the effects of risk factors other than maternal age on the occurrence of trisomy 21. For example, maternal age-matched case-control designs were used by Olshan et al. (1989) to examine the effect of paternal occupation factors and by Cohen and Lilienfeld (1970) and Cohen et al. (1977b) to examine the effects of past radiation exposures (and other factors).

Confounding can also be handled in the analysis by stratification and/or multivariate models (Schlesselman, 1982; Kelsey et al., 1985; Kahn and Sempos, 1989). Some of the basic methods are illustrated here by considering certain specific examples. In a case-control study, Erickson (1978) examined the relationship between advanced paternal age and Down syndrome after adjustment for maternal age using the Mantel-Haenzel procedure. He used different definitions for advanced paternal age (≥ 40 years and ≥ 55 years). For each of these definitions, the relationship between paternal age and case-control status was assessed in a series of 2×2 tables for each year of maternal age. A basic plan for some of these tables is shown in Table 4–13. Although odds ratios can be obtained for each of these tables, an overall odds ratio across maternal ages can also be obtained by using the Mantel-Haenzsel test. In this study, after adjustment for maternal age, there was a moderately increased risk associated with advanced paternal age.

Multivariate methods are increasingly used in epidemiologic analyses to account for several variables (continuous or dichotomous) simultaneously. The logistic model shown in Equation 4-3 can be expanded to include several variables simultaneously

$$\ln \frac{P(Y = 1)}{1 - P(Y = 1)} = a + b_1 x_1 + b_2 x_2 + \ldots + b_n x_n, \qquad (4\text{-}5)$$

where $x_1, x_2 \ldots x_n$ represent n independent variables used to predict the probability of occurrence of the outcome y. Values of the regression coefficients b_i can be obtained using maximum likelihood procedures and these can be interpreted in terms of odds ratios, computed as $OR = \exp(b_i)$, for each risk factor after adjustment for the effects of other variables.

Existing methods are currently available for matched studies as well as unmatched designs; and the model can be applied both in cohort and case-control studies (Schlesselman, 1982; Kahn, 1983). Another example is a study of the relationship of maternal thyroid disorders and the risk of birth defects in offspring (Khoury et al., 1989a). This case-control study, based on the Metropolitan Atlanta Congenital Defects Program registry, examined the

Table 4–13. Illustration of the adjustment for maternal age in the analysis of the association between advanced paternal age and Down syndrome

Maternal age*	Paternal age	Down syndrome	Control	Odds ratio	X^2
20	$\geq$ 40	0	22		
	< 40	104	5817	0	0.39
22	$\geq$ 40	1	40		
	< 40	149	6422	1.08	0.006
24	$\geq$ 40	2	87		
	< 40	121	5564	1.06	0.006
32	$\geq$ 40	18	290		
	< 40	101	2137	1.08	0.30

Data from case-control study by Erickson (1978).
*Only selected maternal ages are shown for illustration.

possible association between maternal hypothyroidism and hyperthyroidism and the risk of birth defects. Analyses were done comparing the history of thyroid disorders in mothers of 218 babies with trisomy 21, 33 babies with other autosomal trisomies, and 3027 normal babies frequency-matched by hospital of birth, race, and period of birth. Logistic regression models were used to adjust for the possible confounding effects of other maternal variables, most notably maternal age (Khoury et al., 1989a). In these data, no association between thyroid disorders and Down syndrome was seen. This finding is also consistent with a more recent study on the lack of association between Down syndrome and thyroid antibodies (Torfs et al., 1990).

Finally, the issue of interaction (or effect modification) has to be considered, since it bears greatly on the process of adjustment for confounding. If the impact of a risk factor on the outcome varies across different values of a third variable, "statistical interaction" or "effect modification" exists. Simple adjustment for such a third variable may mask important biologic relationships. An example of effect modification is pertinent here regarding the association between maternal cigarette smoking and Down syndrome in livebirths. Based on data from the Collaborative Perinatal Project (CPP), Hook and Cross (1988) examined the occurrence of Down syndrome at birth in relation to maternal smoking status. As shown in Table 4–14, the frequency of Down syndrome was 0.87 per 1000 livebirths among smokers and 1.44 per 1000 livebirths among nonsmokers (relative risk = 0.60). This apparent "protective effect" of smoking on the occurrence of trisomy 21 might be explained by prenatal selection, that is, there may have been greater prenatal loss among trisomic fetuses whose mothers are cigarette smokers (Khoury et al., 1989b). When the analysis was performed by maternal race, this apparent "protective effect" was entirely limited to blacks (relative risk = 0.20), however, and was not observed in whites (relative risk = 1.13). Here, adjustment for race could have obscured the apparent effect modification of race. The exact biologic significance of this finding is unclear, and may be related to greater prenatal selection forces among blacks. Methods to deal with interaction in multivariate modeling, such as logistic regression, are reviewed elsewhere (Breslow and Day, 1980; Schlesselman, 1982; Kahn, 1983; Kelsey et al., 1986).

Table 4–14. Association between maternal smoking and the prevalence of Down syndrome in livebirths, by race

Race	Smoking	Prevalence per 1000 livebirths	Difference in prevalence	Relative prevalence
White	Yes	1.35	+0.15	1.13
	No	1.20	0.00 (reference)	1.00 (reference)
Black	Yes	0.37	−1.27	0.23
	No	1.64	0.00 (reference)	1.00 (reference)
All	Yes	0.87	−0.57	0.60
	No	1.44	0.00 (reference)	1.00 (reference)

Adapted from Hook and Cross (1988).

The problem of effect modification is discussed further in Chapter 5 in the context of detecting interactions between genetic and environmental factors contributing to disease.

4.4.4. Statistical Issues and Sample Size Considerations

Sample size issues must be considered both in the design and interpretation of epidemiologic studies of genetic traits. Before launching such studies, investigators need to determine how many subjects are required to address the objectives of the study at hand. Formulas for estimating minimal sample sizes, both for cohort studies and case-control studies, are available for standard study designs (e.g., Rothman and Boice, 1982; Schlesselman, 1982). To improve precision in measuring associations between a mutation and a suspected risk factor, investigators have to deal with a number of variables:

1. The background mutation rate in unexposed individuals in a cohort study, or the frequency of exposure to the risk factor among controls in a case-control study
2. The relative size of the groups (ratio of number of unexposed to exposed people in a cohort study, or ratio number of controls to cases in case-control study)
3. The magnitude of the effect to be detected (e.g., the minimal relative risk or risk difference detectable)
4. The likelihood of finding an association by chance, that is, a type I error
5. The likelihood of missing a real effect, if present, that is, a type II error, which is the complement of statistical power

The interplay between type I and type II errors must always be considered. As shown in Table 4–15, if there is no association between the exposure and the mutation, that is, the true relative risk is 1, estimates of the relative risks obtained in independent and unbiased studies will have a wide distribution and, in some studies, extreme values of estimated relative risks may be obtained. The level of statistical significance is usually set to accept a certain proportion of conclusions as false positives, and this is the probability of a type I error (i.e., rejecting a true null hypothesis). At the conventional 5%

Table 4–15. Statistical issues in epidemiologic studies of genetic traits: type I and type II errors, statistical power, and sample size.

	Truth	
Results of study	*No association* (RR = 1)	*Association* (e.g., RR = 2)
No association	True negative $(1 - \alpha)$	False negative (β), type II error
Association	False positive (α), type I error	True positive $(1 - \beta)$

level, 5% of all tests are expected to show significant associations on the basis of chance alone. The actual critical value used for a given test statistic will depend on whether a one- or two-sided test is desired (Rothman, 1986). An alternative approach is the use of confidence intervals around the point estimate of a rate or relative risk measure. A 95% confidence interval around an estimated relative risk represents the expected variability in that point estimate, that is, 95 of 100 replicates of this analysis would fall within this confidence interval. Type I errors are always of concern when multiple statistical tests are performed. For example, in the Down syndrome case-control study of Olshan and coworkers (1989) described earlier (Table 4–10), 59 categories of paternal occupations were examined as possible risk factors for Down syndrome. Three such associations were found to be statistically significant at the 0.05 level. As acknowledged by the authors, this is entirely consistent with the 5% type I error level since 3 of 59 statistical tests are expected to be significant by chance. This issue must be kept in mind in any hypothesis-generating study, especially case-control investigations of multiple exposures or risk factors (Thomas et al., 1985; Rothman, 1986). Further studies are needed to determine whether such findings persist in other settings as well (i.e., hypothesis-testing studies). Also, the consistency of these significant associations within a biologically plausible framework must be considered. In the Down syndrome study, it is not immediately apparent what might be the common exposures among diverse occupational groups such as janitors, mechanics, and farm managers/workers (Olshan et al., 1989).

As shown in Table 4–15, the counterpart to type I errors are type II or β errors. These occur when an alternative hypothesis is true (i.e., when there exists an underlying association between an exposure and a genetic trait), but it is not detected by the statistical test. The complement of a type II error is statistical power. For example, when one designs a study with 80% power to detect a relative risk of some specified level, the implication is that there is an 80% chance of finding the true association, and a 20% chance of failing to do so, that is, committing a type II error. In general, the smaller the sample size, the less the statistical power to detect a true underlying association.

Table 4–16 illustrates the effects of various parameters on sample sizes required to detect specific levels of relative risk. Here, a hypothetical cohort

Table 4–16. Approximate sample sizes needed in a cohort study to detect excess mutation rates due to exposures by background mutation rate and relative risk from exposure

Background mutation rate	Relative risk from exposure		
	2	5	10
10^{-2}	2,500	300	100
10^{-3}	25,000	3,000	1,100
10^{-4}	247,000	30,000	10,600
10^{-5}	2,400,000	300,000	110,000

Sample sizes based on equal numbers among exposed and nonexposed individuals, α error = 0.05 (two-sided), and statistical power = 0.80.

study is designed with a 1:1 ratio of exposed to unexposed individuals, over a range of background mutation rates. As can be seen, the lower the background mutation rate and the lower the magnitude of the true relative risk to be detected, the larger the sample sizes needed to avoid type I and type II errors at the levels set here. Given that many genetic mutations in humans are very rare (on the order of 10^{-4} or 10^{-5}), usually large numbers of individuals would have to be studied to detect a statistically significant association between an exposure and the mutation rate. This hypothetical situation is plainly illustrated by studies of children of atomic bomb survivors in Japan (Neel et al., 1988b). Based on about 13,052 children of "proximally exposed parents" and 10,609 children of "distally exposed parents" Neel et al. (1988b) found, in each group, 3 mutations affecting electrophoretic mobility (mutation rates of 0.45 per 10^5 in the exposed group and 0.64 per 10^5 in the unexposed group). Obviously, no statistically significant difference could be detected between these two mutation rates. Turning to Table 4–16, one can see that more than 100,000 persons in each group would be required to detect even a 10-fold difference in mutation rates, and about 2,400,000 to detect a 2-fold excess. This example illustrates the difficulty of measuring small changes in human mutation rates.

The lack of statistical power in the atomic bomb studies has to be reconciled with their original objectives. As emphasized by Neel et al. (1988b):

> the studies in Hiroshima and Nagasaki are not designed to test the hypothesis that radiation produced mutations in the survivors of the atomic bombings. Radiation has produced mutations in every properly investigated plant or animal species to which it has been applied. . . . Our challenge, rather, is to treat the results of the various studies . . . as an approximation of the true effect, ultimately combining all these findings to derive a best estimate of the genetic doubling dose of radiation for humans.

The doubling dose method has been widely used in radiation genetics and "refers to the amount of radiation necessary to produce as many mutations as those that occur spontaneously in a generation" (Sankaranayanan, 1988). In other words, it is the dose of radiation needed to produce a relative risk of 2. In the Japanese studies, estimation of the doubling dose is still forthcoming and must eventually take into account the various types of genetic outcomes that were measured, for example, chromosomal abnormalities and adverse pregnancy outcomes, in addition to a more refined estimation of the gonadal dosage.

4.5. ANALYTIC STUDIES: DETERMINANTS OF THE GENETIC STRUCTURE OF POPULATIONS

Thus far, we have been concerned with the study of factors that affect the occurrence of new genetic mutations in human populations as opposed to those transmitted from previous generations. To gain a better understanding of other determinants of the distribution of genes in populations, one must turn to classical population genetic concepts. Although the distribution of new dominant mutations can be understood in terms of the epidemiologic concepts of place/time/person, such an approach is clearly inadequate to understand the basis for population and ethnic variations in the frequency of existing genetic traits. Genetic traits of interest include polymorphisms such as blood groups, HLA antigens, DNA markers, as well as autosomal recessive diseases, such as cystic fibrosis and Tay-Sachs disease. In many autosomal recessive disorders, the homozygous genotype usually occurs because the individual has inherited two abnormal alleles, one from each parent, according to simple Mendelian patterns of transmission, rather than because any new mutations have occurred in either parent. In turn, the abnormal allele in each parent may have been inherited through many generations, completely concealed in the heterozygous state. In this situation, it is usually impossible to pinpoint the timing of a genetic mutation. Consequently, studying exposure characteristics of parents of affected children does not shed any light on the etiology of the genetic trait.

4.5.1. Population Genetics Concepts

As reviewed in Chapter 2, the behavior of genes in populations can be described by the Hardy-Weinberg principle, which predicts genotype frequencies as simple functions of allele frequencies. This allows investigators to make the transition between the measurement of phenotypes in populations to the measurement of allele frequencies at a given locus. Once a new genetic change arises in a germ cell, several factors may operate to allow for the persistence or the elimination of the mutation in subsequent generations and to determine the frequency of the genetic trait at any given point in time. In addition to factors directly affecting recurring mutations, the three main factors acting on new genetic traits in populations are (1) selection, (2) chance fluctuations (also called genetic drift), and (3) deviations from random mating (examples in Table 4-17). These factors are extensively discussed in the population genetics literature (e.g., Haldane, 1961; Cavalli-Sforza and Bodmer, 1971; Crow, 1986; Vogel and Motulsky, 1986). Mathematical models have been developed to evaluate the role of these forces in altering the frequency of genetic traits in human populations over generations and, consequently, in the evolutionary process (Vogel and Motulsky, 1986). A review of these topics is outside the scope of this book. Instead, the impact of these factors on the frequency of genetic traits in populations, and the extent to which epidemiologic approaches can be used to assess their impact on human populations, are discussed here.

4.5.2. Epidemiologic Considerations

Frequently, the first clues to the determinants of the distribution of genetic traits in populations come from simple ecologic observations. An example here is that of the observed correlation between the worldwide geographic distribution of malaria in the early twentieth century and the allele frequencies

Table 4–17. Examples of factors affecting the genetic structure of populations

Factors	Effect on frequency of genetic trait	Examples
Selection		
Mortality		
Increase	Decrease	Trisomy 16, triploidy "sentinel" phenotypes
Decrease	Increase	Sickle cell trait in malaria endemic areas
Fertility		
Decrease	Decrease	Down syndrome, XXY "Sentinel" phenotypes, phenylketonuria
Chance fluctuations		
Random drift/ founder effect	Decrease or increase	Ellis-van Creveld syndrome in the Old Order Amish
Deviations from random mating		
Inbreeding	Increase homozygosity	Autosomal recessive disorders in populations with high inbreeding rates

of certain abnormal hemoglobins (including Hb S, C, and E) (Sutton, 1988). Countries with endemic falciparum malaria were found to have high allele frequencies for these abnormal hemoglobins. Such ecologic designs are also used in epidemiology. For example, when mortality from rectal cancer is plotted as a function of per capita beer consumption over several countries worldwide (Breslow and Enstron, 1974; Kelsey et al., 1986), an increase in the level of rectal cancer mortality with increasing alcohol consumption is noted. Both of these types of observations are ecologic in nature and are subject to the well-known ecologic fallacy, that is, no causal association between alcohol and rectal cancer can be inferred, since alcohol consumption was not measured directly in subjects with disease and those without disease. Such an ecologic association may be entirely due to extraneous or confounding factors associated with both alcohol consumption and the occurrence of rectal cancer. Likewise, the ecologic association between malaria and sickle cell trait, although suggestive of causal connection, cannot be readily interpreted as a cause-effect relationship without conducting further studies that compare directly morbidity and mortality rates in individuals with Hb AA, AS, and SS (in cohort or case-control studies) while also considering other potentially confounding factors. Over the years, however, a compelling body of evidence has been accumulated to document the survival advantage of the Hb AS carriers in malaria-stricken environments (Vogel and Motulsky, 1986). It should be pointed out, however, that it is usually difficult, or impossible, to document such selective environmental effects on genetic mutations, since dramatic changes in the environment have occurred over the last few generations in almost all populations.

Another example of ecologic observation is that of the high frequency of Tay-Sachs disease in Ashkenazi Jews as compared with other populations.

Two alternative explanations have been suggested to explain this observation. The first postulated that the high frequency of Tay-Sachs disease may be due to the effects of chance fluctuations that are the result of founder effect and possibly genetic drift (Wagener et al., 1978). The second explanation proposes that selection factors (in addition to genetic drift) are needed to explain patterns of occurrence of this genetic disease. Selection was postulated to be the result of some advantage in heterozygous individuals (Chakravarti and Chakraborty, 1978), although confirming evidence is quite limited. These seemingly opposing explanations are based on the use of different mathematical models, each of which has inherent assumptions and limitations (Ewens, 1978). Our objective here is to evaluate the extent to which it is possible to use empirical epidemiologic study designs to distinguish among such alternative hypotheses regarding factors influencing the genetic structure of populations.

Beyond the initial ecologic clues, epidemiologic studies can be designed to compare the frequency of a genetic trait among population subgroups and examine factors that might explain such differences. In these studies, issues pertaining to study design (case-control, cohort), selection of study subjects (representativeness, etc.), sample size issues, information collected, and confounding variables have to be considered.

To illustrate the problem of confounding in studies of genetic traits, suppose a study compared two populations for the frequency of blood group A antigen (Table 4–18). In this study, population 1 has a higher frequency of blood group A compared with population 2 (40% versus 28%). In reality, neither of these populations can be considered a truly single random mating population (termed a "deme" in population genetics); and each has a different racial composition, with population 1 consisting predominantly of whites and population 2 of blacks. Because of the known racial difference in the distribution of ABO blood group antigens, this "stratification" effect (Sutton, 1988) leads to different frequencies in blood group A antigen in population 1 compared to population 2, although the race-specific frequencies are identical: 41% for whites and 26% for blacks in both populations. The concept of population stratification is identical to that of confounding and should be taken into account when designing studies that compare frequencies of genetic traits between groups. While this is an obvious example of confounding by race, confounding may be more subtle. For example, blacks in different geographic locations may differ with respect to the extent of genetic admixture

Table 4–18. Example of the effect of race stratification (or confounding) on the comparison of the frequency of blood group A in two hypothetical populations

Race	Population 1			Population 2		
	Total	A	%	Total	A	%
White	18,000	7,380	41	2,000	820	41
Black	2,000	520	26	18,000	4,680	26
Total	20,000	7,900	40	20,000	5,500	28

with whites. Even within a single ethnic group, there may be stratification by socioeconomic class, which, in turn, can affect mating patterns. Likewise, a single broadly defined racial group, such as Caucasians, is more often a mixture of many subgroups with different migration patterns, fertility histories, genetic backgrounds, and likely different allele frequencies at many loci.

4.5.3. Study Approaches to Factors Affecting Population Genetic Structure

This section reviews the impact and available epidemiologic approaches to evaluating factor that affect the genetic structure of human populations over time.

Selection

To study the effects of selection forces on the distribution of genetic traits, one must consider how selection operates. Fitness of individuals with different genotypes is ultimately measured by the number of fertile offspring (Sutton, 1988). As shown in Table 4–17, selection operates at two levels: early mortality and reduced fertility, both of which affect the probability of transmission of genes (and any new mutation) to subsequent generations. A new mutation may be associated with increased risk of early death. For example, sentinel phenotypes are deliberately selected because they are associated with very poor survival; thus, there can be no, or negligible, transmission of the mutation to subsequent generations. On the other hand, a few mutations have been documented to be associated with lowered mortality levels in the presence of certain environmental factors. Again, the best-known example here is the heterozygote advantage of the sickle cell mutation in areas with endemic falciparum malaria, a situation that explains the high frequency of the sickle cell allele in some populations. Finally, many mutations apparently offer no particular advantage or disadvantage to the individual in terms of either survival or reproduction, that is, they are selectively neutral. These include many protein and DNA polymorphisms. The term "polymorphism" has been used to refer to the situation where multiple allelic forms are maintained at population frequencies too high to be solely attributed to recurrent mutation. By convention, a genetic trait is defined as polymorphic if the most common allele has a frequency of .99 or less. There has been considerable discussion in the literature regarding why there are so many polymorphic traits in human populations, and a continuing debate about the importance of selective versus neutral forces in maintaining polymorphisms throughout the evolutionary process (King and Jukes, 1969; Crow, 1986; Vogel and Motulsky, 1986).

Selection can also operate through reduced fertility. If a new mutation is associated with sterility, obviously it cannot be transmitted to subsequent generations and hence qualifies as a "genetic lethal." If carriers of a new mutation have reduced fertility compared with those without the mutation, this results in decreased likelihood of transmission of the genetic trait to subsequent generations. On the other hand, genetic traits associated with increased fertility are preferentially transmitted. For example, a study reported increased number of offspring among cystic fibrosis heterozygotes (Knudson et al., 1967). To evaluate the effect of selection on the frequency of the genetic traits in populations, a sound epidemiologic approach must be used to document genotype-specific mortality and/or fertility.

Usually the reverse question is asked, namely, what is the effect of the genetic trait on mortality and fertility? Thus, the primary use of epidemiologic studies is to compare morbidity, mortality, and fertility outcomes between individuals with a given genetic trait and those without the trait. In particular, if the hypothesis is that of a heterozygote-selective advantage, then investigators would attempt to document directly levels of mortality and fertility among individuals with the various genotypes. This approach essentially involves studying the role of the genetic trait in disease, with the ultimate interest in early mortality and reduced fertility. Early mortality and fertility are emphasized because for genetic traits with delayed age at onset of clinical symptoms until after the reproductive age (such as Huntington's disease), increased risk of mortality will not play an appreciable role in altering the transmission of the genetic mutation to subsequent generations. Such studies are further discussed in Chapter 5.

This reverse approach has its limitations, however. Epidemiologic studies of the relationship between genetic traits and mortality and/or fertility endpoints can be conducted only in current populations where the existing environment is distinctly different from that which prevailed over much of human history. Selection may have operated in the near or distant past via environmental factors that no longer exist today. For example, once malaria is eradicated in a population, heterozygotes carrying the sickle cell allele no longer appear at any selective advantage. Instead, selection operating against individuals with the homozygous sickle cell genotype may gain the upper hand and gradually decrease the frequency of the sickle cell allele over time. The extent and speed of the decline in gene frequency can be predicted, but the length of time involved usually spans scores of generations and thus precludes direct testing (Vogel and Motulsky, 1986). Thus, it is important to note that the absence of selective forces acting on a genetic trait in modern populations does not imply the absence of such selective forces over the full history of the species.

Finally, it is important to realize that selective factors rarely operate alone. Other forces such as founder effects, random genetic drift, and departure from random mating have played, and continue to play, an important role in shaping the genetic constitution of present-day populations. Disentangling these diverse effects is a challenging task in epidemiologic studies of genetic traits in populations.

Chance Fluctuations

Chance fluctuations have an important role in the determination of gene frequencies in populations. In any finite population of individuals, allele frequencies at each genetic locus may or may not be representative of the frequencies in the previous generation. If each generation is considered as a sample of the genes present in the previous generation, the smaller the original population, the wider the fluctuations in allele frequencies. Although sampling variations between two generations may be modest, they lead to significant changes in allele frequencies over many generations (genetic drift). Eventually, genetic drift can lead to either elimination of an allele (allele frequency = 0) or fixation (allele frequency = 1) in the absence of influx from immigration or recurrent mutations. Mathematical models have been used to study the process of genetic drift and make inferences regarding its role in specific situations (Vogel and Motulsky, 1986).

A special case of chance fluctuation is founder effect, which occurs when a new population is formed from a small group of individuals whose gene pool may differ by chance from the originally larger population (Sutton, 1988). Chance fluctuations from ancestral allele frequencies attributable to founder effect have been suggested as the explanation of very high gene frequencies for rare single-gene disorders in selected populations or ethnic groups. Ellis-van Creveld syndrome serves as an example of such a phenomenon in the Old Order Amish (McKusick, 1978). Another example is the very high heterozygote frequency of Niemann-Pick disease (type D) in Nova Scotia, where all cases have been traced to one couple born in the 1600s (Winsor and Welch, 1978; Sutton, 1988).

Are there available epidemiologic methods to address whether the frequency of a genetic trait in a population is due to chance fluctuations? It is difficult to prove that an increase in the frequency of a genetic trait in a specific population is due to chance. "Basically, the argument depends on the failure to identify differences in fitness between heterozygous and homozygous normal persons" (Sutton, 1988). As indicated earlier in the case of Tay-Sachs disease in the Ashkenazi Jews, it is not simple to disentangle the role of selection from random fluctuation. In the case of small populations with available genealogic history, the identification of a single founder couple is a powerful clue to the potential role of founder effect/genetic drift. Nevertheless, for the vast majority of genetic traits, the role of chance fluctuations are not readily recognized in human populations.

Nonrandom Mating

Deviations from random mating can have a profound influence on the frequency of genetic traits both in prevalence studies as well as in its effects on genetic structure over time. Mate selection in human populations is based, to a certain extent, on similarities in phenotypic characteristics of individuals that may well reflect similarities in genotypic characteristics. This too can lead to changes in the distribution of genotypes over time. The net effect is usually to increase the frequency of homozygotes and decrease that of heterozygotes at any genetic locus affecting physical appearance.

Consider the specific example of inbreeding (also briefly reviewed in Chapter 2). Inbreeding corresponds to any mating pattern between two individuals who share one or more common ancestors. The inbreeding level of an individual, measured by the inbreeding coefficient F, refers to the probability that the individual receives at a given autosomal locus two copies of a gene that are identical by descent (Cavalli-Sforza and Bodmer, 1971). For example, the value of F for the offspring of a first cousin mating is 1/16, of second cousins 1/64 and so on. The average inbreeding coefficient in a population refers to the mean level of inbreeding of all individuals and can be estimated from the proportion of marriages between different classes of relatives weighted by their respective inbreeding coefficient.

As discussed earlier, the impact of inbreeding in human populations is to change genotype frequencies rather than allele frequencies. Inbreeding increases the proportion of homozygotes and decreases the proportion of heterozygotes. Because inbreeding increases homozygosity, the appearance of otherwise rare detrimental recessive traits becomes more likely in inbred populations compared to noninbred populations. Although inbreeding does not directly alter allele frequencies, the increased likelihood of appearance of lethal homozygote genotypes in an inbred population leads to a very gradual decline of the frequency of these alleles over several generations. With higher and more prolonged inbreeding, equilibrium frequencies of truly detrimental alleles become very low even in the face of recurrent mutation (Cavalli-Sforza and Bodmer, 1971). Thus, the effect of "washing out" deleterious genes has to be taken into account in interpreting the effect of inbreeding on the frequency of genetic traits (and disease in general). Inbreeding effects can be quite variable, depending on the duration and intensity of inbreeding.

To study the effect of inbreeding on the frequency of genetic traits in human populations, simple epidemiologic concepts and approaches can be applied to derive the magnitude of the effects of inbreeding (e.g., relative risk, risk difference), as well as the contribution of inbreeding to the frequency of the trait under study (i.e., attributable fraction). Since inbreeding effects may vary across populations due to differences in the duration and intensity of inbreeding, it is important to quantitate the impact of inbreeding in each population studied. An epidemiologic approach to study the role of inbreeding in disease is described in Chapter 5.

In general, one can compare the prevalence of a genetic trait among offspring of individuals with various inbreeding levels. Case-control or cohort approaches can be used, but in each situation, appropriate comparison groups must be selected. In many countries, consanguinity is correlated with several sociodemographic variables, such as type of religion, rural residence, social class, educational level, geographic patterns, age at marriage, and fertility rates (Cavalli-Sforza and Bodner, 1971; Lebel, 1983; Khoury et al., 1985). Thus, it becomes crucial when comparing rates of certain genetic traits between inbred and noninbred individuals to control for these potentially confounding variables, either in the study design (matching) or in the analysis (stratification, multivariate analysis).

To illustrate, consider the study of Alfi and colleagues (1980) in which the effect of inbreeding on the prevalence at birth of Down syndrome was evaluated in Kuwait, where close consanguinity occurs in about 40% of all marriages. The study population included all deliveries in a single hospital over one year (11,614 singletons). In this population, 20 trisomy 21 infants were identified (1.7 per 1000 livebirths). Factors associated with variation in the birth prevalence were examined, including maternal age, birth order, gravidity, and previous reproductive history, as well as parental consanguinity. Results of the consanguinity analysis are shown in Table 4–19. Basically, the prevalence at birth in offspring of consanguineous matings (second cousins or higher) was 4.3 times more than the prevalence in offspring of parents who were nonconsanguineous or the degree of consanguinity was less than second cousins. Furthermore, in this analysis, adjustment was made for the effects of other potential confounding variables (most notably maternal age). Adjustment did not alter the magnitude of the crude relative risk, suggesting there was little, if any, confounding. Thus, from these data, one could estimate that close consanguinity may account for over half the cases of trisomy 21 in this population (see attributable fraction calculation in Table 4–19). More recently, Roberts and colleagues (1991) showed that the mean kinship between parents of Down syndrome cases in Shetland is higher than the general population. These observations suggest a possible role for autosomal recessive gene(s) in the genesis of nondisjunction events (Alfi et al., 1980). Such analyses would benefit further from classification of the trisomy 21 cases by parental origin and meiotic stage and evaluation of inbreeding effects in different case groups. Also, when available, data on parental inbreeding (or consanguinity of grandparents) may shed further light on the mechanisms of such potential genetic effects.

4.6 CONCLUDING REMARKS

In summary, the distribution and determinants of genetic traits in populations can be studied, using both epidemiologic methods and population genetic concepts. The ability to study genetic traits as outcomes depends on the level of identification of these traits (ranging from the molecular to the clinical) as well as methods of ascertainment and measurement of these traits. Once a genetic endpoint is defined, studies can be done to evaluate the distribution of such traits in different populations in order to gain insight into factors affecting such distribution. Analytic studies can then be done to examine risk factors affecting mutations in populations as well as to examine determinants

Table 4–19. Example of the effect of inbreeding on the prevalence at birth of Down syndrome in Kuwait

Parental consanguinity	No. of births	No. of cases	Rate per 1000	Relative risk	Risk difference
Close	3,989	14	3.5	4.3	2.7
None/far	7,436	6	0.8	Reference	Reference

Close refers to marriages involving first cousins ($F = 1/16$), first cousins once removed ($F = 1/32$) and second cousins ($F = 1/64$).

Attributable fraction $= f_c(R - 1)/[1 + f_c(R - 1)] = 53\%$, where f_c is the proportion of offspring with close parental consanguinity ($f_c = 3989/(3989 + 7436) = 35\%$) and R is 4.3.

Data from Alfi et al. (1980).

of the genetic structure of populations in relation to specific genetic traits. In both types of studies, epidemiologic issues as to study design, ascertainment of risk factors, measures of effect, handling of misclassification, confounding, and other potential sources of bias must be considered. At the same time, population genetic concepts can provide further insight into factors that alter the genetic structure of populations over time.

5

Study of Genetic Factors in Disease

5.1. INTRODUCTION

This chapter examines epidemiologic concepts and approaches to assessing the role of genetic factors in disease using population studies. The outcomes of interest are not only disease and disease precursors but normal variants of physiologic attributes, such as eye color and facial features. A brief overview of the biologic basis for the role of genetic factors in health and disease is given in section 5.2. Then, clues to the importance of genetic factors in disease that can be obtained from epidemiologic studies of disease occurrence are reviewed in section 5.3. Section 5.4 addresses epidemiologic approaches to evaluating the importance of genetic factors in the absence of defined genetic mechanisms. We focus on three general types of investigations: migrant, admixture, and inbreeding studies. In section 5.5, epidemiologic approaches to studying the role of measured genes in disease occurrence are discussed, including different study designs and analytic issues, as well as interpretations and limitations of these studies.

5.2. BIOLOGIC BASIS FOR THE ROLE OF GENETIC FACTORS IN HEALTH AND DISEASE

The relationship between genes and pathologic conditions can be understood within the larger framework of how genes affect normal biochemical processes. The one gene–one enzyme concept that evolved from experimental studies (Beadle, 1945; Tatum, 1959) implies that

1. Biochemical processes are under direct genetic control.
2. Biochemical processes can be divided into a series of reactions.
3. Each reaction is under the control of a different gene.

4. Mutation of a gene alters the ability of cells to perform the chemical reaction (Beaudet et al., 1989).

With advances in molecular genetics, the one gene–one enzyme concept has now been modified to the one cistron–one polypeptide concept (Beaudet et al., 1989). Not all gene products are enzymes, and not all enzymes are under the control of only one gene. Many functional enzymes are composed of several polypeptide chains, each of which is a product of a distinct gene (e.g., propionyl CoA carboxylase [Rosenberg and Fenton, 1989]). Also, one polypeptide chain may have multiple enzyme activities (e.g., CAD trienzyme protein [Jones, 1980]). Other variations may be due to alternative promotors, splicing, and posttranslational events (Beaudet et al, 1989).

Because gene products are involved in virtually all biochemical processes, it follows that genetic variability initially due to mutation must play a major role in the variability in the structure and function of the organism in health and disease. The extensive chemical individuality of humans was initially recognized by Garrod (1902) in his work on alkaptonuria, the first example of an "inborn error of metabolism." Subsequently, an extensive array of genetic polymorphisms became detectable at the protein level (Giblett, 1977; Harris, 1980). More recently, genetic variation at the DNA level was found to be even more prominent than the variation observed at the protein level (Cooper et al., 1985).

Clearly, mutations are at the basis of genetic involvement in disease processes. DNA changes may lead to abnormal mRNA development, in turn resulting in alterations at the protein or gene product level. The pathogenetic mechanisms by which protein alterations lead to disease processes can be divided into three general classes, depending on the functions of these proteins (Beaudet et al., 1989):

1. *Proteins with direct effects on the biologic system*: These protein effects include, for example, abnormalities in coagulation factors leading to bleeding disorders (e.g., hemophilias), altered cell shape or membrane stability (e.g., spherocytosis), and abnormalities in collagen chains (e.g., osteogenesis imperfecta).
2. *Proteins with effects on the metabolism of other molecules*: Examples here include disorders of metabolic pathways (e.g., phenylketonuria), abnormalities in transport mechanisms (e.g., cystinosis), and abnormal processing of enzymes (e.g., mucolipidosis II).
3. *Regulatory proteins*: Examples here include the estrogen and glucocorticoid receptors (Beaudet et al., 1989).

In assessing the role of a gene in the biochemical process involved in physiologic variation and pathologic conditions, it is essential to recognize that the effect of any one gene is influenced by its interaction with both environmental factors as well as other genes. For example, the epistatic interactions among the biochemical pathways of the ABO blood group antigens with the Lewis and secretor loci illustrate how the ultimate phenotype determined by one genetic locus can be modified or affected by other genetic loci (Sutton, 1988). In addition, the environment at large provides a multitude of factors—physical, chemical, social, and cultural—that interact with genetic systems, leading to alterations in biochemical and physiologic pathways in health and disease states. The most striking examples of the interaction between single genetic and environmental factors are found in the classical pharmacogenetic disorders, where certain drugs have been discovered to lead to specific complications in some individuals, but not others, because of genetically determined differences in metabolism of these drugs, for example, isoniazid and the acetylator phenotype (Vesell, 1979).

The concept of genetic-environmental interaction is crucial in understanding the dynamics of health and disease. The latter could be considered the end product of one or more problems in homeostatic mechanisms leading to deterioration of a part of the biologic system. Just as there is a tendency in the medical sciences to combine the values of individuals and talk about average "normal" values for physiologic measures, and to an "optimal dose" for a given drug, the same tendency exists in epidemiology in the quantification of disease risks and the impact of risk factors, pretending that the average risk applies equally to all individuals. For example, it has been noted that assigning an equal risk of lung cancer to all smokers only reflects "our ignorance about the determinants of lung cancer that interact with cigarette smoking" (Rothman, 1986). Similarly, Beaudet et al (1989) have observed that "the aggregate of our genes determines who dies of myocardial infarction on a high fat diet, who develops cancer upon smoking, (and) who develops postoperative thromboembolism." Thus, the major challenge in genetic epidemiology is to identify which genetic factors interact with which environmental factors in the pathogenesis of disease. The traditional debate of nature versus nurture (or genes versus environment) is replaced by an active search for both genes and environments in disease.

5.3. CLUES TO GENETIC AND ENVIRONMENTAL FACTORS DERIVED FROM EPIDEMIOLOGIC CHARACTERISTICS

Let us evaluate to what extent descriptive epidemiologic characteristics of disease occurrence by time, place, and persons give clues regarding the possible role of genetic factors in disease (Table 5–1).

5.3.1. Geographic Variation

Geographic variation in disease rates has been observed for many acute and chronic diseases. Such variation may be due to differences in case definition and diagnosis, access to medical care, case ascertainment, and mortality as well as errors in determining the population at risk, that is, the denominator population (Lilienfeld and Lilienfeld, 1980). However, even after ruling out artifactual reasons for geographic variation, differences in incidence rates have been observed for many diseases, for example, coronary heart disease (Ep-

Table 5–1. Clues to genetic and environmental factors from epidemiologic characteristics of disease occurrence

Epidemiologic characteristic	Clues to the presence of	
	Genetic factors	Environmental factors
Geographic variation	+	+
Ethnic/racial variation	+	+
Temporal variation	−	+
Epidemics	+/−	+
Social class variation	−	+
Gender	+	+
Age	+/−	+
Family variables		
History of disease	+	+
Birth order	+/−	+
Birth interval	−	+
Cohabitation	−	+

stein, 1989; Marmot, 1989), stomach cancer (Howson et al., 1986), insulin-dependent diabetes mellitus (LaPorte et al., 1985), and neural tube defects (Elwood and Elwood, 1980; Greenberg et al., 1983). While such variation is usually construed as a strong indicator for the presence of environmentally induced variation, it is consistent with a genetic contribution as well. In fact, geographic variation has been demonstrated in the gene frequencies for many genetic traits (Mourant et al., 1978; Barrai et al., 1984; Barbujani, 1987, 1988; Sokal, 1988; Sokal et al., 1989). Such variation is often monotonically changing on a continental scale (Sokal and Menozzi, 1982; Barbujani, 1987, Barbujani et al., 1989) and depends on selective pressures, reproductive isolation, founder effects, inbreeding, and so on. To the extent that these forces influence the frequencies of genetic factors conferring disease susceptibility, they will partly explain some of the geographic differences in disease frequency. For example, because HLA-DR3 and -DR4 antigens have been found to be associated with insulin-dependent diabetes mellitus (IDDM), LaPorte and coworkers (1985) examined the correlation between IDDM incidence and the frequency of these high-risk HLA antigens across populations. This ecologic analysis did not give conclusive results (Trucco and Dorman, 1989). More recently, a strong association was found between the absence of aspartic acid at position 57 of the HLA-DQ β chain and IDDM (Morel et al., 1988). Preliminary studies suggest that geographic differences in the incidence of IDDM could be due, in part, to geographic difference in this genetic trait (Bao et al., 1989). Another example is the decreasing east to west gradient in the birth prevalence of neural tube defects reported in North America (Elwood and Elwood, 1980). This trend is consistent with environmental factors in disease etiology, but does not rule out genetic contribution to risk.

5.3.2. Racial/Ethnic Variation

Nearly all epidemiologic studies of disease examine and often find racial/ethnic variation in disease occurrence. Many studies also find racial/ethnic differences in drug response (e.g., Zhou et al., 1989) and in physiologic measures (e.g., Pratt et al., 1989). Nevertheless, the interpretation of racial/ethnic variation in terms of genetic and environmental causation is not straightforward (Miller, 1988). As pointed out by Polednak (1987), racial groups should be viewed as dynamic and are constantly undergoing evolutionary change. While the major racial groups (caucasoid, mongoloid, and negroid) may differ little in the frequencies of polymorphic genetic traits (Chakraborty, 1984), substantial genetic variation can be seen within each group, depending on geographic location, patterns of migration, reproductive isolation, and so on. In addition, racial and ethnic variation is almost always associated with socioeconomic differences, life-style variation, cultural factors, and numerous other factors that indicate environmental exposures. Therefore, a major challenge in epidemiologic studies is the interpretation of disease variation by race and ethnicity in terms of specific and measurable genetic and environmental mechanisms.

5.3.3. Temporal Variation

The existence of temporal trends in disease occurrence, such as short-term declines or increases in the disease frequency, is a strong clue to the presence of environmental determinants of risk (Barbujani et al., 1989). As gene frequencies change more slowly in populations over generations, any abrupt changes in disease occurrence, seasonal variation, epidemics, or other changes in frequency over a period of a few years or decades are difficult to explain on the basis of genetic factors alone. For example, the long-term decline in the birth prevalence of neural tube defects in many parts of the world, which preceded widespread utilization of prenatal diagnosis, strongly suggests changes in environmental factors (Elwood and Elwood, 1980; Windham and Edmonds, 1982). Several epidemiologic studies have pointed to improvements in nutritional status, in particular the periconceptional intake of multivitamin preparations as possible reasons for this decline (Mulinare et al., 1988; Milunsky et al., 1989). The presence of temporal changes, however, does not rule out the possible role of genetic factors that might interact with changing environmental determinants.

5.3.4. Socioeconomic Variation

The existence of socioeconomic variation in disease occurrence is a strong indicator for the importance of environmental determinants of risk (Susser and Susser, 1987a, 1987b). However, it is not always clear what social class or socioeconomic status actually mean in terms of exposures, access to medical care, ascertainment, and so on. (Marmot et al., 1987; Liberatos et al., 1988; Marmot, 1989). Socioeconomic factors are numerous, including occupational and environmental exposures, nutritional factors, and life-style patterns. Because of the interrelatedness of these factors, it is important to disentangle as clearly as possible the specific factors that can account for socioeconomic differences and relate them directly to disease processes. Socioeconomic differences could be indirectly related to genetic factors, as these differences are often associated with race and ethnicity that, in turn, may have a genetic basis. It is therefore essential to examine socioeconomic variation in disease occurrence within each racial and ethnic group and within each geographic location.

5.3.5. Gender Differences

The existence of gender differences in morbidity and mortality was long recognized, and by itself sheds little light on the underlying biologic processes involved (Polednak, 1987). Some disorders occur more frequently among men (e.g., certain cancers, coronary heart disease, chronic obstructive pulmonary disease), while others occur more frequently among women (e.g., autoimmune diseases and musculoskeletal disorders). The finding of a gender difference in any disease or trait provides only the initial step toward unraveling the underlying genetic and environmental factors involved.

Genetic factors contributing to disease with large gender differences include not only X and Y chromosome-linked genes but also autosomal genes influencing risk indirectly through hormonal and other physiologic actions. As discussed in Chapter 2, simple recessive X-linked disorders are more common in males because of the lack of compensatory effect of a second X chromosome. X-linked disorders, such as the fragile X syndrome, may partially explain the higher frequency of mental retardation in males (Gustavson et al., 1986; Kahkonen et al., 1987). An example of an autosomal recessive condition manifesting only in females is the Kaufman-McKusick syndrome, which manifests with hydrometrocolpos and other malformations (Robinow and Shaw, 1979).

Although most of the genome is shared by both males and females, hormonal, physiologic, psychological, and morphologic differences can play important roles in pathophysiologic processes leading to various diseases (Polednak, 1987). For example, a large component of the higher neonatal mortality in males compared with females is related to the higher incidence of respiratory distress syndrome in males, which, in turn, may suggest a slower process of lung maturation in the developing male fetuses (Khoury et al., 1985a).

On the other hand, environmental factors may also play an important role in gender differences in disease frequencies. For example, the higher prevalence of cigarette smoking in men for many years could explain the higher lung cancer incidence and mortality in men compared with women (Fielding, 1986). As the prevalence of smoking has increased in women over the past few decades, the rates of lung cancer in women have steadily climbed and the gender gap has become narrower over the past few years (Stolley, 1983; Fielding, 1986). In addition to differences in smoking patterns and alcohol and drug use, numerous other gender differences exist with respect to occupational, life-style, sociocultural, and psychological factors that could explain gender differences in disease occurrence. Thus, the documentation of gender differences in disease is consistent with both genetic and environmental mechanisms.

5.3.6. Age Effects

Age variation in morbidity and mortality rates is nearly universally observed. For many chronic diseases, such as coronary heart disease, certain cancers, and chronic obstructive pulmonary disease, incidence and prevalence increase with advanced age (Polednak, 1987). For other conditions, disease risk is highest in infancy and childhood, and in some diseases, no age effects are seen. The biologic basis for age effects is complex and largely unknown. Increasing risk of disease associated with advanced age may be due to cumulative environmental, occupational, and personal exposures, in addition to changes in physiologic, psychological, immunologic, and endocrine function, some of which are, at least in part, under genetic control.

Many Mendelian disorders, especially recessive diseases such as cystic fibrosis, phenylketonuria, and hemoglobinopathies, are associated with early age at onset (Costa et al., 1985; Childs and Scriver, 1986), while many dominant disorders tend not to manifest until later in life (e.g., Huntington's disease, porphyrias). For some common chronic diseases, there may well be a small proportion of the cases due to simple Mendelian mechanisms. Such cases typically manifest at an earlier age than the more common type. For example, cases of premature coronary heart disease are overrepresented with the autosomal dominant disorder, familial hypercholesterolemia (Goldstein and Brown, 1989). While an early onset form of any disease may suggest an important role for genetic factors and represents a fruitful area for investigation, this does not imply that genetic factors do not operate in cases with later age of onset. As discussed by Sing and Moll (1989), genotypic differences may influence the extent of phenotypic variation and the rate of change in the level of phenotypic traits with age. Moll et al. (1984a) used the example of familial hypercholesterolemia (FH) to illustrate genotypic-dependent changes in cholesterol levels with age, and showed that heterozygotes for the *FH* gene had a more rapid increase in cholesterol levels with age compared with their homozygous normal relatives.

Even for early-onset genetically mediated diseases, however, environmental factors may still play an important role in the occurrence of disease. In the example of FH, R. R. Williams and colleagues (1986) showed evidence that healthy life-style factors may protect against the expression of the genetic defect among male heterozygotes in Utah. Thus, while changes in disease frequency with age are usually indicators of environmental components in disease, they do not rule out important contributions of genetic factors in disease pathogenesis. On the other hand, the existence of early-onset genetic forms of a disease does not rule out a role for environmental factors in improving or aggravating morbidity.

5.3.7. Familial Variables

Familial variables (Table 5–1) may provide initial clues to the relative importance of genetic factors in disease occurrence. As commented by Susser and Susser (1987a), the discovery of familial aggregation "is a universal signal for geneticists to begin investigation of genetic causes." The documentation of familial aggregation is equally consistent with both genetic and environmental hypotheses, and both should be seriously pursued (see Chapter 6).

From an epidemiologic perspective, several familial variables tend to point toward environmental components rather than genetic factors (Susser and Susser, 1987a). These include the following:

1. *A birth interval effect*: The risk of disease in siblings of affected individuals changes with the interval from the birth of the case, as has been observed for neural tube defects (Yen and MacMahon, 1968; Khoury et al., 1982b).
2. *A cohabitation effect*: A disease or trait shows evidence of household aggregation rather than familial aggregation. For example, this effect might be seen when the risk of a disease in a genetically unrelated spouse of an affected person is increased over the risk of disease in a spouse of an unaffected person. Confounding related to assortative mating has to be carefully considered, however (Susser and Susser, 1987a, 1987b).
3. *Birth order effects*: Where the risk of disease varies according to the birth order of the individual or when the risk of familial recurrence of disease after an affected person changes by birth order, it is usually difficult to evoke simple genetic mechanisms to explain birth-order effects. Maternal-fetal Rh incompatibility provides a counterexample, however, where a disorder with strong birth-order effect can be traced to a genetically controlled process.

5.4. EPIDEMIOLOGIC APPROACHES TO THE EVALUATION OF GENETIC FACTORS IN THE ABSENCE OF MEASURED GENETIC TRAITS

In this section, we discuss three types of population studies of the role of genetic factors in disease in the absence of measured genetic traits. These include migrant, admixture, and inbreeding studies.

5.4.1. Migrant Studies

Migrant studies provide one approach that theoretically can help refine geographic variation in disease frequency in terms of the relative importance of genetic factors. However, inferences from migrant studies are only tentative and subject to potential biases and limitations (Lilienfeld and Lilienfeld, 1980; Howson et al., 1986; Susser and Susser, 1987a; 1987b). Given that the geographic variation in the frequency of a disease or trait between two countries is real and not due to artifactual differences, investigators can compare the mortality or morbidity experiences of individuals who migrate from one country to another with the experience of individuals in the two countries, respectively. In the event of a strong genetic influence on the disease, it is expected that the disease frequency among migrants would be similar to the disease frequency in the country of origin rather than the disease frequency in the host country. On the other hand, in the presence of a strong environmental influence, it is expected that the disease frequency among migrants would be similar to the disease frequency in the host country rather than the disease frequency in the country of origin. Migrant studies have been utilized for a variety of conditions, including cancer and other chronic diseases (Reid, 1966; Haenzel and Kurihara, 1968; Haenzel, 1970; Modan, 1980; McMichael et al., 1980, 1989; King et al., 1985; Elford and Phillips, 1989; Prentice and Sheppard, 1989; Salmond et al., 1989; Ward, 1990).

Migrant studies, however, rarely give unequivocal findings. Migrants are usually self-selected. Often they may not be representative of either population of origin or migration. Differences may include factors such as age, gender, level of education, occupation, religion, social and economic factors, and, most importantly, general health status. To the extent that these and other unmeasured factors play a role in the etiology of disease, they could affect comparisons of disease frequencies among the three groups. Every effort should be made in migrant studies to measure and adjust for such potential confounding factors.

Furthermore, there are other inherent difficulties in separating genetic and environmental effects. The fact that migrants manifest the disease rates of the country of origin is consistent not only with a genetic component of the disease but with early environmental components that operate before migration (e.g., childhood exposures). In this situation, the age at migration can be helpful in evaluating the role of early environmental factors. For example, if migrants who moved as adults have a disease frequency similar to that of the country of origin, but those who migrated early in life have a different disease frequency, that is more consistent with early environmental effects rather than with a clear-cut genetic component (Spielman, 1982). Also, evaluation of disease frequency in successive generations of migrants can shed further light on the role of environmental factors. For example, in the case of gastric cancer, first-generation Japanese migrants do manifest incidence rates of the country of origin (Howson et al., 1986). However, second-generation migrants, unlike their parents, manifest rates of gastric cancer that are more similar to those of the host country rather than the country of origin (Howson et al., 1986), suggesting the role of environmental changes, since large genetic differences do not usually occur over the span of a single generation. Although changes in environmental factors do occur with migration, first-generation migrants tend to maintain to a certain degree the sociocultural, dietary, and life-style habits that are similar to their premigration environment (Kato et al., 1973; Kelsey, 1979), making it difficult to separate genetic from environmental effects.

Finally, migrant studies must be interpreted in the larger context of other types of studies. As Ward (1990) points out, migrant studies of blood pressure in populations recently adopting western life-style underscore the importance of environmental factors such as diet, physical activity, and psychological stress in the development of hypertension. However, family studies in both westernized and tribal populations consistently show patterns of familial correlation consistent with genetic control of blood pressure. Thus, both environmental and genetic factors contribute to the distribution of blood pressure and associated hypertension (Ward, 1990).

Thus, while migrant studies can provide some clues to the relative importance of genetic factors, to be useful, such studies should strive to make comparison groups as similar as possible with respect to potentially confounding variables. In addition, it is important to evaluate specific pre- and post-migration factors (e.g., dietary factors) and the age of migration.

5.4.2. Admixture Studies

When a disease or a trait manifests racial/ethnic variation, admixture or out-crossing studies provide one population-based approach to evaluate the relative importance of genetic factors. Theoretically, if two populations differ in their gene pools, then mating between persons from these populations could lead to two broad consequences (Vogel and Motulsky, 1986; Sutton, 1988):

1. There could be a disruption of combinations of genes that have been previously favored by selection ("coadapted genotypes") with potential deleterious effects on health.
2. There is increased likelihood of heterozygosity in the hybrid offspring.

While there is no evidence of a detrimental effect of outcrossing in humans, it is a theoretical possibility (Morton, 1982). There is ample evidence of a positive effect of hybridity in animals and plants (termed "hybrid vigor"), but, in general, human studies of outcrosses tend to show that offspring lie between the parental racial values for most perinatal outcomes (e.g., birth-weight). The health effects of racial admixture on a variety of perinatal outcomes have been examined in observational studies in humans using data on offspring of interracial matings in different populations, but these are limited by the availability and quality of records on the outcome in the child and the racial identity of parents. Examples of studies in this area include the following:

1. Evaluation of the effects of interracial crossing in Hawaii on perinatal outcomes (birthweight, infant mortality, etc.) and birth defects such as cleft lip and palate (Morton et al., 1967; Ching and Chung, 1974; Chung et al., 1987)
2. Evaluation of the extent of racial admixture in Brazil and its effect on morbidity and mortality (Morton, 1964; Krieger et al., 1965; Santos and Azevedo, 1981; Helena et al., 1982)
3. Admixture studies in American Indians and their effects on the prev-

alence of non-insulin-dependent diabetes mellitus (R. C. Williams et al., 1986; Knowler et al., 1988)
4. Studies of white-black admixture in the United States and their effects on disease such as insulin-dependent diabetes mellitus (Reitnauer et al., 1982) and some perinatal conditions (Khoury and Erickson, 1983, 1984)
5. Admixture studies in Mexican-Americans and their effects on gall-bladder disease and non-insulin-dependent diabetes mellitus (Weiss et al., 1984; Chakraborty and Weiss, 1986; Hanis et al., 1986)

The extent of racial admixture can be measured in a variety of ways including (1) reported admixture (Khoury et al., 1983; 1983; Knowler et al., 1988; Moy et al., 1989), (2) the use of surnames (Azevedo et al., 1983), and (3) the use of polymorphic genetic markers (Reitnauer et al., 1982; R. C. Williams et al., 1986; Knowler et al., 1988). To illustrate the general epidemiologic approaches to racial admixture studies, let us consider the study of Knowler and coworkers (1988) on the prevalence of non-insulin-dependent diabetes mellitus (NIDDM) in American (Pima) Indians. This study examined the determinants of the high prevalence of non-insulin-dependent diabetes mellitus in the Pima Indians (Bennett, 1971). If the excess in diabetes in the Pima Indians were related even in part to genetic factors, then one would expect to find variation in the prevalence of diabetes, depending on the extent of racial admixture with non-Indians. Individuals with a greater proportion of non-Indian genes should have a lower than expected prevalence of NIDDM. In this study the index of Indian heritage was determined by using interview data on individuals and their relatives, and ranged from 0 to 8. For example, a person who has one parent who is full-blooded Amerindian (8/8) and one parent who is Caucasian (0/8) was assigned a value of 4. This index of Indian heritage gave close agreement with a single genetic marker (Gm haplotype 3;5,13,14) that is frequent in Caucasians and virtually absent in Amerindians (R. C. Williams et al., 1986). The prevalence of NIDDM by the index of Amerindian heritage is shown in Table 5–2 (for persons over 35 years of age). Despite the small sample sizes for some categories, a clear trend of increasing prevalence can be seen, ranging from 15% in persons with an index of 0, to 39% in persons with an index of 4, and 60% in persons with an index of 8. Because of the known effects of age on diabetes prevalence, the authors conducted all analyses stratified by age (Knowler et al., 1988). Another interesting observation was that the relationship between the Gm haplotype marker and diabetes in this population was entirely due to this effect of admixture. In other words, since racial admixture was related to both the genetic marker and the prevalence of the disease, it acted as a confounding variable. After stratification of the results (Table 5–3), the association between the genetic marker and the prevalence of NIDDM disappeared, indicating that its association with diabetes was a proxy for racial admixture rather than a true biologic effect. The issue of confounding is further discussed in section 5.5.4.

It should be noted that the interpretation of the effects of racial admixture

Table 5–2. Prevalence of type II diabetes in a sample of American Indians age 35 years and over, by the index of reported Indian heritage

Index* Indian heritage	Sample size	Number with diabetes	Percent
0	20	3	15.0
1	0	0	—
2	0	0	—
3	0	0	—
4	23	9	39.1
5	0	0	—
6	26	11	42.3
7	11	3	27.2
8	1781	1068	60.0

Type II diabetes: non-insulin-dependent diabetes mellitus.

*Index is calculated using the reported Indian heritage on the parents' grandparents. A full-blooded Indian has a value of 8, while a Caucasian has a value of 0. A person with one parent who is a full-blooded Indian (8/8) and one who is Caucasian (0/8) is assigned a value of 4.

Adapted from Knowler et al. (1988).

is still subject to the usual limitations of confounding and selection. For example, in the study of Knowler and colleagues (1988), while the finding of a strong effect of racial admixture is entirely consistent with a genetic component, it does not entirely rule out environmental and other cultural confounding factors if these unmeasured factors vary with increasing admixture and are associated with the prevalence of diabetes. Such confounding factors, however, have to show a trend in prevalence with increasing admixture.

In the case of a true genetic basis for observed admixture effects, the quantitative relationship between disease frequency and the amount of admixture in a population depends on the number of loci affecting disease risk

Table 5–3. Association of type II diabetes with haplotype Gm 3;5,13,14 in American Indians, by the index of reported Indian heritage

Index of Indian heritage	Gm marker	Percent* with diabetes
0	Present	17.8
	Absent	19.9
4	Present	28.3
	Absent	28.8
8	Present	35.9
	Absent	39.3
Total (not stratified)	Present	8.0
	Absent	29.0

Type II diabetes: non-insulin-dependent diabetes mellitus.

*Adjusted for age.

Adapted from Knowler et al. (1988).

and allele frequencies (Chakraborty and Weiss, 1986). Estimation of the amount of racial admixture usually is based on frequencies of polymorphic genetic markers from two parent populations and the "hybrid" group. To be useful, such markers should not themselves be causally associated with disease risk, and should be able to discriminate between the two parent populations (i.e., rare in one population and common in the other). Consider a diallelic genetic marker with frequencies of $P(A)$ and $P(B)$ in the parent populations (A and B), with $P(H)$ in the hybrid population formed by one-way migration from A to B. The amount of genetic admixture m, or the fraction of alleles contributed by population A (for example) can be computed as

$$m = \frac{P(H) - P(A)}{P(B) - P(A)} \qquad (5\text{-}1)$$

(Bernstein, 1931; Cavalli-Sforza and Bodmer, 1971).

When dealing with multiple genetic systems at different loci, or with more than two alleles at any given locus, maximum likelihood methods have been developed to estimate the amount of overall admixture as well as admixture at each specific locus (Krieger et al., 1965; Elston, 1971). The relationship between the estimated fraction of admixture and disease risk can then be incorporated into epidemiologic studies of disease. For example, in a case-control study of IDDM in U.S. blacks, Reitnauer and coworkers (1982), using four polymorphic genetic markers, found 21.4% of white gene admixture among black IDDM cases as compared with 17.9% white gene admixture among black control subjects. This suggests some role for genetic influences in the increased risk of IDDM in U.S. blacks. Again, the possibility of confounding cannot be entirely ruled out. The increasing number of DNA markers becoming available should improve estimates of racial admixture; and this may increase the popularity of admixture studies in epidemiologic investigations (Moy et al., 1989).

Finally, admixture studies can be used to distinguish between maternal and paternal determinants of disease etiology. For example, dizygotic twinning is a phenomenon related to multiple ovulation and shows substantial racial variation, with blacks having higher rates than whites, who in turn have higher rates than orientals. Because the event is of maternal origin (possibly related to hormonal levels), it follows that maternal race should be a more important determinant of the frequency of dizygotic twinning than paternal race. In fact, data on offspring of interracial crosses in different populations (Morton et al., 1967; Khoury et al., 1983) confirm the strong maternal race effect independent of paternal race. Data from the study of Khoury and colleagues (1983) are presented in Table 5–4. Here, only information on the frequency of unlike-sex twin (all dizygotic) deliveries are shown. The higher frequency of unlike-sex twinning is observed for black mothers (regardless of the father's race) compared with white mothers (regardless of the father's race). This finding persisted after adjustment for sociodemographic factors. No difference was observed for like-sex twinning (a mixture of mono- and dizygotic twins) (Khoury et al., 1983). While this observed maternal race

Table 5–4. Maternal and paternal race effects on the frequency of unlike-sex twin delivery in interracial crosses in the United States

Parental races mother–father	Number of births	Number of twins	Proportion per 1000 deliveries
Black–black	948,756	3,777	4.0
Black–white	7,576	38	5.0
White–black	33,703	81	2.4
White–white	7,090,871	17,166	2.4

Adapted from Khoury and Erickson (1983).

effect is consistent with a strong genetic component, environmental factors should not be ruled out, especially those that could relate to differential prenatal survival by race. Similar analyses for maternal factors in cleft lip and palate did not yield consistent results in studies from different populations (Khoury et al., 1983; Chung et al., 1987).

5.4.3. Inbreeding Studies

The overall impact of inbreeding is to increase the likelihood of homozygosity at each autosomal locus, at both the individual and the population levels. For fully penetrant autosomal recessive disorders, the effects of consanguinity are readily apparent. More generally, inbreeding studies can be used to evaluate a recessive genetic component in any disease with complex etiology and pathogenesis. However, because the prevalence of consanguineous marriages has declined to very low levels in most European and North American countries in recent years (Lebel, 1983), it has become increasingly difficult to apply this study approach to evaluate the role of genetic factors in disease occurrence in these areas. Despite declining trends, however, there continues to be a relatively high prevalence of consanguineous marriages in several countries such as Israel, Lebanon, Egypt, Algeria, Kuwait, India, Japan, as well as certain religious isolates in the United States (Khlat and Khoury, 1991). Consequently, the study of inbreeding effects in these populations can provide a valuable approach in the search for genetic factors in disease.

The general aim of inbreeding studies is to assess whether there is an association between the level of inbreeding of individuals and patterns of morbidity (Freire-Maia and Elisbao, 1984) and mortality (Khoury et al., 1987a). Instead of focusing on nonspecific and etiologically heterogeneous outcomes (e.g., mortality, all birth defects), such studies are likely to be more rewarding for clinically well-defined conditions. Accordingly, inbreeding studies can be used to investigate a nonspecific recessive genetic component to disease, and to assess the genetic load due to genes that are lethal or detrimental in the homozygous state (Morton, 1982). The limitations of using inbreeding studies for the purposes of estimating genetic load have been recently summarized (Khlat and Khoury, 1991), and will not be addressed further.

From an epidemiologic perspective, inbreeding studies can be conducted by using the usual designs (cohort, case-control, or cross-sectional), with the exposure variable of interest being the coefficient of inbreeding of each individual (Wright, 1922), which is known for the common types of consanguineous marriages (Table 5–5). However, when there are multiple genealogic connections (as occurring in the multigeneration genealogies of isolated populations, such as the Old Order Amish) inbreeding coefficients must be computed directly. Several methods may be used, including (1) the path method of Wright (1922) (see Table 5–5 for a simple illustration of the method for common relatives), (2) iterative computation (Rostron, 1978), and (3) graph methods (Marayuma and Yasuda, 1970).

In a cohort study, the frequency of a disease outcome is compared among individuals with different levels of the inbreeding coefficient, whereas in a case-control study, individuals with disease are compared to those without disease regarding their level of inbreeding. In designing such studies, however, it is crucial to have appropriate comparison groups (Roberts, 1985). Since inbreeding patterns tend to be differentially distributed in the population, and are usually correlated with socioeconomic levels, education, religion, occupation, and geography, these factors can be potential confounders and should be considered in the design of the study, in the analysis, or in both. For example, in a cohort study, inbred and noninbred individuals should be chosen carefully to be of similar socioeconomic background, education, and so on. Moreover, in the analysis, these variables should be examined by using stratification and adjustment.

Inbreeding coefficients can be used either as continuous variables or categorized into groups (e.g., noninbred, inbred at the level of first-cousin mat-

Table 5–5. Inbreeding coefficients for offspring of common consanguineous marriages, and method of calculation using the path method of Wright

Parental consanguinity	Number of common ancestors (c)	Values of		Inbreeding coefficient
		m	n	
Full siblings	2	1	1	1/4
Uncle–niece	2	2	1	1/8
First cousins	2	2	2	1/16
First cousins once removed	2	3	2	1/32
Second cousins	2	3	3	1/64
Second cousins once removed	2	4	3	1/128
Third cousins	2	4	4	1/256

m and n refer to the number of paths from a common ancestor; c refers to number of common ancestors. Inbreeding coefficient:

$$F = \sum_{i=1}^{c} \left(\frac{1}{2}\right)^{(n_i + m_i + 1)}$$

Adapted from Wright (1922).

ing, inbred at the level of second-cousin mating). Measures of absolute and relative risks as well as those of attributable fraction can be computed as for other risk factors (Khoury et al., 1987a). Absolute and relative risks can be used to assess the strength of the association between inbreeding and the disease, and these may be useful in genetic counseling. As pointed out by Freire-Maia (1990), such relative risk measures may be artificially low for outcomes such as mortality, wherever the overall level of mortality is high. An index called the genetic effects of inbreeding (GEI) is suggested as an alternative and is calculated as

$$GEI = \frac{P_i - P_0}{1 - P_0},$$ (5-2)

where P_i is the probability of the event (e.g., death) in an inbred person, and P_0 is the probability of the event in a noninbred person (Freire-Maia, 1990). In addition, the public health impact of inbreeding can be evaluated with the concept of attributable fraction, which refers to the proportion of deaths (or any other relevant outcome) in the population that could be prevented if consanguinity were absent. To illustrate various epidemiologic parameters of inbreeding effect, Table 5–6 presents data derived from the WHO collaborative study of congenital malformations (Chakraborty and Chakravarti, 1977), showing the effects of first-cousin marriage on the prevalence at birth of all major defects in terms of absolute and relative risks and attributable fraction. In these populations, a relatively modest effect of inbreeding on the frequency of all birth defects (which is no doubt a highly heterogeneous group) can be seen. More generally, because of the low prevalence of inbreeding in many populations, the public health impact of inbreeding in terms of attributable fraction is likely to be very small (Khoury et al., 1987a). Finally, it is noteworthy that epidemiologic measures of absolute and relative risks can be

Table 5–6. Illustration of the measurement of inbreeding effects on the prevalence at birth of major birth defects: WHO survey on birth defects

	Sao Paulo, Brazil	Bombay, India	Singapore, Malaysia
Number of births	14,394	39,49	15,699
% children of first-cousin marriage	1.70	8.38	3.89
% major birth defects in noninbred group	1.02	1.58	1.04
% major birth defect in offspring of first cousins	1.69	2.03	1.31
Relative risk	1.66	1.28	1.26
GEI	0.68	0.46	0.27
Attributable fraction %	1.11	2.29	1.00

GEI, genetic effects of inbreeding (Freire-Maia [1990]).
Data adapted from Chakraborty and Chakravarti (1977).

reconciled and interpreted along with indicators of genetic loads (Khlat and Khoury, 1991; Freire-Maia, 1990).

5.5. EPIDEMIOLOGIC APPROACHES TO THE STUDY OF THE ROLE OF SPECIFIC GENES IN DISEASE OCCURRENCE

This section addresses epidemiologic approaches to the study of genetic factors in diseases; study designs and analytic issues, as well as potential pitfalls and limitations are considered.

5.5.1. Strategies for Finding Disease-Susceptibility Genes

Given that most common diseases have complex etiologies and pathogenesis, it is important to address the role of specific genes in the occurrence of these diseases. The search for disease-susceptibility genes is conducted using two main methods: the association approach in which evidence is sought for a statistically significant association between an allele and a disease, and the linkage approach in which evidence is sought for cosegregation between a locus and a putative disease locus, using family studies. The incorporation of the linkage approach in epidemiologic studies is further discussed in Chapter 9.

In conducting association studies, two general types of methods can be distinguished: (1) the first is based on analysis of gene products or their direct phenotypic expression and their relationship to clinical and subclinical parameters of disease, and (2) the second is based on direct analysis of the DNA. Until recently, specific alleles at marker loci were measured exclusively by examining gene products. This method relied on the analysis of proteins, enzyme systems, antigens, and other biochemical measures. The 1960s and the 1970s witnessed a plethora of studies that sought to relate specific diseases to genetic polymorphisms, including blood groups (ABO, Rh, MNS, secretor, etc.), HLA systems, serum proteins, and polymorphic enzyme systems (Vogel and Motulsky, 1986). Although numerous "associations" had been described, many findings have not contributed to the understanding of the etiology and pathogenesis of the diseases studied. Because of problems and biases related to confounding, misclassification, and selection, as well as the lack of a biologic model to explain many of these associations (see section 5.5.4), this study design became less favored than the linkage approach where investigators use genetic markers in family studies to localize specific disease-susceptibility genes. While the linkage approach is even more popular with the increasing availability of DNA polymorphisms, there has been a resurgence of interest in studies of association between disease and DNA markers.

It is important to view studies of genetic marker–disease associations within the larger framework of epidemiologic studies of risk factor–disease associations. In epidemiologic studies, the tendency to do a "fishing expedition" for risk factors without prior biologic knowledge of disease has been criticized (Gordis, 1988). Similarly, in the context of genetic marker studies, it is important to address meaningful biologic hypotheses, with appreciation of the limitations of the study design and the inferences regarding the genetic marker of interest. Nevertheless, as indicated by Vogel and Motulsky (1986, p. 205, and Chapter 1), it is likely that the approach of relating specific genes to disease occurrence will become very useful in situations where "the genotype-phenotype relationships are so complex that a clear analysis from the phenotype down to the genes by Mendelian methods is barred, so that methods of quantitative genetics have to be relied upon. . . . This strategy will help in applying Mendelian approaches to situations where Galtonian techniques now are the only applicable methods."

Thus, an emerging strategy in the search for genetic factors in disease is the evaluation of "candidate genes" and their products that may play a role in disease pathogenesis. An example of such a single-gene system is the α_1-antitrypsin polymorphism that has been related to pulmonary emphysema. The presence of the *PiZ* allele in the homozygous state leads to a deficiency in α1-antitrypsin, a protein that has a protective function against protease-mediated destruction of lung tissue during inflammatory processes (Tockman et al., 1985; Kimbel, 1988). Thus, it appears that the pathogenesis of chronic obstructive pulmonary disease (COPD) associated with α_1 antitrypsin deficiency results from the lack of protection from proteases released as a result of bronchial irritation from infections, smoking, and other factors. This is an example of a genetic polymorphism analyzed at the gene product level, with the clinical consequences of gene action described in the context of epidemiologic studies. α_1-Antitrypsin deficiency could be considered an autosomal recessive disorder with incomplete penetrance for COPD, as not all *PiZ* homozygous individuals will develop COPD. However, with the recognition of multiple factors involved in the etiology and pathogenesis of COPD, as well as the rarity of *PiZ* homozygosity, it has become clear that the *PiZ* system can account for only a small fraction of COPD in the population (Tockman et al., 1985).

Another example of a genetic polymorphism that may play a role in the pathogenesis of disease is the cytochrome P-450 enzyme system, a supergene family involved in the oxidative metabolism of steroids, fatty acids, and prostaglandins, as well as innumerable drugs, environmental contaminants, chemical carcinogens, and mutagens (Gonzalez et al., 1986). Recent evidence has been accumulating regarding the role of these polymorphisms and their interaction with environmental factors, such as cigarette smoking and occupational exposures, in the genesis of certain cancers (Ayesh et al., 1984; Caporaso et al., 1989a). Other genetic polymorphisms involved in the metabolism of drugs and chemicals that have been described include the acetylator phenotype (Cartwright et al., 1982), alcohol dehydrogenase (Shibuya et al., 1989), and paraoxonase (Mueller et al., 1983). Genetic variation in these and other enzyme systems may play a role in genetic susceptibility to diseases associated with environmental exposures.

Another challenging area of interest for epidemiologic studies is the study of possible adverse health effects in heterozygotes for many of the rare autosomal recessive diseases, such as PKU, homocystinuria, and cystic fibrosis

(Vogel, 1984; Boers et al., 1985; Vogel and Motulsky, 1986; Lemma et al., 1990). While classical autosomal recessive disorders are individually quite rare in populations, heterozygotes for these disorders account for a substantial fraction of individuals in many populations. Many autosomal recessive diseases are associated with enzyme deficiencies in homozygotes and intermediate levels of these proteins are seen in heterozygotes. While intermediate levels of proteins and enzymes can adequately fulfill their intended functions most of the time, it is unclear whether such levels may be inadequate when the biologic system is stressed by exogenous or other endogenous factors. Vogel (1984) postulates that heterozygosity for autosomal recessive diseases could account for an appreciable fraction of what are apparently multifactorial diseases.

Table 5–7 summarizes the major characteristics, as well as the relative merits and limitations, of the gene product approach and the molecular approach in epidemiologic studies of disease. While DNA is universally available in all nucleated cells and thus is readily accessible for study, many enzymes and proteins are not always detectable in accessible tissues and fluids. For example, phenylalanine hydroxylase enzyme, which is deficient in PKU, is found only in the liver, as are most cytochrome P-450 enzymes. Instead of relying on direct measurement of gene products, investigators must use other indirect methods for genotype assignment. In the case of the acetylator phenotype, which is under the control of a single autosomal locus, Cartwright and coworkers (1982) used a dapsone loading test with subsequent measurement of the ratio of monoacetyldapsone/dapsone in plasma. This test was then used in a case-control study of bladder cancer. Another example is the debrisoquine metabolizing enzyme, a cytochrome P-450 enzyme involved in the metabolic oxidation of debrisoquine (and a variety of drugs and chemicals). This enzyme is under single-locus control at an autosomal locus. Individuals can be fast or poor metabolizers, depending on the presence or absence of several different coding mutations within this gene (Gonzalez et al., 1988; Skoda et al., 1988). To classify individuals into fast or poor metabolizers, investigators have thus far relied on a drug loading test with subsequent urine measurement of the metabolic ratio of debrisoquine to 4-hydroxydebrisoquine (Ayesh et al., 1984; Caporaso et al., 1989a). Different methods of analyses of the distribution of the metabolic ratio were shown to lead to different phenotypic and genotypic assignments (Caporaso et al., 1989b). Because fast metabolizers have been suggested to have an increased lung cancer risk (Ayesh et al., 1984; Caporaso et al., 1989a), genotype misclassification will affect estimates of relative risks associated with lung cancer (see section 5.5.4).

Likewise, the molecular approach may not always lead to a correct classification of the underlying susceptibility allele. Under ideal conditions, if the gene of interest has been completely sequenced, the presence and location of one or more mutations within the gene can be correlated with altered gene products to detect abnormal biologic function, and these may then be compared between affected and unaffected individuals in epidemiologic studies. If a mutation in a susceptibility allele involves the restriction site itself, the ensuing restriction fragment length polymorphism (RFLP) will be different

Table 5–7. Comparison of the characteristics of the gene products approach and the molecular approach in epidemiologic studies of genetic factors in disease

Characteristic	Gene products approach	Molecular approach
What is measured?	Proteins, enzymes	DNA
Relative accessibility to measurement	Less accessible, as only certain tissues and cells may express gene products	More accessible, as DNA is universally available in cells
Accuracy of measurement of underlying genotype	Subject to issues of metabolic pathways such as absorption, excretion, control from multiple gene loci, and inaccuracies of laboratory measurements	Some methods, such as restriction enzyme analysis, may not accurately measure underlying genotype unless RFLP is involved directly or is in linkage disequilibrium
Extent of polymorphism in populations	Less extensive	More extensive
Use in epidemiologic studies	Association between disease and marker (case-control/cohort)	Association between disease and marker (case-control/cohort)
Limitations		
Confounding	By unmeasured genetic factors	By unmeasured genetic factors
Misclassification	Due mainly to incorrect genotype assignment	Due mainly to linkage disequilibrium
Type I errors	Likely	More likely because of extensive polymorphisms
Biologic interactions	Nearer to functional effects of the gene and its interaction with other factors	Farther from functional effects of the gene and interaction with other factors

RFLP, restriction fragment length polymorphism.

between the normal and the susceptibility allele. For example, in sickle cell disease (Figure 5–1), a nucleotide substitution in the β-globin chain gene obliterates the recognition site of the enzyme MSt2 leading to a variation in the RFLP between normal and abnormal alleles (Beaudet et al., 1989). Thus, direct analysis of the RFLP pattern indicates the presence of the abnormal allele, that is, here the 1.15-kb segment indicates the normal allele, while the 1.30-kb segment indicates the sickle cell allele. However, it is important to keep in mind that this direct approach can thus far detect only mutations that lead to deletions, rearrangements, and point mutations affecting the restriction site itself (Gibbs and Caskey, 1989). The majority of point mutations, however, do not occur at recognition sites for restriction enzymes and thus cannot be detected using this approach. With improvements in recombinant

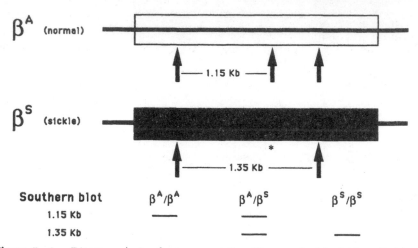

Figure 5–1. Direct analysis of a gene mutation illustrated with sickle cell disease.

DNA technology, other methods are being developed to detect all known mutations within sequenced genes. These methods include, for example, the use of synthetic oligonucleotide probes, and enzymatic amplification and direct genomic sequencing (Yandell and Dryja, 1989). Recent applications of these technologies have led to the detection of mutations in the cystic fibrosis gene (Lemma et al., 1990) and the retinoblastoma gene (Yandell et al., 1989).

Even though the actual sites of mutations that are involved in the disease process may not always be detectable with restriction enzyme analysis, RFLP patterns in the region of the gene can still be extremely useful in identifying putative susceptibility loci. Figure 5–2 shows a hypothetical example in which the site of the mutation for a disease-susceptibility gene is closely linked to a RFLP site for an anonymous DNA probe (see Chapter 9 for more details on linkage analysis). The 2-kb segment in this example cosegregates with the susceptibility mutation, with some fixed rate of recombination. In another family, perhaps the 1-kb segment will cosegregate with the susceptibility allele, however. Therefore, no association should be expected between the disease and the 2-kb segment (or the 1-kb segment) in general population studies. Instead, one should be able to demonstrate that multiply affected relatives within the same family are more likely to share the same RFLP segment (or haplotype) than expected, based on chance. Evidence for genetic linkage is thus accumulated, one family at a time; and results are pooled over several families to derive measures of recombination fraction. Sometimes, one may be able to find an association in population studies between a closely linked DNA marker and the disease. This can arise from "linkage disequilibrium" (Morton, 1984), and occurs if the mutation has arisen relatively recently, if there is a founder effect, or if there is selective advantage for specific haplotypes (Gibbs and Caskey, 1989). In general, there will be considerable linkage disequilibrium among markers in small regions of the chromosome, and various RFLP markers in the immediate region of a single locus can

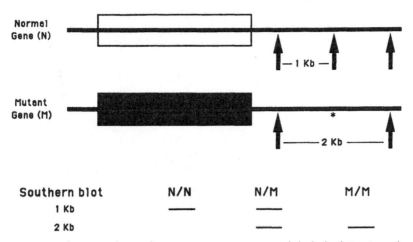

Figure 5–2. Indirect analysis of a gene mutation using tightly linked DNA markers.

constitute distinct haplotypes that are unique to given alleles. Such haplotypes can mark the distinct origin of certain mutant alleles. For example, the *PiZ* allele appears to have arisen as a single mutation on a specific haplotypic background (Cox et al., 1985), while the sickle cell mutation appears to have arisen several times independently (Hill and Wainscoat, 1986). Presently, most associations between RFLPs and diseases should be viewed in the context of linkage disequilibrium rather than interpreted as direct cause-effect relationships. As discussed by several authors (Ferns et al, 1986; Cooper and Clayton, 1988), RFLPs are simply DNA markers for the actual alleles involved in disease etiology; and any association between DNA markers and diseases should be complemented with family studies that seek to demonstrate genetic linkage between these markers and disease-susceptibility loci.

One example of using DNA markers in epidemiologic studies is the case-control study of Ardinger and coworkers (1989) in which an association was seen between two RFLPs at the transforming growth factor α locus (TGFA) and the occurrence of cleft lip and palate. TGFA and four other candidate loci were investigated using one or more RFLPs because of their suspected role in palate formation in rodents. The biologic basis of this association remains to be explained, but it offers possibilities for further analyses of the TGFA gene activity in affected and unaffected individuals, as well as family studies to look for evidence of possible linkage. Linkage disequilibrium is not unique to DNA markers and has been observed in associations detected at the level of the gene product. Many of the associations between specific HLA alleles and various diseases may be due to linkage disequilibrium among alleles in the HLA region. One example is that of hemochromatosis, an autosomal recessive condition whose locus is linked to the HLA region. The disease itself is also associated with certain HLA alleles because of linkage disequilibrium (Lin et al., 1985). The effect of linkage disequilibrium on detecting associations is further discussed in section 5.5.4.

5.5.2. Study Design

Study designs for examining associations include cohort, cross-sectional, and case-control approaches. A review of these types is provided in Chapter 3. General applications of these approaches are discussed here, using examples from the literature.

The basic goal for all these studies is to examine the relationship between disease occurrence and the gene(s) of interest. This is shown in Table 5–8. For simplicity, it is assumed that the susceptibility gene has two alleles: N, the normal allele, and S, the disease-susceptibility allele. As shown in Table 5–7, investigators can use either gene products or DNA markers to classify individuals into genotypes of interest (i.e., NN, NS, and SS). In a cohort approach, individuals with various genotypes are thus followed for disease or other relevant biologic endpoints. Some measure of disease risk (e.g., disease incidence or cumulative incidence) is compared among the three groups, and measures of relative risks comparing NS and SS individuals with a baseline risk (for NN). In a cross-sectional study, the prevalence of one or more clinical outcomes is measured at the same time as the genetic markers are.

Sometimes both cross-sectional and longitudinal components can be used in the same study. For example, in the investigation of chronic obstructive pulmonary disease conducted by Cohen (1980), a cross-sectional evaluation included examining the relationship of simple genetic systems (i.e., α_1-antitrypsin deficiency genotypes, ABO blood groups, ABH secretor status, and PTC taster ability) to the prevalence of pulmonary function abnormalities as measured by spirometry. A longitudinal follow-up component was then added to this study, in which deterioration in pulmonary function and mortality were examined over a five-year period (Beaty et al., 1982; Menkes et al., 1984). Here, the measures of cumulative risks of these outcomes were examined in relation to the genetic markers of interest. Both in the cross-sectional and longitudinal components of this study other familial and environmental risk factors were considered in the analysis (Cohen, 1980; Menkes et al., 1984).

In a case-control study, the frequency of the different genotypes is compared between individuals who have the outcome of interest (cases) and a sample of individuals who do not (controls). Measures of odds ratios shown in Table 5–8 closely approximate those of relative risks for a cohort study for when the disease is rare (Lilienfeld and Lilienfeld, 1980; Rothman 1986).

Table 5–8. Cohort and case-control approaches to examine the relationship of disease with specific genetic traits

Genotype	Cohort study		Case-control study		
	Disease risk	Relative risk	Frequency in cases	Frequency in controls	Odds ratio
NN	I_1	1	A_1	B_1	1
NS	I_2	I_2/I_1	A_2	B_2	A_2B_1/A_1B_2
SS	I_3	I_3/I_1	A_3	B_3	A_3B_1/A_1B_3

Simple gene system with two alleles; N, normal allele; S, susceptibility allele.

Case-control studies also provide a practical approach for evaluating several genetic factors at once and are generally less expensive than cohort studies. In designing case-control studies, however, it is important to consider several issues that can lead to potential biases, as discussed elsewhere (Schlesselman, 1982; Kelsey et al., 1986; Rothman, 1986).

First, controls should be chosen to represent the population from which the case group was derived. Much has been said about population-based case-control studies where cases are chosen to include all affected individuals with a disease in a particular population. In such situations, controls must then be a representative sample of nondiseased individuals in the same population. Such studies permit direct inferences regarding the determinants of disease in that population. Such population-based studies, however, are often expensive and difficult to implement. Valid case-control studies can be mounted, using cases from one or a few hospitals or clinics, provided that controls for these kinds of studies are chosen carefully to reflect the population from which cases were derived (Rothman, 1986). Frequently, however, controls are chosen from convenient samples of individuals that are available to the investigators and on whom blood samples have been drawn. When the sampling frame for controls is ill defined, investigators may introduce selection and confounding biases that interfere with the results of the study (Chapter 3). In a hypothetical case-control study of the association between a certain birth defect and several candidate genes, suppose that cases were patients recruited from a medical genetics clinic at a university hospital. On the other hand, suppose that control subjects are chosen as a convenient sample of individuals (such as hospital workers) on whom blood samples were available. The investigators proceed to examine differences in cases and controls with respect to DNA haplotypes for several candidate genes. Clearly, the sampling frame for controls in this hypothetical study is ill-defined both in time and space. Controls may not be ethnically similar to the population from which cases were derived. Differences in the distribution of DNA haplotypes between cases and controls could be due to population stratification (i.e., confounding) with respect to the genes of interest and possible effects of the genes on survival rather than the etiology of the condition.

Second, it is preferable to chose incident rather than prevalent cases for a case-control study. Incident cases are new cases with recent onset that come to the attention of investigators. For example, in the hypothetical study referred to above, cases could be a mixture of new and old cases. This mixing should not lead to a bias in the results, provided that the duration of illness is not related to the exposures (here the genes) of interest. This may not always be true, however, if polymorphic genetic systems are related to morbidity from other conditions that can alter the clinical course and/or survival of affected individuals. Prevalent cases represent a subset of incident cases that have survived long enough to be in the study, and thus could be different from the original case group with respect to the risk factors of interest as well as the type and natural history of the disorder.

Third, in designing and analyzing case-control studies, it is important to consider factors that could potentially act as confounders, other than the genetic traits of interest. A simple example of a confounder is race/ethnic group. Because the frequencies of many polymorphic genetic markers differ among various racial and ethnic groups, as does overall disease occurrence, race/ethnicity can act as a potential confounding variable if it is not considered in the design and the analysis of the study. In situations where the case group may come from a racially mixed population, one might consider a control group that is matched to the case group by a race/ethnic group, and perform all analyses stratified by the race/ethnic group. Matching can be done individually or for groups (i.e., frequency matching). An example of individual matching would be a case-control study of a birth defect where cases are ascertained in the newborn period from numerous hospitals scattered over a large geographic area. For each case, one or more controls could be chosen from subsequent births in the same hospital with the control infant of the same race as the case. This design provides individual matching by hospital of birth, time of birth, and race. An example of frequency matching is provided by the large case-control study of birth defects conducted by the Centers for Disease Control in the early 1980s to assess whether men who served in Vietnam have an increased risk of fathering babies with birth defects (Erickson et al., 1984). In this study, cases were ascertained from a population-based registry for birth defects, comprising babies born between 1968 and 1980 with serious birth defects diagnosed in the first year of life. Controls constituted a 1% random sample of all births in this same population during the same period. Because this study extended over a relatively long period of time, investigators sought to assure comparability between cases and controls with respect to tracing and interviewing parents, as well as the quality of information obtained regarding risk factors. A frequency-matched design was adopted. The design variables were hospital of birth, race, and time of birth, resulting in 120 strata corresponding to all combinations of these variables. Controls were chosen to ensure that their distribution across these strata matched that of cases.

Another method for matching is the use of relative controls, which ensures homogeneity between cases and controls with respect to ethnic background. Although cases and controls drawn from the same family have a tendency to share common familial environmental factors as well as genes, Goldstein and colleagues (1990) have shown that selection of controls from relatives of cases does not per se introduce bias in the estimate of effects (odds ratios) unless the risks of exposure-specific disease change over time. This finding held whether exposure was defined as a specific genetic trait or an environmental factor that may cluster in families.

Fourth and finally, in designing studies of genetic factors in disease, it is important to consider environmental risk factors that have been previously implicated in pathogenesis or where there is reason to suspect a biologic interaction with the genetic factor of interest. For example, in the COPD study referred to earlier (Cohen, 1980), information was collected not only on the genetic markers of interest (e.g., α_1-antitrypsin phenotypes and others), but also on cigarette smoking and other factors. Cigarette smoking is the most important risk factor for COPD described to date. Thus, in such a study, the objective of the investigators is not only to adjust for the effects of smoking as a potential confounder, but to study whether the effects of smoking on pulmonary function differ among individuals who carry various genetic traits of interest. In other words, the effects of the presence of a genetic trait on the disease outcomes may be modified by exposure to cigarette smoking (Khoury et al., 1986). In studying the association between oral clefts and candidate genes, for example, it is important to collect data on other risk factors for clefts that could interact with the candidate genes examined. One such factor is maternal cigarette smoking. Some studies have suggested an excess risk of oral clefts in offspring of women who smoked during pregnancy (Ericson et al., 1979; Khoury et al., 1989b). Thus, it is possible that smoking might interact with genetically susceptible hosts (e.g., persons with polymorphisms in transforming growth factor genes, or a cytochrome P-450 gene) in causing clefts in a subgroup of exposed fetuses. Various aspects of interaction are discussed further in section 5.5.3.

5.5.3. Analytic Issues

This section deals with issues related to the analysis of epidemiologic studies of genetic trait-disease associations.

Measures of Association

Referring to Table 5–8, the goal for the analysis is to compare disease frequency among individuals with different genotypes. In a cohort study, the measures of frequency are incidence rate and cumulative incidence, while prevalence is used in a cross-sectional study. In a case-control study, the measures of interest are the frequency of the different genotypes in cases versus controls. Such comparisons lead to measures of absolute risks, relative risks (or odds ratios), and attributable fraction (Woolf, 1955; Green, 1982a, 1982b; Payami et al., 1989). For case-control studies, however, absolute risks can be inferred only indirectly from knowledge of disease frequency in the population. In the event that the susceptibility allele increases risk only in homozygotes (i.e., susceptibility acts as an autosomal recessive), the risk of disease in persons with the SS genotype will be increased over that of persons with either NN or NS genotypes. When the susceptibility allele acts as a dominant trait, persons with either the NS or SS genotypes have an equally increased risk over those with the NN genotype. In the absence of complete dominance or recessivity, the risk of disease in persons with the NS genotype may be intermediate between disease risks of NN and SS individuals, respectively. For rare diseases with NN persons as a reference group, the magnitude of the relative risks in Table 5–8 should be almost identical to the corresponding odds ratios.

By computing the magnitude of absolute, relative, and attributable risks, the expected impact of various types of single-gene models for susceptibility can be quantitated (Table 5–9). For a purely Mendelian disease with full penetrance and no heterogeneity (where carrying the susceptibility allele is both necessary and sufficient for the disease), the risk of disease in people

Table 5–9. Quantitative evaluation of a disease susceptibility genotype in terms of absolute, relative risks, and attributable fraction

Type	Disease risk		Relative risk	Attributable fraction
	With genotype	Without genotype		
Genotype with complete penetrance for disease and no heterogeneity	1	0	∞	1
Genotype with incomplete penetrance and no heterogeneity	$P(D|G_1)$	0	∞	1
Genotype with complete penetrance for disease and heterogeneity	1	$P(D|G_0)$	$1/P(D|G_0)$	AF
Genotype with incomplete penetrance and heterogeneity	$P(D|G_1)$	$P(D|G_0)$	R	AF

$P(D|G_1)$ = disease risk in persons with the genotype (penetrance).
$P(D|G_0)$ = disease risk in persons without the genotype.

Relative risk: $R = \dfrac{P(D|G_1)}{P(D|G_0)}$

$P(G_1)$ = frequency of the susceptible genotype in the population.

Attributable fraction: $AF = \dfrac{P(G_1)(R - 1)}{1 + P(G_1)(R - 1)}$

with the susceptible genotype is 1; the risk of disease in people without the genotype is 0; the relative risk is infinity; and the attributable fraction is 1. Even for single-gene diseases with incomplete penetrance but no etiologic heterogeneity (i.e., the susceptibility allele is necessary but not sufficient), relative risk is infinity and the attributable fraction is 1. At the other end of the spectrum are disease-susceptibility genotypes that are neither necessary nor sufficient for the development of disease, for which various measures of risk can be estimated in epidemiologic studies. These calculations assume that the association between the genotype in question and the disease is causal. Such associations might also occur due to confounding, selection bias, linkage disequilibrium, or could be totally spurious (see section 5.5.4).

It is important to attempt to estimate all of these measures in any epidemiologic study. Each gives a slightly different type of information regarding the role of the susceptibility gene. To illustrate, refer to the examples of genetic trait-disease associations listed in Table 5–10. Consider the association between α_1-antitrypsin deficiency and COPD. By relative risk standards, this is a strong association (relative risk of 20). Also, by absolute risk standards, it is also a very strong association. The vast majority (>90%) of individuals with the genetic trait eventually develop COPD. However, from an attributable fraction perspective, α_1-antitrypsin accounts for very little of COPD in the population (<1%). Any prevention or intervention effort to reduce COPD by targeting this high-risk group alone will have little impact on the

Table 5-10. Illustration of various measures of association between diseases and single-gene traits

	Ankylosing spondylitis	Chronic obstructive pulmonary disease	Bladder cancer
Disease risk	0.002	0.05	0.019
Allele	*HLA-B27*	*PiZ*	Slow acetylator
Allele frequency	0.036	0.02	0.75
Genotype associated with disease risk	Homozygous and heterozygous	Homozygous *PiZ*	Homozygous slow acetylator
Relative risk	100	20	1.6
Attributable fraction %	88	0.8	25
Absolute risk (penetrance %)	2.5	99	2.3

Adapted from Khoury and Flanders (1989).

risk of COPD in the general population, largely due to the etiologic heterogeneity of this group of conditions (Tockman et al., 1985). Similarly, the relationship between familial hypercholesterolemia and coronary artery disease, while causal with a high relative risk among carriers of the *FH* allele, accounts for very little of the total burden of the common disease (Moll, 1984). On the other hand, if one considers the association between the *HLA-B27* allele and ankylosing spondylitis, another observation emerges. Here, not only is the association strong in terms of relative risk (about 100), it seems that the vast majority of cases in the population may be attributable to the *B27* allele (about 90%). However, when one examines the association from an absolute risk perspective, it is apparent that only a small fraction of individuals with the *B27* allele will contract the disease during their lifetime. This suggests the presence of other susceptibility cofactors that are needed to produce disease. Other genetic and infectious agents (such as *Klebsiella*) have been suggested as possible interacting cofactors (Ahearn and Hochberg, 1988).

These examples illustrate rather extreme situations. For many risk factor–disease associations reported in the literature, relative risks may be even smaller (e.g., the acetylator phenotype in bladder cancer with an estimated relative risk of 1.5 as shown in Table 5–10). Absolute risks are also not elevated, and attributable fractions may be low. These observations point to the extreme etiologic heterogeneity in common diseases and the biologic interaction among numerous factors that contribute to the development of disease.

Interaction

In addition to assessing the role of a specific susceptibility allele in a disease using epidemiologic methods, it is important to consider in the analysis the possible impact of other genetic and environmental factors that could interact with the gene in question. Although the concept of genetic-environmental interaction is central to ecogenetics (Brewer, 1971; Omenn and Motulsky, 1978; Motulsky, 1978; Calabrese, 1984; Mulvihill, 1984) and has long been recognized by geneticists (Haldane, 1946), studies in this area have examined primarily the relationship between genetically determined enzyme systems and disease without considering environmental determinants (e.g., Ayesh et al., 1984; Barbeau et al., 1985). An epidemiologic framework can be useful in evaluating genetic-environmental interactions in the context of ecogenetic studies (Khoury et al., 1988a; Ottman, 1990). The failure to consider environmental components of the disease, in addition to the measurement of the susceptibility genotype, may lead to erroneous inferences concerning the role of genes in disease etiology.

In Table 5–11, a simple genotype-environment interaction model is examined in the context of both cohort and case-control designs. Both the susceptibility genotype at a single locus and the environmental exposure are considered dichotomous (either present or absent). This model, of course, is simplistic because it considers only a single-gene locus and a single environmental factor without regard to dose of exposure. Nevertheless, it helps to illustrate the complexities of interpreting associations between alleles and diseases, especially when the magnitude of the association is relatively modest (e.g., relative risk < 2). As shown in Table 5–11, it is assumed that, among unexposed individuals without the susceptible genotype, there exists a certain background risk of disease, I, reflecting etiologic heterogeneity. Exposed individuals without the genotype have a disease risk IR_e (where R_e refers to the relative risk of disease for the exposure in the absence of the susceptibility genotype, i.e., the risk due to the environmental factor in nonsusceptible genotypes). If $R_e = 1$, then the exposure is not a risk factor in the absence of the genotype, whereas if $R_e > 1$, then exposure exerts an effect even among individuals without the genotype (i.e., it has a deleterious effect not specific to individuals with the susceptible genotype). Also, unexposed individuals with the genotype have a disease risk IR_g (where R_g refers to the relative risk associated with the susceptibility in the absence of the environmental exposure). If $R_g = 1$, then the genotype requires an environmental trigger to increase disease risk. If $R_g > 1$, then the genotype alone produces excess risk through some mechanism independent of the environmental exposure. If $R_g < 1$, then, in the absence of the specific environment exposure, the genotype is protective against the disease. Individuals with both the genotype and exposure have a disease risk IR_{ge} (where R_{ge} is the ratio of disease risk in exposed individuals with the susceptibility genotype to disease risk in unexposed people without the genotype; this reflects the strength of interaction). R_g, R_e, and R_{ge} are relative risks estimated in case-control studies from the corresponding odds ratios as shown in Table 5–11. In studies of genotype-disease associations in which environmental effects are not considered, only the marginal genotypic effects can be estimated. The observed relative risk of disease R for individuals with the susceptible genotype, compared to those

Table 5–11. A simple genotype-environment interaction model in the context of epidemiologic studies

Genotype-environment	Cohort study		Case-control study		
	Disease risk	Relative risk	Frequency in cases	Frequency in controls	Odds ratio
$-,-$	I	1	A_1	B_1	1
$-,+$	IR_e	R_e	A_2	B_2	A_2B_1/A_1B_2
$+,-$	IR_g	R_g	A_3	B_3	A_3B_1/A_1B_3
$+,+$	IR_{ge}	R_{ge}	A_4	B_4	A_4B_1/A_1B_4

From Khoury et al. (1988a).

without it, can be written as a function of R_g, R_e, R_{ge}, and P_e (population exposure frequency to the environmental factor),

$$R = \frac{(1 - P_e)R_g + P_eR_{ge}}{(1 - P_e) + P_eR_e} \tag{5-3}$$

The relative risk of disease for the susceptibility genotype can also be estimated using odds ratio estimates of R_g, R_e, and R_{ge} obtained from the case-control design (Table 5–11). The relationship among R_{ge}, R_g, and R_e depends on the particular pattern of interaction between the susceptibility genotype and the exposure. In epidemiologic studies, two commonly considered statistical models are the additive model where $R_{ge} = R_g + R_e - 1$ and the multiplicative model where $R_{ge} = R_g \times R_e$ (Kahn, 1983). However, a biologic model of interaction might differ from these simple forms of interaction.

The effects of six biologically plausible patterns of genotype-environment interaction on the relative risk of the genotype R are summarized in Table 5–12, and Figure 5–3. In each situation, it is assumed that the combination of the genotype and the exposure is deleterious ($R_{ge} > 1$), the exposure alone increases risk ($R_e > 1$), but the genotype may be associated with either increased or decreased risk ($R_g < 1$, or $R_g > 1$).

In the *first pattern of interaction*, neither the genotype alone nor the exposure alone causes excess risk (i.e., $R_g = 1$, $R_e = 1$). Two examples can be given. One example is that of a very rare environmental exposure, succinylcholine administration during anesthesia, and its interaction with pseudocholinesterase deficiency in producing postoperative apnea (Evans, 1983). Another example involves a universal environmental exposure such as phenylalanine in the diet and its interaction with phenylalanine hydroxylase deficiency responsible for phenylketonuria (PKU) and its accompanying mental retardation. In both examples, neither exposure alone nor genotype alone produces excess risk, but only the combination results in increased risk of disease. Under this type of interaction, the relative risk associated with the genotype (R) as measured in the population tends to increase with increasing strength of interaction (R_{ge}) and frequency of exposure to the environmental

Table 5–12. Some patterns of genotype-environment interaction that could be observed in epidemiologic studies

Patterns	Effect on disease risk of	
	Genotype in absence of environment	Environment in absence of genotype
1	No effect $R_g = 1$	No effect $R_e = 1$
2	No effect $R_g = 1$	Increases risk $R_e > 1$
3	Increases risk $R_g > 1$	No effect $R_e = 1$
4	Increases risk $R_g > 1$	Increases risk $R_e > 1$
5	Decreases risk $R_g < 1$	No effect $R_e = 1$
6	Decreases risk $R_g < 1$	Increases risk $R_e > 1$

component (f) (Table 5–13). With infrequent exposures ($<1\%$ of the population), however, the relative risk associated with the genetic factor is close to unity, implying no measurable genotypic effect. Even in the face of strong interaction ($R_{ge} = 100$), the relative risk is still less than 2. Thus, a low relative risk for the genotype does not negate the importance of the genotype in the etiology of the disease, if there is interaction with an environmental trigger and if the exposure frequency is low. Alternatively, high relative risks imply either a frequent environmental exposure, strong genotype-environment interaction, or both. Under this scheme, it would be easy to detect PKU as a risk factor for mental retardation in the general population because of the universality of the environmental trigger (i.e., normal diet).

A *second pattern of interaction* (Table 5–12) is that of a relatively innocuous genotype in the absence of the specific exposure ($R_g = 1$), but an environmental exposure that increases risk in individuals without the corre-

Table 5–13. Relative risks associated with a susceptibility genotype in type 1 interaction, by exposure frequency and the magnitude of interaction R_{ge}

Exposure frequency	R_{ge}		
	5	10	100
0.001	1.004	1.009	1.099
0.01	1.04	1.09	1.99
0.10	1.40	1.90	10.9
0.50	3.0	5.5	50.5
1.0	5.0	10.0	100.0

From Khoury et al. (1988a).

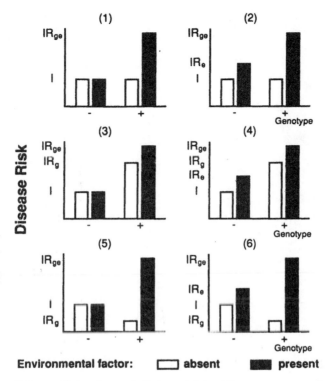

Figure 5–3.   Patterns of genotype-environment interaction.

sponding genotype ($R_e > 1$). An example of this type of interaction might
be xeroderma pigmentosa (XP), exposure to ultraviolet light, and the production of skin cancer (Mulvihill, 1984). In this case, $R_g = 1$ because the
genotype requires an environmental trigger (i.e., sun exposure) but actually
$R_e > 1$ because sunlight is a more general risk factor for skin cancer among
individuals without XP (Frank and Slesis, 1986). As shown in Table 5–14,
under a type 2 interaction, where the environmental effect is seen for all
genotypes (i.e., $R_e > 1$), the relative risk R associated with the genotype will
decline with increasing strength of the environmental effect (R_e), at any given
exposure frequency. The impact of R_e is larger at higher exposure frequencies.
This effect can be intuitively understood by noting that the probability of
disease among individuals without the genotype will be inflated by an excess
risk due to the exposure to the environmental factor in a fraction of all
individuals. Thus, the nonspecificity of the environmental effect vis-à-vis the
susceptible genotype will tend to dilute the measured effect of the susceptibility genotype in the general population.

In the *third pattern of interaction*, the genotype alone is associated with
excess disease risk, whereas the exposure alone is not ($R_g > 1$, $R_e = 1$). An
example of this type of interaction may be glucose-6-phosphate dehydrogenase (G6PD) deficiency and fava beans (Table 5–15). In this example, eating
fava beans alone does not produce hemolytic anemia, whereas G6PD defi-

Table 5–14. Relative risks associated with genotype in type 2 interaction, by exposure frequency and R_e

Exposure frequency	R_e		
	2	5	10
0.001	1.098	1.095	1.089
0.01	1.97	1.91	1.83
0.10	9.91	7.79	5.74
0.50	33.7	16.8	9.1
1.0	50.0	20.0	10.0

Assumption: $R_{ge} = 100$.
From Khoury et al. (1988a).

ciency alone without ingestion of fava beans can lead to hemolytic anemia if there is exposure to certain antimalarial drugs (Evans, 1983).

In the *fourth pattern of interaction*, both the genotype and the environment are each associated with excess risk of disease ($R_g > 1$, $R_e > 1$). An appropriate example here is α_1-antitrypsin deficiency and cigarette smoking, which both contribute to risk of emphysema. Individuals with the PiZ phenotype have a very high risk of emphysema even if they do not smoke ($R_g > 1$), and smokers have a high risk of emphysema even if they do not have the deficiency gene ($R_e > 1$). When the genotype confers excess disease risk in the absence of the environmental component ($R_g > 1$), the net effect is to increase the measured effect of the genotype in the population R at any given R_{ge}, R_e, and f. Thus, if the genotype confers excess risk of disease regardless of the environmental exposure, a genotypic effect is easier to detect in the population, especially with increasing levels of R_g. Type 4 interaction is a combination of types 2 and 3 interactions.

The *fifth and sixth patterns of interaction*, listed in Table 5–12, occur when there is a reversal of the genotype's effect, depending on the presence or absence of the environment. In this case, the genotype is protective in the absence of the environment ($R_g < 1$), but is deleterious in the presence of the environment ($R_{ge} > 1$). Although no clear-cut examples in human genetics

Table 5–15. Relative risks associated with genotype in type 3 interaction, by exposure frequency and R_g

Exposure frequency	R_g		
	2	5	10
0.001	2.098	5.095	10.09
0.01	2.98	5.95	10.9
0.10	11.8	14.5	19.0
0.50	51.0	52.5	55.0
1.0	100.0	100.0	100.0

Assumption: $R_{ge} = 100$.
From Khoury et al. (1988a).

can be cited, a related example is that of the sickle cell trait and its selective advantage in malarial environments, but its possible disadvantage in the absence of falciparum malaria (Calabrese, 1984). These types of interactions are included to illustrate that, under this reversal of a genotypic effect in different environments, the failure to consider environmental components will lead to serious errors in assessing the role of the genotype in disease etiology. As shown in Table 5–16, measured values of R can vary from less than unity (protective effect) to more than unity (risk factor effect) depending on values of P_e and R_g. At a given exposure frequency, the more protective the genotypic effect (R_g), the lower the measured R in the population. On the other hand, at a given R_g effect, the higher the exposure frequency, the higher the measured R in the population. Thus, in this situation, if the environmental component is neglected, some studies might find a protective effect of the genotype, while others will find a detrimental effect, and confusion will ensue.

The effects of genetic-environmental interactions on the measured phenotype are further complicated by the number of genetic loci involved, the nonadditivity of the genetic effects (Ward, 1985), the dose of the environmental exposure, and the presence of etiologic heterogeneity (Sing et al., 1985). Nevertheless, numerous studies have examined the relationship between genetic traits and disease entities without considering environmental factors. Examples range from HLA studies to studies of specific enzyme systems. As shown in these illustrations, because of the pattern of interaction, the frequency of exposure to the environmental component (that can vary among different populations), and the strength of interaction, the importance of the genotype in disease etiology may not be appropriately assessed. This problem can be illustrated using the example of bladder cancer and the slow acetylator phenotype (Table 5–10). In this study, Cartwright and colleagues (1982) found a modest relative risk of 1.6 by comparing all cases and controls. However, when this association was examined among workers possibly exposed to aryl nitrite compounds, the magnitude of the relative risk became much stronger (about 17), suggesting a biologic interaction between the carcinogen and the acetylation pathway. In general, a stratified analysis for

Table 5–16. Relative risks associated with genotype in type 5 interaction, by exposure frequency and R_g

Exposure frequency	R_g		
	1/2	1/5	1/10
0.001	0.60	0.30	0.20
0.01	1.50	1.20	1.10
0.10	10.4	10.2	10.1
0.50	50.2	50.1	50.0
1.0	100.0	100.0	100.0

Assumption: $R_{ge} = 100$.
From Khoury et al. (1988a).

disease risk (odds ratio) to estimate values of R_e, R_g, and R_{ge}, as shown in Table 5-11, could potentially clarify whether an interaction exists between a genotype and an environmental factor, as well as the type of interaction. However, sample size limitations often become severe in such stratified analyses. Adjustment for potential confounding variables can be achieved either by study design (such as matching) or via appropriate statistical procedures (such as the Mantel-Haenzel procedure for stratified analyses or by multivariate analysis [Kahn and Sempos, 1989]). In addition, case-control designs allow evaluation of duration and multiple levels of the environmental exposure and its interaction with the genotype (dose-response effects), and permit several genes to be considered as well.

Finally, the contribution of genotype-environment interaction to disease risk can also be measured in terms of attributable fraction. As indicated by several authors (Walker, 1981; Rothman, 1986), one can estimate the proportion of disease due to the interaction of any two factors. In the examples above such a proportion would be

$$AF_{ge} = \frac{p_{ge} \times (R_{ge} - R_e - R_g + 1)}{R_{ge}}, \tag{5-4}$$

where p_{ge} is the proportion of all cases with both the genotype and the environmental factor. In type 1 interaction, for example, because R_g and R_e are equal to 1, this quantity reduces to

$$AF_{ge} = \frac{p_{ge} \times (R_{ge} - 1)}{R_{ge}} \tag{5-5}$$

which is the familiar Miettinen's formula discussed earlier (see Table 3-10). In this situation, one can show that the attributable fraction of disease due to the interaction is equal to the attributable fraction from the genotype AF_g (without regard to the environmental factor) because all the genotypic effect is due to interaction with the environmental factor, that is,

$$AF_g = \frac{p_g \times (R - 1)}{R}. \tag{5-6}$$

5.5.4. Pitfalls and Limitations

This section reviews some potential pitfalls and limitations in inferring causality from studies of associations between disease and genetic traits. These problems are common to epidemiologic studies in general.

Confounding

The demonstration of a statistical association between an allele and a disease does not mean that such an association is causal in nature. Unmeasured confounders associated with both the disease outcome and the genetic trait create spurious associations or mask true underlying biologic relationships. In the more general epidemiologic setting, confounders are usually thought of in terms of other risk factors. For example, if one wanted to study the risk of Down syndrome in the offspring of older fathers, it is important to consider maternal age, as advanced maternal age is associated both with advanced paternal age and the risk of Down syndrome (see Chapter 4). In genetic studies, however, unmeasured confounders can be either genetic or environmental factors that are likely to produce differences in allele frequencies. Racial, ethnic, and other reasons for population stratification are major sources of confounding with genetic factors.

To illustrate, Table 5–17 presents a hypothetical example of a disease that manifests racial variation in risk, where the disease risk is 5% in whites and 1% in blacks. In this example, the alleles at the marker locus are also associated with race, with whites having a higher frequency of the allele compared with blacks (50% versus 20%). In a total sample composed of a mixture of whites and blacks, the risk of disease appears to be elevated among individuals with the marker allele compared with individuals without the allele (4.3% versus 2.4%). However, when the analysis is stratified by race, it can be seen that there is no association between the allele and the disease within each group.

While this is a relatively straightforward example of confounding that can be corrected for by simple stratification of the data, confounding by race, ethnic groups or other population subgroups can be quite subtle. Because there is variation in the frequency of many genetic traits within population groups, it becomes even more important to have groups that are as homogeneous as possible, and this must be considered in the design and analysis phase. For example, as discussed earlier, racial groups may be genetically heterogeneous because they have different genetic histories. These genetic differences may not be as marked due to recent admixture. One example of confounding is the study of Knowler and associates (1988) regarding the prevalence of diabetes in the Pima Indians and its relation to the Gm 3;5,13,14 haplotype over different categories of genetic admixture (see Tables 5–2 and 5–3). In this study the absence of this particular Gm haplotype was associated with a higher prevalence of diabetes (29% versus 8% in Table 5–3); however,

Table 5–17. A hypothetical example of a disease-allele association confounded by race

Race	Presence of allele	No. of persons	No. affected	% Affected
White	Yes	500	25	5.0
	No	500	25	5.0
	All	1000	50	5.0
Black	Yes	100	1	1.0
	No	900	9	1.0
	All	1000	10	1.0
Total sample	Yes	600	26	4.3
	No	1400	34	2.4
	All	2000	60	3.0

this particular Gm haplotype turned out to be an index for white admixture. When the analysis was stratified according to an index of admixture (Table 5–2), no association was found between diabetes and the Gm haplotype within each category, indicating that this polymorphic trait is merely a nonspecific genetic marker and likely does not play a true biologic role in the pathogenesis of the disease. Thus, it is important to minimize confounding in the design of studies: whenever possible, comparison groups should be drawn from the same population, and stratified by subpopulation.

Misclassification

The effects of differential and nondifferential misclassification on the measurement of associations between risk factors and genetic traits are discussed in Chapter 4. Whenever indirect methods of genotype assignment are used (e.g., identifying carriers based on loading tests), a certain amount of genotype misclassification must be expected. If such misclassification is nondifferential (i.e., not different between cases and controls), the estimated association between disease and a measured genotype is likely to underestimate the magnitude of the true underlying association. However, if genotype assignment is differential (i.e., the accuracy varies between cases and controls) spurious associations could result. Differential misclassification might occur, for example, whenever the test gives different results for cases and controls. In the example of debrisoquine metabolic phenotypes and lung cancer, this could occur if individuals with lung cancer have an altered metabolism and handle the drug differently than from nondisease controls. Given the current knowledge of metabolism of debrisoquine, this does not seem to be a problem.

When dealing with polymorphic alleles that are part of a complex of closely linked loci (e.g., the HLA complex or the more general situation of several RFLPs around candidate genes), genotype misclassification can occur because of linkage disequilibrium. Whenever the measured marker allele is closely linked to the true susceptibility allele and is in disequilibrium with it, one can consider that the marker allele can serve as a proxy for the underlying susceptibility allele. As shown in Table 5–18, the relationship between the marker allele and the susceptibility allele can be characterized quantitatively in terms

Table 5–18. Relationship between a susceptibility allele and a closely linked marker allele

Marker allele	Susceptibility allele		
	Present	Absent	Total
Present	a	b	$a + b$
Absent	c	d	$c + d$
Total	$a + c$	$b + d$	$a + b + c + d$

Sensitivity of the marker allele: $a/a + c$.
Specificity of the marker allele: $d/b + d$.
Under Hardy-Weinberg equilibrium odds ratio: $ad/bc = 1$.
Under linkage disequilibrium: $ad/bc > 1$.

of sensitivity, specificity, and odds ratio. When there is no disequilibrium between the two loci (i.e., the two loci are in Hardy-Weinberg equilibrium in the population), the odds ratio is essentially unity. This implies that no association will be found between the marker allele and the disease in any epidemiologic study. Whenever there is complete linkage (i.e., no recombination), the presence of the marker allele is always associated with the susceptibility allele (odds ratio of infinity), and, therefore, there will be no genotype misclassification. In the more general case of linkage disequilibrium, the marker allele and the disease susceptibility allele will be associated (odds ratio > 1). This results in a misclassification of the underlying susceptibility allele if the marker allele is used to classify individuals instead. An indirect association between the marker allele and the disease will occur. Whenever there is a nondifferential misclassification problem, the odds ratio between a marker allele and the disease is likely to underestimate the true odds ratio relating disease to the unmeasured susceptibility allele. For example, in the study of Ardinger and colleagues (1989), using RFLPs around the TFGA locus and cleft lip and palate (CLP), the association between CLP and the 3.0-kbp RFLP obtained, using TaqI restriction enzyme analysis (shown in Table 5–19 as the $C2$ allele), is likely due to a misclassification within the area of the $TGFA$ gene due to linkage disequilibrium between this RFLP and the putative susceptibility locus. Thus, the magnitude of the odds ratios and attributable fractions found in that study may underestimate the true biologic role of the $TGFA$ gene locus in cleft lip and palate. One approach to address the issue of linkage disequilibrium is to look for evidence of association between the disease and a specific haplotype composed of alleles at tightly linked loci within the area of the candidate gene. Table 5–20 shows the results of the haplotype analysis performed by Ardinger and colleagues (1989) from this same study. In this situation, the presence of the haplotype $C_2A_2B_2$ (both in the homozygote and heterozygote state) appears to be associated with a higher risk of clefts, strengthening the idea of a biologic association between the $TGFA$ gene locus and clefts. Nevertheless, it would be crucial to confirm and extend the results of this suggestive association in linkage studies of families ascertained through affected probands (see Chapter 9).

Table 5–19. The association between transforming growth factor alpha alleles and the risk of cleft lip and palate

	Genotypes			
	C_1C_1	C_1C_2	C_2C_2	Total
Cases	59	17	2	78
Controls	89	8	1	98
Odds ratio	1.0	3.2	3.0	

C_1 allele is 3.0 kbp restriction fragment length polymorphism (RFLP) segment, while the C_2 allele is 2.7 kbp RFLP segment using Taq1 restriction enzyme analysis of the transforming growth factor alpha (TGFA) gene probe.
Data adapted from Ardinger et al. (1989).

Table 5–20. The association between a transforming growth alpha RFLP $C_2A_2B_2$ haplotype and the risk of cleft lip and palate

| | Genotype (no. of $C_2A_2B_2$ haplotypes) | | | |
	0	1	2	Total
Cases	54	11	2	67
Controls	75	4	1	80
Odds ratio	1.0	3.8	2.8	

RFLP, restriction fragment length polymorphism.
C_2 allele is 1.7 kbp RFLP segment using Taq1 restriction enzyme.
A_2 allele is 4.0 kbp RFLP segment using BamH1 restriction enzyme.
B_2 allele is 1.2 kbp RFLP segment using Rsa1 restriction enzyme.
Data from the study of Ardinger et al. (1989).

Type I Errors

Type I errors were discussed in the context of epidemiologic studies of genetic traits (see Chapter 4). These errors apply to epidemiologic studies of genetic trait-disease associations as well. Type I errors have been discussed in the context of HLA-disease associations (Svejgaard et al., 1974; Kaslow and Shaw, 1981). When the relationship between a disease and an *HLA* allele is explored, it is important to recognize that multiple comparisons are examined involving multiple *HLA* alleles at multiple loci. Therefore, by default, multiple statistical tests are performed. At the conventional 0.05 level, 5% of all tests for association between a disease and a particular allele will be statistically significant by chance alone (i.e., false positives). Although some investigators have suggested lowering the critical value for significance to some equally arbitrary cutoff (say a p value of 0.01 or 0.001), or dividing the critical value by the number of tests performed, it is more likely that demanding replication in other studies and other populations will provide a better way to confirm a biologically meaningful association between a genetic marker and a disease (Rothman, 1986).

Type I errors are especially important in the context of using multiple DNA markers to search for susceptibility genes in common disease. As researchers clone and sequence more genes, and as more restriction enzymes are used in conjunction with multiple gene probes, more polymorphisms in small regions of the genome will be detected. A major challenge in the coming decades will be to differentiate the spurious from the biologically meaningful relationships among a multitude of associations between disease and DNA markers that will be found over many epidemiologic studies. Clearly, the establishment of true cause-effect relationships, as in all other areas of epidemiology, depends on many issues, including replicability and the presence of some biologically plausible model to explain these findings.

5.6. CONCLUDING REMARKS

In summary, epidemiologic methods provide important contributions to evaluating the role of genetic factors in disease distribution in populations. While limited clues can be obtained regarding genetic factors from the characteristics of disease distribution by time, place, and persons, several study approaches can suggest important genetic contribution to disease in the absence of specific and measurable genetic traits. The approaches include migrant, admixture, and inbreeding studies. Nevertheless, results from such studies should be cautiously interpreted because of potential problems of confounding and selection.

When specific genes can be measured at the DNA or gene product level, the candidate gene approach can provide a useful methodology to assess the association between specific alleles and disease occurrence using standard epidemiologic designs (cohort, case-control, and cross-sectional studies). In these studies, it is important to collect information on environmental risk factors that could interact with the genetic trait of interest in predicting disease. Evidence for genotype-environment interaction should be specifically examined in the analysis. Like all epidemiologic studies, several pitfalls and limitations should be considered. In particular, associations between genetic traits and diseases could be due to confounding (specifically population stratification), misclassification of genotype (commonly associated with linkage disequilibrium), as well as chance (type I errors that arise from multiple testing). Population study approaches should thus be complemented with family study approaches, which would incorporate specific genetic traits and environmental factors in testing for different modes of inheritance.

Epidemiologic Approaches to Familial Aggregation

6.1. INTRODUCTION

The study of familial aggregation is a central theme in genetic epidemiology in which major methodologic and statistical advances have been recently made. As King and colleagues (1984) pointed out, family studies encompass three approximately sequential steps of scientific investigation. First, researchers attempt to determine whether or not there is evidence of familial aggregation in a disease or trait. If familial aggregation is found, the second step is to discriminate among environmental, cultural, and/or genetic factors that may contribute to this clustering. Third, when evidence of a role for genetic factors is found, analyses designed to test for specific genetic mechanisms are carried out. This chapter reviews some basic epidemiologic principles and approaches that can be applied (1) to detect the presence of familial aggregation and (2) to evaluate whether familial aggregation can be attributed to genetic or environmental factors. Note that unraveling the causes of familial aggregation does not constitute an end in itself in genetic epidemiology, but it is an important step in defining the role of genetic factors contributing to disease occurrence in the population at large. Epidemiologic principles and approaches are crucial not only for detecting the presence of familial aggregation, but they also pave the road for sound application of specific genetic models.

6.2. EPIDEMIOLOGIC CONCEPTS APPLIED TO FAMILIES

Traditional epidemiologic concepts of disease definition, classification, natural history, and pathogenesis (reviewed in Chapter 3) are also critical in family studies. Such concepts, however, must be slightly modified or extended for family data. In particular, treating family information as a potential risk factor for disease in the individual requires some adaptation of the traditional concepts of causation. Also, standard statistical approaches used to test for clustering must be modified in family studies because observations on family members cannot be considered to be independently distributed. Furthermore, the boundaries between the two main study designs of classic epidemiology (i.e., case-control and cohort studies) become blurred in family studies (Susser and Susser, 1989).

6.2.1. Epidemiologic Concepts of Disease

Familial aggregation studies provide a unique framework for evaluating epidemiologic concepts of disease, for assessing the spectrum for expression of a disease, and for identifying heterogeneity. As in all epidemiologic studies, the case definition is an important prerequisite. Traditionally, studies of familial aggregation begin by identifying a group of individuals with a specific disease (index cases) and determining whether relatives have an excess frequency of the same disease when compared to an appropriate reference population. While most often the phenotype of interest is a disease (i.e., affected versus nonaffected), it can also be a physiologic trait that has a continuous distribution (e.g., cholesterol levels). Table 6-1 shows some examples of studies that have examined familial aggregation of various diseases or traits. These include breast cancer (Sattin et al, 1985), rheumatoid arthritis (del Junco et al., 1984), and myocardial infarction (ten Kate et al., 1982), as well as studies that estimate familial correlations for continuous traits, such as birthweight (Beaty et al., 1988b) and peak newborn bilirubin levels (Nielsen et al., 1987).

The study of family members of index cases can provide an opportunity for understanding the familial nature of disease or its precursors and risk factors. These risk factors are frequently quantitative measures of traits associated with a chronic disease. For example, as shown in Table 6-1, family studies have been used to evaluate clustering in disease risk factors (e.g., the twin study of risk factors for cardiovascular disease by Feinleib and colleagues [1977]). Such studies can point out that risk factors, such as cholesterol and blood pressure, may themselves be under genetic control and, therefore, may indirectly contribute to the familial aggregation of the disease. Indeed, it has been argued that aggregation of such risk factors for heart disease may be responsible for most of the familial aggregation of heart disease itself (Perkins, 1986). This remains a topic of debate, however.

Also, familial aggregation studies can be used to point out common etiologic and pathogenetic mechanisms between different diseases. For example, Cohen and coworkers (1977a) found a common familial component in chronic obstructive pulmonary disease and lung cancer, and suggested that impaired pulmonary function may be important in the pathogenesis of lung cancer (Cohen, 1980). Linet and associates (1989) found that relatives of patients with chronic lymphocytic leukemia have an excess frequency of other lymphoproliferative malignancies, again suggesting common pathogenetic mechanisms. Conversely, family studies can reveal underlying heterogeneity within

Table 6−1. Some examples of familial aggregation studies illustrating various aspects of disease definition, pathogenesis, and classification in probands and relatives

Author (year)	Disease/trait in index case	Disease/trait in relatives	Comments
Sattin et al. (1985)	Breast cancer	Breast cancer	Familial aggregation of a disease
del Junco et al. (1984)	Rheumatoid arthritis	Rheumatoid arthritis	Familial aggregation of a disease
ten Kate et al. (1982)	Myocardial infarction	Myocardial infarction	Familial aggregation of a disease
Beaty et al. (1988b)	Birthweight	Birthweight	Continuous trait in sibs
Nielsen et al. (1987)	Peak bilirubin in newborn	Peak bilirubin in newborn	Physiologic trait associated with neonatal jaundice
Feinleib et al. (1977)	Cardiovascular risk factors	Cardiovascular risk factors	Risk factors for a disease
Cohen (1980)	Chronic obstructive pulmonary disease and lung cancer	Impaired pulmonary function	Etiologic similarities for different diseases
Linet et al. (1989)	Chronic lymphocytic leukemia	Lymphoproliferative cancers	Etiologic and pathogenic similarities
Khoury et al. (1982b)	Neural tube defects	Neural tube defects	Etiologic heterogeneity within a malformation
Tokuhata and Lilienfeld (1963)	Lung cancer	Lung cancer	Interaction between family history and smoking

a disease. For example, siblings of children with isolated neural tube defects (NTD) have an excess risk of NTD compared to siblings of NTD cases with other malformations, a finding that suggests an underlying etiologic heterogeneity among infants with NTD (Khoury et al., 1982b).

Familial Factors as Risk Factors for Disease

Although epidemiologists have long been interested in familial factors as risk factors for disease (Lilienfeld, 1965), most epidemiologic studies do not collect or analyze family history data. For example, in a literature review, only 25% of cancer case-control studies included a family history component (Phillips et al., 1991). In case-control studies, a positive family history for disease is often treated as a risk factor, that is, as an exposure variable often dichotomized into yes/no categories, although other approaches are also available (see section 6.4). Positive family history is usually defined as the presence of disease in one or more first-degree relatives (parents, siblings and offspring) for both cases or controls. The analytic strategy is to then test whether or not a positive family history confers any excess risk of disease. However, relying exclusively on casual family histories obtained from an interview of cases and controls has serious limitations and can lead to erroneous interpretations (Weiss et al., 1982).

In general, family history of disease should not be considered as a simple attribute of a person, comparable to age or cigarette smoking. Family history depends on many factors, such as the number of relatives, their biologic relationship to the index case, their age distribution, and the disease frequency in the population. The impact of the number of relatives on the frequency of a positive family history is illustrated in Figure 6–1a. Even for a disease without any genetic etiology whatsoever, that is, where the risk to a relative of a case is equal to the population risk k, the probability of a positive family history in a case must increase with the observed number of such relatives (here only one type of relatives was considered, i.e., sibs). For example, the probability of an index (case or control) having a negative family history (i.e., no sibs affected) is $(1 - k)^n$ where n is the number of sibs. Clearly, when n is large, the probability of having a negative family history is lower than when n is small. As the disease frequency in the population increases, the risk for any one sib is higher and the proportion of cases (or controls) with a positive family history reaches its maximum more quickly. For diseases with a frequency of 5% to 10%, then it would be quite possible to find one or more affected relatives by chance alone in large sibships.

When the disease is purely genetic (e.g., autosomal dominant [Figure 6.1b] or autosomal recessive [Figure 6.1c]), the proportion of cases with a positive family history, that is, probability that a case has at least one affected relative, also increases with the number of such relatives. Here k becomes a function of allele frequencies (for an autosomal dominant disease $k = p^2 + 2p(1 - p)$, where p is the frequency of the disease allele, while for an autosomal recessive disease, $k = p^2$). The probability of a sib of a case (or another type of relative) being affected is easily calculated using the ITO matrices of Li and Sacks (1954). Such conditional probabilities are shown in Table 6–2 for various types of relatives of an affected individual (i.e., the case) under the two simplest Mendelian models, autosomal dominant and autosomal recessive. Using these formulas, Figures 6.1b and 6.1c show the expected proportion of cases with one or more affected sibs for autosomal dominant and recessive diseases. The expected proportion of cases with a positive family history is, of course, higher for dominant diseases compared with recessive ones. Even given the higher baseline risk expected for simple dominant diseases with complete penetrance; however, there will be some cases with no affected sibs.

Another consideration when using positive family history as a risk factor is that different types of relatives have different patterns of risk. While Figure 6–1 considered only risk in sibs, Table 6–2 shows the probability that relatives other than sibs of a case are also affected. As seen here, among first-degree relatives, offspring and siblings have quite different risks for purely genetic diseases, and these risks are again functions of the allele frequency. For

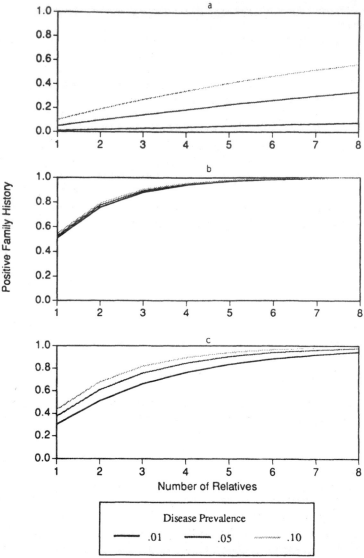

Figure 6–1. Proportion of cases with positive family history by number of first-degree relatives and disease prevalence when the disease: (a) has no genetic etiology; (b) is inherited as autosomal dominant; and (c) is inherited as autosomal recessive.

example, for autosomal recessive diseases, offspring of an affected person generally do not manifest disease unless it is extremely common, because the other parent is unlikely to contribute a rare disease allele.

Other limitations on the use of family history as a risk factor include any condition that affects the observed patterns of transmission and expression of genes in families. These include, for example, incomplete penetrance, variable expressivity (which contributes to misclassification), variation in the age at onset, the presence of etiologic heterogeneity, gene-environment in-

Table 6–2. Probability that a relative of an affected individual (case) is also affected for a simple autosomal dominant and recessive disease, respectively, for different types of relative

Type of relative	Probability of being affected	
	Autosomal dominant	Autosomal recessive
Offspring	$\dfrac{1 + p - p^2}{2 - p}$	p
Sibling	$\dfrac{4 + 5p - 6p^2 + p^3}{4(2 - p)}$	$\dfrac{(1 + p)^2}{4}$
Niece/nephew	$.5\left[(1 - q^2) + \dfrac{p}{(1 - q^2)} + \dfrac{pq}{(1 + q)}\right]$	$\dfrac{p(1 + p)}{2}$
First cousin	$\dfrac{p}{4(1 - q^2)}[4p^3 + q(15p^2 + 14pq + 1)]$	$\dfrac{p(q + 4p)}{4}$

p = frequency of disease allele, and $q = 1 - p$ = frequency of the normal allele.
Adapted from Weiss et al. (1982), based on Li and Sacks' (1954) ITO matrix method.

teraction and epistasis (see Chapter 2). In general, these factors decrease the probability that a relative of an individual with a simple genetic disease will also be affected.

6.2.3. Overlap Between Case-Control and Cohort Approaches

When epidemiologic concepts are applied to the analysis of family data, an unavoidable overlap is seen between the two main types of epidemiologic designs: namely, the case-control and cohort designs. To illustrate, assume that in a case-control study of a disease, each case and control have one and only one relative. Family history in this situation can be analyzed in two ways. Positive family history can be considered as an exposure attribute of cases and controls themselves (see Table 6–3) where the odds ratio represents the ratio of odds of exposure (i.e., having an affected relative) in cases over the odds of exposure in controls. On the other hand, the family history could also be viewed from a cohort perspective where relatives of cases and controls become the focus of analysis, and the relationship to either a case or a control becomes the exposure. The disease frequency in relatives of cases can then be compared with that in relatives of controls, using an appropriate measure (see section 6.4.2). In this situation, if the odds of disease is chosen as the measure, then the case-control and the cohort approaches yield identical estimates of the odds ratio (Table 6–3). In reality, however, this scheme is complicated by several factors, including the methods of ascertainment, variation in the number of relatives per case and control, their exact relationship to the index (case or control), the lack of statistical independence among

Table 6-3. Family history viewed from both a case-control and cohort approach perspective

	Disease in index persons	
Disease in a relative	Case	Control
Disease	*a*	*b*
No disease	*c*	*d*
Total	*a* + *c*	*b* + *d*

Either the case-control or cohort design can be adapted to family studies. The status of relatives of both cases and controls is summarized in a single 2 × 2 table, where *a* is the number of affected relatives of cases, *b* is the number of affected relatives of controls, etc.

Case-control approach: The exposure is having an affected relative. The odds of having an affected relative for a case is *a/c*, and the corresponding odds among relatives of controls is *b/d*. Thus, the odds ratio is *ad/bc*.

Cohort approach: The exposure is being a relative of a case. Disease frequency in relatives of an exposed person (i.e., relative of cases) is *a/a* + *c*. Disease frequency among relatives of unexposed persons (i.e., relatives of controls) is *b/b* + *d*. The relative risk is then (*a/a* + *c*)/(*b/b* + *d*). If odds of disease is taken as measure of frequency then the odds ratio for disease becomes *ad/bc*.

these relatives, variation in age distribution of the two groups of relatives, and the availability of information on other risk factors in relatives themselves.

6.3. SAMPLING DESIGNS IN FAMILY STUDIES

Both case-control and cohort study designs can be adapted to include family studies either as an integral part or as a small component of a larger study. Since many genetic diseases are rare, it is frequently easier to adapt the case-control design for family studies, although cohort studies can often provide valuable insights into the public health impact of genetic or familial diseases. Using epidemiologic principles to design family studies provides specific measures of secular, geographic, and other environmental factors that may also influence risk. Variation due to such nongenetic forces should not be ignored, for they may provide important clues about disease etiology, and some environmental factors may be amenable to intervention.

6.3.1. Epidemiologic Studies with a Familial Component

The case-control method is deeply rooted in epidemiology, and it provides a natural extension for studying familial aggregation. Case-control studies with a familial component follow the same general rules and guidelines for design, conduct, and analysis reviewed in Chapter 3. There are two broad categories of familial aggregation studies based on this design: the family history method and the family study method (Andreasen et al, 1986). These terms have been used mainly in the psychiatric literature in the context of validating clinical diagnostic entities. A summary of the features, advantages, and limitations of the two approaches is presented in Table 6-4.

Family History Approach

In the family history method, investigators usually obtain information from the cases and controls themselves concerning the presence of disease (or any

Table 6–4. Various approaches to the study of familial aggregation that may be incorporated into a case-control design

	Family history approach		Family study approach
	Abbreviated	Detailed	
Features	Asking about the presence of disease in relatives of cases and controls	Detailed inquiry about relatives of cases and controls with and without disease	Detailed evaluation of relatives of cases and controls with and without disease
Sources of data	Usually cases and controls	Usually cases and controls	Relatives of cases and controls
Measures of disease frequency in relatives	No direct measure	Prevalence, incidence,* cumulative incidence*	Prevalence, incidence,* cumulative incidence*
Measures of familial aggregation	Odds ratio	Odds ratio, relative risk, family history scores†	Odds ratio, relative risk, family history scores†
Advantages	Quick and inexpensive	Provides a direct measure of risk in relatives	Provides a direct measure of risk in relatives; examines risk factors for disease in relatives; evaluates outcomes in relatives
Limitations	No measure of disease risk in relatives; may be biased by family size and recall differences	More involved, requires validation of outcomes in relatives; no assessment of exposures in relatives	Most involved and expensive, possible selection bias in participation
Limitations common to all designs	Ascertainment bias, selection bias, fertility effects, lack of statistical independence, statistical power, etiologic heterogeneity		

*Requires age-of-onset data.
†Also used to detect heterogeneity.

other trait) in their relatives. When cases and controls are not available (e.g., patients may be deceased), information can be obtained from other individuals such as spouses or parents. For childhood onset diseases (such as birth defects and mental retardation), family history information is usually obtained from parents. As shown in Table 6–4, two main subclasses can be recognized along the spectrum of the family history approach in case-control studies: an abbreviated approach and a detailed family history evaluation. Although each subtype is considered separately here, there is overlap between them, and many epidemiologic studies start with a detailed family history evaluation but publish their final results in abbreviated form (e.g., Bourguet et al., 1985; Sattin et al., 1985).

Abbreviated Family History Approach. The abbreviated family history approach entails the addition of only a few questions regarding the presence of disease in relatives to an interview given to cases and controls regarding their own past exposures and experiences. It essentially summarizes familial information into one or two pieces of data, and offers only limited opportunity for rigorous assessment of familial aggregation. For example, it may include a question on the presence or absence of a similar disease in one or more first-degree relatives (and possibly other classes of relatives), but does not involve obtaining any detailed information on all relatives. While providing a quick way to screen for the overall impact of positive family history, this approach provides no measure of disease risk among relatives. A positive family history is essentially treated as merely another exposure variable in the case-control study; and the odds ratio is the resulting measure testing for familial aggregation by comparing frequency of a positive family history among cases and controls.

As noted in section 6.2, since family history is not truly an attribute of the cases and controls, this estimated odds ratio can be affected by differences in family size and structure. For example, if cases generally come from larger families than controls, the probability of finding at least one affected relative of a case will intrinsically be greater than that of controls, even in the absence of any underlying difference in risk. Conversely, controls may come from larger families because the disease present in the case influences family size, resulting in downward bias in frequency of positive family history among cases. Consider the extreme situation where the disease is associated with complete infertility, so that cases have no offspring. In this situation, the probability of finding at least one affected first-degree relative of a case is automatically lower than that for a control because cases have fewer numbers of first-degree relatives compared to controls. Even when the disease itself does not influence fertility directly, the burden of caring for an affected family member (i.e., the case) may lead to smaller sibship sizes. Alternatively, if the disease is a severe childhood disease that is commonly lethal, there may be larger family sizes among case families as the parents of an affected child attempt to "replace" the case with another child.

The family history approach is also affected by potential differential recall between cases and controls. If cases remember more affected relatives than do controls, the estimated odds ratio will be inflated. This may be especially critical in collecting information on more distant relatives (e.g., first cousins), where the knowledge of their own disease status may lead to better recognition and reporting of the disease in the extended family. The magnitude of recall bias in obtaining family history in case-control studies is difficult to measure. However, several studies have suggested that the ability of individuals to recall the presence of disease in their own relatives may be quite limited (e.g., Schull and Cobb, 1969; Napier et al., 1972; Hastrup et al., 1985). Therefore, misclassification of the true status with respect to family history could occur. If the rate of misclassification in reporting family information were the same between cases and controls (i.e., if it were nondifferential), the estimated odds ratio would be underestimated (if the true odds ratio is >1), as with any exposure variable in case-control studies (Flegal et al., 1986).

This is illustrated in the hypothetical example given in Table 6–5, where the odds ratio measuring the association between a positive family history and risk of disease is calculated, assuming the ability of both cases and controls to recall accurately the presence of family history is imperfect but equal, that is, *nondifferential* recall. In this example, when there is no misclassification of the true family history, the estimated odds ratio is at its true value of 9.0. However, with decreasing sensitivity and/or specificity, the estimated odds ratio drops. Here, sensitivity is a measure of the rate of correctly reporting a positive family history, while specificity is a measure of correctly reporting a negative family history. As shown in Table 6–5, the observed odds ratio is always less than its true value when there is some misclassification of either positive or negative family history by either cases or controls. A low specificity has a greater effect on the estimated odds ratio when there is completely accurate reporting of positive family histories (i.e., when sensitivity is 1.0), but the combined effect of both types of misclassification will quickly mask any association between positive family history and risk of disease.

Table 6–6 illustrates the situation of *differential* recall of family history between cases and controls. To make this example simple, here the specificity is fixed at 1.0 and only sensitivity of recall is varied between cases and controls, that is, no one with a negative family history mistakenly reports a positive family history, but not all positive family histories are accurately reported. When there is a higher sensitivity in cases than controls, the estimated odds ratio associated with positive family history is higher than its true value. On the other hand, if cases underreport positive family history compared to controls, the odds ratio would be lower than its true value.

Table 6–5. Expected odds ratio for the impact of a positive family history on risk in a case-control study at different sensitivity* and specificity† levels

Specificity	Sensitivity			
	0.40	0.60	0.80	1.00
0.40	0.72	1.00	1.43	2.25
0.60	1.00	1.38	1.91	2.74
0.80	1.52	2.11	2.85	3.86
1.00	6.00	6.71	7.67	9.00

Assumptions: Based on 100 cases (50 with + family history and 50 without) and 100 controls (10 with + family history and 90 without), so the true odds ratio is 9.00.

*Sensitivity: proportion of cases and controls with a positive family history correctly identified through interview.

†Specificity: proportion of cases and controls with a negative family history correctly identified through interview.

The same sensitivity and specificity is assumed for both cases and controls. Note the distinct weakening of the observed association due to the nondifferential recall.

Table 6–6. Effect of differential recall on estimated odds ratio for the impact of a positive family history on risk in a case-control study at different sensitivity* levels

Sensitivity of controls	Sensitivity of cases			
	0.40	0.60	0.80	1.00
0.20	12.3	21.0	32.7	49.0
0.40		10.3	16.0	24.0
0.60			10.4	15.7
0.80				11.5

Assumptions: Here, the same disease frequencies given in Table 6–5 are used, and the true odds ratio is 9.00. However, the sensitivity of cases is more than that of controls in recalling a positive family history, however, the specificity is fixed at 1.0.

*Sensitivity: proportion of cases or controls with a positive family history correctly identified through interview. The odds ratio is inflated due to the differential recall bias.

Detailed Family History Approach. As part of the family history approach, investigators can gather detailed information on the status of all relatives of a specified type (e.g., first-degree) from both cases and controls, regardless of their disease status (Table 6–4). Often a chronologic listing of all siblings and offspring is collected as part of a case-control study. For each person, information is gathered on certain demographic information such as sex, birth order, and dates of birth. Then, questions are asked about the vital status of the person (and, if deceased, the cause of death and age). If the person is alive, inquiry is made into his or her medical history. If the person has the disease of interest, information is then asked about age at onset and diagnosis. This rather involved interviewing process obviously is more time-consuming than the collection of casual family history (positive or negative). Nevertheless, it is a standard practice in the evaluation of patients in genetics clinics where complete family histories are routinely collected, and is becoming more popular in epidemiologic studies. Note, however, that in a typical case-control study of disease, interviews can last an hour or more, even when not collecting family information, usually because a wide variety of exposures is of interest to researchers (including occupational history, residential data, and past exposures and illnesses). Therefore, the inclusion of a detailed family history evaluation is not always feasible.

The most important advantage of using a detailed family history evaluation in case-control studies of disease is that cohorts of relatives can be constructed with "exposure" to either a case or a control noted. Measures of disease frequency can thus be calculated and compared between these two groups (see section 6.4.1 below). If complete information on the age of onset is available, survival analysis may be appropriate, although standard survival models do not consider the lack of independence among relatives in a family. Initial assessment of disease outcomes in individual relatives is achieved by obtaining a full disease history from the cases and controls or by interviewing the relatives directly. However, either approach is subject to potential recall bias as discussed above. To overcome this problem, it is sometimes possible to add a step to validate reported outcomes on affected relatives from available hospital or medical records, rather than relying solely on interview data. Clearly, there are limits on exposure and other risk-factor information that can be obtained from each relative, and this restricts the search for the underlying causes of familial aggregation (see section 6.6). Nonetheless, this extended family history method is an important step in confirming evidence of familial aggregation.

Family Study Approach

In the family study method, investigators use the case-control design to enroll relatives for more detailed evaluation usually including direct interview, obtaining medical records to validate reported disease, and possibly clinical and laboratory evaluation for physiologic traits or genetic markers associated with the disease. This study design is the most expensive and requires considerable resources for tracing and assembling cohorts of relatives. Nevertheless, this scheme has numerous advantages. It allows (1) a direct examination of the disease outcomes in relatives, (2) collection of both risk factor and exposure data on each relative, and (3) when coupled with laboratory measures (e.g., biochemical analysis and genetic markers), it permits a more complete assessment of genetic and environmental factors, as well as, ultimately, segregation and linkage analysis of the family data (see Chapters 8 and 9). One potential problem is ascertainment bias (discussed in section 8.3) because all families are ascertained via affected or unaffected individuals, and this must be considered in the analysis of genetic models. Another potential problem is selection and participation bias among the relatives choosing to participate. A preferential participation rate by affected compared to unaffected relatives can lead to an overestimation of true disease frequency. There also exists the possibility of a differential participation rate among relatives of cases compared to relatives of controls.

An example of the family study approach is the Johns Hopkins study of chronic obstructive pulmonary disease (COPD) (Cohen et al., 1975; Cohen, 1980). In this study, COPD cases, lung cancer cases, and hospital and community controls were interviewed regarding a variety of demographic and exposure data potentially related to the etiology of pulmonary disease, as well as family history. The case-control design was used as a starting point for detailed family studies in which relatives of cases and controls were invited to participate in an evaluation of exposure data, pulmonary function testing, and measurements of certain genetic markers. This multidisciplinary study also provided data for several investigations of risk factors for COPD itself (Cohen, 1980), studies of interaction between smoking and certain genetic markers in increasing the prevalence of airways obstruction (Khoury et al., 1986), analyses of family data on the genetic and environmental mechanisms for airways obstruction (Khoury et al., 1985a), and mechanisms of genetic control of pulmonary function (Astemborski et al., 1985; Beaty et al., 1987; Cotch et al., 1990; Rybicki et al., 1990).

6.3.2. Case Studies with Population Comparison

When cases come from a well-defined population where rates of disease are known (perhaps due to an ongoing disease registry or other surveillance efforts), measures of disease frequency in case families can be directly compared with the expected disease frequency for this population. For rare conditions (disease frequency of 1% or less), the disease frequency in the general population is almost identical to the disease frequency in relatives of unaffected individuals who could serve as controls. As the disease frequency in the population increases, however, this approximation becomes less valid.

One example of this approach is the study of the incidence of rheumatoid arthritis in 1631 biologic relatives of 78 cases ascertained from the population-based registry of Rochester, Minnesota. Here incidence in relatives was compared to age- and sex-adjusted rates of rheumatoid arthritis for this same population (del Junco et al., 1984). This population-based design is becoming more popular because of the following:

1. For many diseases, including cancer and birth defects, reasonably accurate registries are now available in various populations.
2. There is a rapid proliferation of automated record linkage systems that provide the ability to link disease information on relatives drawn from the same population.
3. This approach provides the opportunity to search for certain nongenetic sources of clustering, such as geographic and secular variation.

A number of methods have been developed to compare observed individual risks to appropriate expected values, both in sibships and in families of arbitrary structure, as described in section 6.4 in this chapter.

6.3.3. Fixed Clusters of Relatives

Another approach to the study of familial aggregation of disease is sampling fixed sets of relatives, regardless of their disease status. The best-known fixed design is the twin method, although others such as the family set method have been developed. The advantages to a fixed cluster sampling design are (1) all sampling units are of the same size and all are equally informative, (2) they allow greater control over observable environmental risk factors, and (3) statistical methods for balanced designs can be tailored to the question at hand. The primary disadvantages of relying on fixed clusters of relatives are (1) the cluster design may restrict inferences to the general population because the clusters themselves may not be representative, and (2) clusters are often difficult to identify and recruit resulting in differential participation rates. Twins reared together have a unique social and behavioral development experience merely because they grow up with a co-twin, while twins reared apart are not only exceptionally difficult to find but are likely to have been involved in unusual situations leading to their separation.

Twin Studies

Twin studies have been popular in medical research for decades, although their utility and limitations continue to be debated (Schull and Weiss, 1980;

Hrubec and Robinette, 1984). Theoretically, twin studies provide a simple way to separate genetic from environmental factors by study design rather than by analysis only (see Table 6–7). Since monozygotic (MZ) twins share 100% of genes, while dizygotic (DZ) twins on average share only 50% of their genes (just as do full sibs), one can assess the relative importance of genetic and environmental factors by comparing MZ to DZ twins for concordance of disease (when dealing with a qualitative trait) or for correlation (when dealing with a quantitative trait). Studies of twins raised apart are appealing because they permit (in theory) less ambiguous identification of genetic factors. In practice, however, analysis of separated twins is hampered by nonrandom assignment of the co-twins to similar environments, and by substantial undocumented biases in recruitment and tracing of separated co-twins. A more detailed discussion of the role of twin studies in quantitative genetics is given in Chapter 7.

Concordance can be viewed as the conditional probability (or cumulative incidence) of the second twin's being affected given that the first is affected. If MZ twins have a higher concordance than DZ twins, there is suggestive evidence for a genetic basis for the disease. On the other hand, any discord-

Table 6–7. Comparison of disease frequency measures in different types of familial aggregation studies and comments about interpretation

Study	Comparison of disease frequency		Excess disease frequency suggests
	Group 1	Group 2	
Case-control	Relatives of cases	Relatives of controls	Genetic and/or environmental
Case-population	Relatives of cases	Population frequency	Genetic and/or environmental
Twin study	Member of an affected MZ twin pair	Member of an affected DZ twin pair	Genetic component
	Member of an affected DZ twin pair	Sibling of an affected person	Environmental component
Family sets	Spouses of cases	Spouses of controls	Environmental component
	Cousins of cases	Cousins of controls	Genetic component
Adoption study	Natural parent of adopted cases	Natural parent of adopted controls	Genetic component
	Adoptive parent of adopted cases	Adoptive parent of adopted controls	Environmental component
	Natural parent of adopted cases	Adoptive parent of adopted cases	Genetic and/or environmental

MZ, monozygotic; DZ, dizygotic.

ance between MZ twins automatically leads one to conclude there must be some role for environmental factors in risk. Since DZ twins and full sibs share on average 50% of their genes, a higher concordance rate in DZ twins compared with full sibs further points to a role for shared environmental factors (Susser, 1985). In reality, however, interpretation of twin concordance rates is rarely straightforward.

In addition to difficulties in accurate determination of zygosity, other potentially confounding problems arise in twin studies. Some biases may be prenatal in origin, while others could be postnatal (Price, 1950; Scarr, 1982). For example, compared to DZ twins, MZ twins may have differences with respect to implantation patterns, intrauterine positions, timing of fission, patterns of prenatal circulation and survival, as well as differences in labor and delivery events. Some of these discrepancies could lower concordance in MZ twins, even when genetic factors are of primary importance in determining risk to disease. On the other hand, postnatal biases could include a greater similarity in environmental exposures among MZ twins compared to DZ twins because of their overall greater physical resemblance. This potential bias may lead to an inflated concordance rate in MZ twins when compared with that reported for DZ twins, even when there is little genetic involvement in risk.

A variety of sources have been used in ascertaining twins for genetic epidemiologic studies (Allen, 1965; Hrubec and Robinette, 1984); and twin registries are now available in several countries (Hrubec and Neel, 1978; Kaprio et al., 1978; Hauge, 1980). Analysis of families of monozygotic twins drawn from such registries allows separate identification of shared maternal factors contributing to phenotypic variation not otherwise possible (Nance et al., 1978). However, whenever twin registries are voluntary, there will be substantial self-selection, and more MZ twins may be recruited than DZ twins. In addition, when twins are recruited, female pairs tend to volunteer more often than male pairs. These selection biases may also minimize the environmental variation between twins, and inflate the apparent role for genetic factors.

Other Fixed Clusters

Fixed clusters of relatives other than twins can also be used as a study design to separate genetic and environmental factors. For example, use of "family sets" as a sampling strategy is one approach that can yield much information about the role of genetic factors in complex diseases, particularly in diseases of late onset (Schull and Weiss, 1980; Susser, 1985). Briefly, this approach takes samples of fixed relationships, usually matched for age, race, and certain environmental factors. One common family set consists of an index (proband), a spouse, a sibling, a first cousin, and one unrelated individual where all are within a defined age range. The unrelated individual is typically matched to the index for certain demographic characters (sex, race, etc.). This family set method was originally designed for studies of late onset chronic diseases where parents of index cases are either likely to be dead or may be a select group of survivors free of disease, and children of cases are likely to be too young to be at appreciable risk (Harburg et al., 1970; Schull et al., 1970). Within each family set, the spouse provides information on household environment, the sibling and the cousin provide differing degrees of genetic information, and the control is matched for observable environmental factors outside the household. The family set method has been used in population surveys (Harburg et al., 1970; Schull et al., 1970; Moll et al., 1983), and its advantages and limitations have been discussed (Schull et al., 1977).

6.3.4. Adoption Studies

Adoption studies provide another approach for studying familial aggregation, which can separate, by design, genetic from environmental factors (Susser, 1985). The design of adoption studies may take on several possible forms, but such studies are most successful in populations where adoption records are systematically kept. For example, such studies can begin by identifying natural parents whose children have been adopted. Affected parents and control parents who have given up children for adoption can be identified, and the frequency of disease in the adopted away children is then compared between these two groups. If children of parents with the condition have an excess disease frequency when compared with children of parents without the condition, then an effect of genetic factors can be inferred, since the role of environmental factors is partially eliminated by the adoption process. Another approach is retrospective, where adopted children are identified first, and those adoptees with and without disease serve as cases and controls. When the natural parents of both case and control adoptees are traced, the frequency of disease in parents can be compared directly.

In either situation, one should also compare the frequency of disease between adoptive parents of both cases and controls (who are biologically unrelated to their adopted children). If adoptive parents of cases have a higher frequency of disease than adoptive parents of controls, environmental factors may predominate in determining risk (Table 6–7). Adoption studies have been successfully used in investigations of psychiatric disorders (e.g., Heston, 1966; Rosenthal et al., 1971; Goodwin et al., 1973), blood pressure and obesity (Annest et al., 1979a, 1979b; Stunkard et al., 1986), and even premature death (Sorensen et al., 1988; Williams, 1988).

The success of adoption studies depends heavily on the availability of records and the ability to reconstruct biologic relationships. When such records are not kept systematically, selection biases favoring identification of affected sets of adoptee, adoptive parent and biologic parent may inflate the observed rates of disease in these three groups. Variations of adoption studies include twins reared apart and half-sibs reared apart (Susser, 1985). The advantages and limitations of adoption studies have been debated and discussed (Gottesman and Shields, 1976; Kessler, 1976; Susser, 1985). In addition to regulations regarding confidentiality of records and intrinsic limits on information about true parental status, there remain problems with adoption studies (e.g., small numbers, lack of adjustment for confounding factors, and selection biases). The question of representativeness should also be considered in studies of adoptees, their adoptive, and their biologic parents, especially in studies of behavioral traits and psychiatric disorders.

6.3.5. Genealogies

An expanding area in genetic-epidemiologic methodology is the use of population-based genealogies (Schull and Weiss, 1980). Such an approach is currently feasible in only selected populations where documented or potentially obtainable genealogic records exist. These include such diverse groups as the Mormons in Utah (Skolnick, 1980; Bishop and Skolnick, 1984), Mexican-Americans in Laredo, Texas (Schull and Weiss, 1980), and the Old Order Amish in Lancaster County, Pennsylvania (McKusick, 1978; Khoury et al., 1987a). This approach relies on the identification of genetic links among all or most living individuals in the community, and places each person into one or more multigenerational pedigrees. Genetic distance between two individuals can then be measured in terms of kinship coefficients which specify the probability of an allele being shared by two individuals identical by descent.

The genealogical approach has the appeal of providing the ability to follow a total population over time without having to sample through affected individuals, as done in all case-control studies. The requirements of this approach include the ability to do the following:

1. Identify the population of interest and all genealogic links between individuals
2. Identify health outcomes, for example, by direct observation or by record linkage with health registries such as the cancer registry in Utah (Bishop and Skolnick, 1984)
3. Collect information on individuals regarding vital events and pertinent risk factors for the disease or trait to be studied (Schull and Weiss, 1980)

Such genealogical information allows coefficients of genetic relationship to be calculated for both cases and controls from these populations, and these genealogical indices can also be useful in studies of familial aggregation. If, for example, there were strong familial aggregation of a rare disease in a closed population, all or most cases might share a common genetic defect. This should be reflected in a higher kinship coefficient among cases compared to controls, although familial clustering due to environmental defects could mimic this pattern of shared genes among cases. Jorde and colleagues (1983) reported that the mean kinship coefficient among 249 cases of neural tube defects who were in the Utah Genealogical Data Base was an order of magnitude greater than a series of controls drawn from this same genealogical database (which encompassed 1.2 million individuals). More detailed examination of these kinship coefficients showed that most of the differences between cases and controls could be attributed to a relatively small number of affected sib pairs among the cases, however. This raises the possibility that an environmental factor common to sibs may be contributing to the apparent familial aggregation reflected in the analysis of kinship coefficients.

Similar studies utilizing the Utah Genealogic database and the statewide tumor registry have been used to examine the degree of genetic relatedness among cases of various types of cancer (Bishop and Skolnick, 1984). Again, a modified case-control design was used, in which the average kinship coefficients between all case pairs was compared with the average kinship coefficient between all control pairs. Consistent evidence for genetic factors was seen for several common cancers. Population-based geneologic data offer opportunities for studies which pull together genetics, epidemiology, and demography (Bean, 1990).

While measures of genetic relationship, such as the kinship and inbreeding coefficients, are appealing when found to be associated with a particular disease, caution must be exercised in interpreting such observations. For example, if cases with a rare disease were found to have a high inbreeding coefficient (or equivalently, found to come from consanguineous matings where the parents had nonzero kinship coefficients), it is critical to have appropriate controls before inferring that a genetic mechanism is operating. For example, Roberts (1985) found that 12% of patients with multiple sclerosis in an Orkney Island population were inbred to some extent. While this was significantly higher than the general population of the British Isles, it was *not* higher than controls drawn from this same Orkney population. When detailed comparisons of Orkney cases and controls were carried out, the cases were found to be even more inbred than Orkney controls (Roberts, 1991). It is important to note that the structure of the population determines the degree of genetic relationship among individuals, and that this changes over time and may involve migration patterns among several populations (Castilla and Adams, 1990). A properly designed case-control study should reflect this when employing measures of genetic relationship to identify familial aggregation.

6.4. MEASURES OF FAMILIAL AGGREGATION

The goal of family studies is, first, to determine whether a given disease shows familial aggregation, and second, to identify possible causes of such clustering. In a case-control setting, the null hypothesis is that the disease has the same frequency in families of cases compared to families of controls. In a cohort setting, the null hypothesis is that there is no clustering of disease within families identified in a defined cohort. The specific measures of disease frequency are similar to those in population studies reviewed in section 3.4, and include incidence, cumulative incidence, and prevalence.

6.4.1. Relative Measures and Difference Measures

To measure the disease frequency in families ascertained through cases and controls, cohorts of case relatives and control relatives must be constructed. Such reconstructed cohorts can be summarized into a single 2 × 2 table as shown in Figure 6-2. A simple count of the frequency of disease history among relatives of cases and controls may not be appropriate for late-onset

Affected   Nonaffected

	Affected	Nonaffected	
Case Relatives	n_{11}	n_{12}	$n_{1.}$
Control Relatives	n_{21}	n_{22}	$n_{2.}$
	$n_{.1}$	$n_{.2}$	N

Figure 6–2. A two-by-two table summarizing disease status in reconstructed cohorts of relatives of cases and relatives of controls. A total of $n_{1.}$ relatives of cases and $n_{2.}$ relatives of controls were identified ($n_{1.} + n_{2.} = N$), of which $n_{.1}$ were affected and $n_{.2}$ were nonaffected.

diseases, where there is substantial censoring of the data (i.e., where many individuals have not yet passed through the age of risk). Ideally, estimates of lifetime risk from life tables (Chase et al., 1983) or other survival models would be used (Self and Prentice, 1986).

Measures of association include *relative measures* such as odds ratios ($OR = n_{11}n_{22}/n_{12}n_{21}$) or relative risks ($RR = (n_{11}/n_{.1})/(n_{21}/n_{.2})$); and *difference measures* such as risk difference ($RD = (n_{11}/n_{1.}) - (n_{21}/n_{2.})$). Such measures should always be calculated separately for different classes of relatives (e.g., sibs, offspring, uncles/aunts, and first cousins). However, such simple analysis conceals much of the variation among families and ignores the natural dependence among members within the same family. When computing the conventional odds ratio from such a 2×2 table, for example, it is assumed that all observations contributing to any cell are independent, identically distributed random variables. Obviously, this is true *only* under the null hypothesis that risk is independent of biologic or cultural relationships among relatives.

Weiss and colleagues (1982) have shown that the expected value of both the odds ratio and the relative risk obtained from this type of table is a function of prevalence in the general population, the particular mechanism of inheritance, and the type of relationship involved. Even for simple Mendelian disorders, summary measures of familial aggregation obtained from a simple 2×2 table such as this can be surprisingly low. This may explain why, for many chronic diseases, consistent evidence for familial aggregation has been reported but the odds ratios (or relative risks) obtained from most case-control studies have been unimpressive, showing only a 2- to 3-fold increase in risk associated with being ascertained through a case.

For example, Table 6–8 shows expected values of relative risk for sibs of cases compared to the disease frequency in the population for an autosomal dominant disease with incomplete penetrance and in the presence of sporadic (or nongenetic) cases. The attributable fraction given here refers to the proportion of cases in the population which are genetic in origin. As can be seen whenever penetrance of the disease gene is less than 100%, the expected value of this relative risk is reduced, even when all cases of disease are due to a simple Mendelian mechanism (i.e., even when the attributable fraction is 100%). Similarly, the lower the attributable fraction (i.e., proportion of

Table 6–8. Ratio of risk of disease in sibs of cases to disease frequency in the population, for a dominant trait with variable levels of penetrance and attributable fraction (etiologic heterogeneity), for different disease frequencies

Disease frequency	Attributable fraction*	Penetrance†		
		50%	75%	100%
0.001	1%	2.3	3.9	6.0
	50%	121	189	249
	100%	251	374	500
0.01	1%	1.1	1.3	1.5
	50%	13.6	19.9	25.5
	100%	25.8	37.9	50.4
0.1	1%	1.02	1.03	1.04
	50%	2.3	2.8	3.2
	100%	3.3	4.3	5.4

*Attributable fraction refers to the proportion of cases in the population due to the genetic trait (see Chapter 3).
†Penetrance refers to the probability of disease for an individual carrying the disease allele (i.e., either homozygote or heterozygote) being affected. This may be a function of other environmental and genetic factors.
Adapted from Weiss et al. (1982).

disease due to the genetic mechanism), the lower the relative risk will be regardless of penetrance (Majumder et al., 1983). Finally, as the disease frequency in the population increases, the relative risk also drops. As shown in Table 6–8, in some situations the expected relative risks are very close to unity, and therefore it may often be difficult, if not impossible, to detect the presence of familial aggregation using overall measures of relative risks even when Mendelian mechanisms are operating.

When cases and controls are individually matched, pooling families of all cases and controls into a single table will bias downward the estimated odds ratio by ignoring stratification across each case-control pair. In reality, matching cases and controls generates an individual 2×2 table for all relatives from each matched pair, and an overall estimate of the odds ratio is needed. Since the investigator has no control over the number of relatives any given case or control has, many matched pairs may be uninformative in that they have too few relatives or lack a mixture of both affected and unaffected relatives. For this type of individual 2×2 table to be informative and contribute to the estimator for the overall odds ratio, both affected and unaffected relatives must be available for any matched pair. Given informative tables from each of $i = 1 \cdots I$ matched pairs, however, a regression model for the odds ratio (OR) from this type of table can be written as

$$\ln (OR) = \alpha + \beta Z_i, \qquad (6\text{-}1)$$

where the vector Z_i represents a vector of covariates observed on the ith stratum (e.g., matching variables for the case-control pair), and the intercept represents the baseline or common odds ratio. Liang and coworkers (1986) have shown how an unbiased estimator for the odds ratio can be obtained for sparse data without assuming complete independence among the relatives contributing to each row of the tables. This approach reduces to the usual Mantel and Haenszel (1959) estimator for the odds ratio when there is no effect for the covariates (i.e., $\beta = 0$). The importance of obtaining unbiased estimates for β arises when the odds ratio can vary with observable characteristics of the case or control, for example, race and sex. A slightly different parameterization of the same underlying statistical model permits a more detailed analysis that takes into consideration observed covariates on the relatives themselves (see the subsection "Extensions to Matched Case-Control Studies," later in this chapter).

Difference measures of increased risk can also be used to quantitate familial aggregation, where the difference in disease frequency among relatives of cases and relatives of controls is estimated. In this context, simple recurrence risks for congenital and early-onset diseases can be used, or lifetime risk measures obtained from life table analysis of late onset disease. Such difference measures may provide additional insight into biologic mechanisms. To illustrate, Table 6–9 shows both relative and difference measures of sibling aggregation for several diseases. For example, for phenylketonuria, a rare autosomal recessive disease, the relative effect measure is astronomically high (2500) and the absolute measure is practically identical to the actual recurrence risk in siblings of cases (25%). The risk difference of 25% is more useful, since it points toward a single gene mechanism for phenylketonuria.

The situation becomes more complex for disorders of unknown etiology, however. For example, if we compare neural tube defects (NTD) to rheumatoid arthritis (RA) with respect to the relative and difference measures of sibling aggregation, interesting contrasts arise. The relative risk measure is much higher for NTD than RA, (20 versus 1.5), while the difference measure for NTD and RA are virtually identical (about 2%). Because RA is much more common than NTD in the general population, a much smaller relative-risk measure translates into similar risk difference. The interpretation of such a difference measure of risk depends on the underlying etiologic model(s). For example, 2% excess risk in sibs is consistent with environmental risk

Table 6–9. Illustration of relative and difference measures of familial aggregation in siblings, for various diseases

| Disease | Disease frequency in sibs* | | Relative measure A/B | Difference measure A − B |
	Cases (A)	Controls (B)		
Phenylketonuria	25%	1/10000	2500	25%
Neural tube defects	2%	1/1000	20	2%
Rheumatoid arthritis	5.7%	3.7%	1.5	2%
Breast cancer	18.4%	8.0%	2.3	10.4%

*Lifetime risk (cumulative incidence) of disease estimated from the literature. Disease frequency in the population was used when available instead of disease frequency in siblings of controls.

From Khoury et al. (1982b) for neural tube defects, del Junco et al. (1984) for rheumatoid arthritis, Sattin et al. (1985) and Zdeb (1977) for breast cancer.

factors shared among sibs, with a single gene disorder having reduced penetrance (perhaps where the disorder requires the presence of some environmental factor), with a multifactorial model for liability, with etiologic heterogeneity among different families, or practically any combination of the above. Further analytic approaches (both epidemiologic and genetic) are required to distinguish among these competing explanations.

6.4.2. Family History Scores

Although it is not always simple to stratify family history information, it is imperative to quantitate the risk associated with having different configurations of affected relatives. For example, it is intuitive that an individual (age 45) whose father died of heart disease at age 56, and whose only sister developed coronary heart disease before the age of 60, has a greater risk than an individual (also age 45) whose father died of heart disease at age 75, and who has 4 of 5 older sibs who are healthy, but one sister, age 68, who has been diagnosed with angina. Both have a positive family history with two affected first-degree relatives, but some consideration should be given to the age distribution of those relatives.

A more systematic approach to quantitating family history involves calculating the expected number of affected family members based on demographic information (age, sex, race, and possibly birth cohort). Estimates of cumulative incidence rates derived from appropriate population surveys or registries are multiplied by the total person-years at risk for the family to calculate the expected number of cases for a family. If gender is a risk factor for the disease, the person-years for females would be separated for the person-years for males. Person-years at risk should be based on the age at data collection (examination or interview) for unaffected persons, the age at diagnosis for affected family members, or the age at death for deceased relatives, as appropriate. If possible, gender, race, and perhaps time-specific incidence rates should be used to compute the expected number of cases. This expected number (E_i) for the ith family is then compared to the observed number (O_i) to give a summary family history (FH) score for this family as

$$FH_i = \frac{O_i - E_i}{(E_i)^{1/2}},$$ (6-2)

where $O_i = \Sigma O_{ij}$ and $E_i = \Sigma E_{ij}$ for all j members of the ith family. This is a standardized form of a Poisson variable, where the mean and variance are identical (A.G. Schwartz et al., 1988). The distribution of family history scores is typically centered around zero, but with a skewed tail composed of families with higher than expected rates of disease. A.G. Schwartz and colleagues (1988) used this family history score also to identify low-risk families for confirmed cancers, where the observed disease risk appeared substantially less than expected. Reed and colleagues (1986) used this same FH score in a study of lipids in young adults, and found an excess frequency of heart disease in families of individuals with high-risk lipid profiles.

Williams and associates (1983) proposed a slightly different form of this family history score, which is

$$FH_i^* = \frac{|O_i - E_i| - 0.5}{(E_i)^{1/2}} \cdot \frac{|O_i - E_i|}{O_i - E_i} \quad \text{if } |O_i - E_i| > 0.5$$

$$= 0 \qquad\qquad\qquad\qquad\qquad \text{if } |O_i - E_i| \leq 0.5.$$

(6-3)

Note the 0.5 in the numerator is merely a correction for small cell sizes, while the second term of this formula merely preserves the sign of the deviation from expected. These modified FH_i^* values can still become unstable when the expected number of events (E_i) is small due to small families, a young age distribution among relatives, or both. Therefore, the computed FH_i^* is often recoded to be less than 1 if a single affected member were responsible for a high score.

Family history scores directly quantitate the disease risk in a family, but they can also be categorized into groups of essentially negative family history $(FH < 0.5)$, mild positive family history $(0.5 \leq FH < 1.0)$, definite positive family history $(1.0 \leq FH < 2.0)$, and very strong family history $(FH \geq 2.0)$. Hunt and colleagues (1986) grouped FH^* scores into categories to identify subsets of families at high risk for developing coronary heart disease in a retrospective cohort study of families ascertained through high-school students in Utah. They concluded that the family history scores could serve to identify families or individuals at highest risk for developing disease over short-term periods. Furthermore, they showed that the FH^* scores themselves showed a dose-response relationship with risk over time in a reconstructed cohort, suggesting they can also serve as a quantitative measure of risk to individuals. Reed and colleagues (1990) showed that family history score is a useful predictor for risk to heart disease, one which is independent of observed lipid levels.

Williams et al. (1983) note that the majority of families in the population have FH scores near zero for a wide variety of chronic diseases (including coronary heart disease, diabetes, and hypertension), and this brings up the problem of assessing the statistical significance of a particular FH score. A small family, with one or two cases of a disease in a sex or age group that normally has very low risk, may in truth be a "high-risk" family, while a large family with several cases of disease in sex or age groups that normally have high risks should not be classified automatically as "high-risk." A.G. Schwartz and colleagues (1988) used a bootstrap approach to generate a distribution of FH scores for permuted "families" of identical structure to the observed families. Here the age-sex-cohort structure of the family was preserved, but unrelated individuals were randomly assigned to be members over a series of replicates to give a sense of the possible distribution of the FH score under the null hypothesis. Comparing the observed FH values to these generated values provides a test of the null hypothesis that disease risk is completely uniform across families. Using data on confirmed cancers in families of fertile women, A.G. Schwartz and colleagues (1988) showed that not only was there a significant deviation from this null hypothesis, but there were distinct groups of *both* "high-risk" and "low-risk" families that could be identified. In another study of breast cancer among families ascertained through cases and controls, Schwartz and colleagues (1991) confirmed that case families were at higher risk of disease overall. In addition, there was evidence for significant heterogeneity in risk among case families. This heterogeneity in risk among case families suggests a small fraction of all breast cancer may be due to a genetic factor segregating in some families.

In another approach to testing for excess risk in families proposed by Chakraborty and associates (1984), the observed vector of outcomes (affected or not) on a family of size n is compared to the baseline risks and standardized by the expected variance in risk. Specifically, this T-statistic is computed for every family with observed vector $\mathbf{Y'} = (Y_1, Y_2, \ldots, Y_n)$ as

$$T(\mathbf{Y}) = \sum_{i=1}^{n} \frac{(Y_i - p_i)^2}{p_i(1 - p_i)}, \tag{6-4}$$

where p_i is the expected risk for the ith member of the family based on population based estimates of risk (usually age-, sex-, and race-specific rates). The probability of any observed $T(\mathbf{Y})$ value can be computed by assuming that the n observed outcomes are completely independent events, and this is merely the probability that a given vector $(\mathbf{Y})$ of binomial variables is observed, that is,

$$P(T(\mathbf{Y})) = P(\mathbf{Y} = \mathbf{y}) = \prod_{i=1}^{n} p_i^{y_i} (1 - p_i)^{(1 - y_i)}. \tag{6-5}$$

Even though it is simple to compute this test statistic and its associated probability for a family of size n, there is no well-recognized distribution for these T-statistics to establish a critical cutoff value for rejecting the null hypothesis of no excess risk. Therefore, it becomes necessary to generate the distribution of all possible T-statistics for each individual family. There are 2^n possible combinations of binary outcomes for any family of size n, ranging from no affected members to all members affected. By computing the T-statistic and its corresponding probability for all such outcomes and then ranking them by their probability, a cumulative probability cutoff value can be assigned (e.g., the 95th percentile or the 99th percentile). Families whose observed $T(\mathbf{Y})$ values fall beyond the cut-point can then be identified as having higher than expected risk of disease.

The T-statistics are relatively easy to compute, especially for small families (where 2^n does not become computationally burdensome), and have been applied in several studies of familial risk to cancers. Bale and colleagues (1984) identified groups of families at excess risk for colon cancer, and Chakraborty et al (1984) showed an excess risk for certain cancers in families ascertained through a patient with retinoblastoma. These T-statistics rely exclusively on group-specific disease rates (either prevalences or cumulative incidences), however, and calculation of the baseline risks (p_i) are critical. Relying on population-derived risks appropriate for sex, age, and race-specific groups does not take into account censoring of observations on family members either from competing causes of death or simple loss to follow-up (Chakraborty, 1985). While appropriate use of cumulative incidence rates among age and sex groups can alleviate the first problem, the latter is more difficult and likely would demand either external information on rates of loss to follow-up or more explicit models. Lubin and Bale (1987) point out that when appropriate baseline risks (usually cumulative incidence rates) are available, these T-statistics have the expected rates of type I error in testing the null hypothesis of no excess risk, even for small families. However, when only crude group-specific prevalence rates are used, the null hypothesis will be rejected more often than expected, and T-statistics can erroneously indicate the presence of families at excess risk.

While both the family history scores and the T-statistics have appealing features, it is important to recognize their limitations. Because of the complexity of family structures possible in any data set, and due to the critical reliance on incidence rate information, it may not always be feasible to adopt either of these measures. Furthermore, there is the limitation of not having a convenient expected distribution for either of these statistics. The bootstrap approach developed by A. G. Schwartz and colleagues (1988, 1991) is computationally intensive and somewhat cumbersome. In the end, while these approaches are not designed to identify specific causal mechanisms, they can be useful in identifying subgroups of families at highest risk for a disease for either more detailed study to define etiology or as part of a planned intervention study.

6.4.3. Lack of Independence Among Relatives

From an epidemiologic perspective, statistical analysis of family data is always hampered by the intrinsic lack of independence among relatives, a situation that invalidates many of the assumptions of standard statistical tests. While it is feasible to select subsets of relatives that do not lead to the violation of a particular model (e.g., pairs of spouses are usually genetically unrelated, or a single pair of biologic relatives from each family can be used to predict one individual's outcome, given the other), this approach is generally wasteful in that it does not utilize all family members. New statistical methods have recently been developed that modify classic analytic models and relax the assumption of strict independence among family members.

For simple analyses of binary outcomes, the classic chi-square test for independence can still be used to test for independence in disease status in pairs of relatives. A simple 2×2 table can be constructed as shown in Table 6–10, where the cells contain the counts of all unique, unordered pairs of relatives in a single class (e.g., sets of twins or all unique pairs of sibs). In Table 6–10, O_A is the observed number of affected pairs, O_D is the number of unaffected pairs, while O_B is the number of discordant pairs where one relative is affected and the other is not. Since the ordering of individuals within a pair is irrelevant in this situation, $O_B = O_C$ and, thus, there are only three independent observations for any set of data. When all the data come as independent pairs (i.e., k, the number of individuals in a class, is fixed at

2, as in twin studies), the classic chi-square test of independence, as shown in Table 6–10, can be used to test for familial aggregation in risk. If there is aggregation within families, such that members of a family tend to be alike, there will be fewer discordant pairs than expected under the null hypothesis (Hunt et al., 1986).

If the size of a set of relatives is greater than 2, however, obtaining all unique, unordered pairs of relatives entails multiple counting of individuals, and this can create an intrinsic dependence among the pairs in such a 2×2 table. For example, for a sibship of size 3, there are 3 possible pairs (sib 1 and sib 2, sib 1 and sib 3, sib 2 and sib 3). Clearly, these pairs are not independent, because each individual appears in 2 distinct pairs. As the num-

Table 6–10. Calculating a chi-square test statistic testing for independence in the disease status in a single class of relatives

A 2×2 table is constructed containing all unique unordered pairs of sibs from N sibships each of size k. Cell A contains all concordant affected pairs, cell D contains all concordant unaffected pairs, while cell B contains all discordant pairs (since ordering within a pair is not considered, $O_C = O_B$).

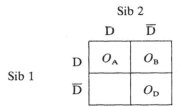

There are N (k choose 2) pairs, thus the overall probability of being affected, p, is estimated as

$$p = \frac{O_A + O_B/2}{N \binom{k}{2}} \tag{1}$$

Denoting $q = 1 - p$, this can be used to compute expected values for each cell as

$$E_A = p^2 N \binom{k}{2} \qquad E_B = 2pqN \binom{k}{2} \qquad E_D = q^2 N \binom{k}{2}$$

under the null hypothesis of complete independence. The usual chi-square goodness-of-fit statistic is

$$\chi^2 = \frac{(O_A - E_A)^2}{E_A} + \frac{(O_B - E_B)^2}{E_B} + \frac{(O_D - E_D)^2}{E_D}$$

$$= \frac{(O_B - E_B)^2}{N \binom{k}{2} 4p^2q^2}$$

Thus, this statistic is solely a function of the observed deviation of discordant pairs from their expectation and the marginal probabilities of disease. As the degree of clustering within family increases, there will be fewer discordant pairs of either type.

Adapted from Hunt et al. (1986).

ber of sibs (k) increases, more of the resulting pairs will be nonoverlapping (i.e., when a pair of pairs is examined, it will more often represent 4 unique people), but there will always be some multiple counting of individuals. For example, even when $k = 7$, fully 50% of all pairs of pairs of sibs will represent only 3 unique people.

Nonetheless, if the null hypothesis *is* true and sibs are independent of one another with respect to risk, then using the usual formula shown in Table 6–10 would still produce a test statistic that approximates a chi-square distribution with 1 degree of freedom (for large N). While this may seem counterintuitive, it is reasonable to say that, if sibs are truly independent of one another in risk, it will not matter if any one sib appeared in several pairs when constructing the final table. Under the null hypothesis, therefore, the test statistic is *not* affected by this multiple counting of individuals within a family, and it is thus perfectly valid to compute the statistic shown in Table 6–10 to test for clustering of a disease within a single class of relatives.

Hunt and coworkers (1986) extended this approach to consider two classes of relatives from each family, for example, parents and offspring. When dealing with a test for independence between two separate classes of relatives, the 2×2 table now contains counts of affected parents and offspring, affected parent–unaffected offspring pairs, unaffected parent–affected offspring pairs, and pairs where neither member is affected, respectively. Using the marginal probability of being affected in the two separate classes, and the marginal probability of having a discordant pair within the two separate classes (that is itself a measure of familial aggregation within a class), Hunt and colleagues (1986) developed a weight for the usual goodness-of-fit statistic which provides a valid test of independence in risk across two classes of relatives.

While this approach for testing the null hypothesis of independence in risk using simple goodness-of-fit statistics is a useful tool for identifying familial aggregation of a disease, it cannot go beyond accepting or rejecting this single null hypothesis. The odds ratio of being affected, given an affected relative, can, of course, be estimated but it is not straightforward to compute valid standard errors in the presence of dependent observations. Furthermore, this approach cannot discriminate among the effects of observable risk factors, unobserved genetic factors, or unobserved environmental factors. More specific statistical models are required, and these too must account for the dependence among relatives (see section 6.5.3.).

6.5. EPIDEMIOLOGIC APPROACHES TO CAUSES OF FAMILIAL AGGREGATION

Once evidence of familial aggregation is found, the next step is to identify the causes of such clustering. Since both genes and environmental factors cluster in families, investigators must keep an open mind regarding causes of familial clustering. Both genetic and environmental factors seem to be operating in most common chronic diseases, and some effort must be made to sort out their independent effects. In the presence of differential genetic susceptibility to the effects of environmental factors, measures of relative risk associated with exposure to that observable environmental factor and measures of familial aggregation can both be diluted toward unity (see Chapter 5). Thus, it is possible to overlook both genetic and environmental effects even when they are operating. Such dilution of the relative risk measure in relatives is also illustrated in Table 6–8, where the incomplete penetrance of an autosomal dominant gene (which could be related to the presence of the environmental factors) leads to a marked lowering of the expected relative risk in sibs. The ability to distinguish between effects of genetic and environmental factors depends, in part, on study design as well as how specific genetic and environmental factors are treated in the analysis.

6.5.1. Study Design

Epidemiologic studies can address, to some extent, the underlying causes of familial aggregation by design, analytical approach or a combination of both. Family studies can attempt to separate the effects of genetic from environmental factors. Although the excess familial risk found in family studies based on the traditional case control design cannot be directly separated into that due to genetic or environmental factors, other study designs are more useful in separating those effects. As discussed in section 6.3 and shown in Table 6–7, twin studies and adoption studies provide clues to the relative importance of genetic factors, and the family set design can provide measures of familial aggregation while controlling for specific environmental risk factors.

As an example, Stunkard and associates (1986) examined the role of genetic factors in a sample of 540 adult adoptees from the Danish adoption register, and reported a strong relationship between the weight class of the adoptees (grouped into five classes ranging from thin to obese) and the body mass index of their biologic parents, but not that of their adoptive parents. Selection bias in terms of preferential placement of adoptees could be ruled out in this study. These findings suggest important genetic determinants for body size and obesity. However, these authors note "the demonstration of a genetic influence tells us little about possible correlation and interaction between heredity and the environment. We do not know, for example, how a genetic predisposition to fatness may be affected by environmental factors." The advantages of separating the genetic from environmental effects by study design are not always apparent. For example, in the case of twin studies, as discussed in the subsection "Twin Studies" above, there may be unexpected biases built to the study design that make the separation of genetic from environmental factors quite difficult.

6.5.2. Analytic Approaches

In addition to trying to sort out genetic factors by some of the designs described above, it is important to collect information on specific, observable environmental risk factors from each relative. Such factors may explain part of the observed familial aggregation of a disease, either by acting as confounders vis-à-vis genetic factors, or by interacting with specific genetic mechanisms in causing disease among susceptible individuals. Statistical modeling on family data without regard to such environmental factors cannot satisfactorily consider, adjust for, or rule out the presence of specific environmental agents affecting risk unless such information is systematically collected and examined for relatives as well as probands.

Environmental Factors in Relatives

For example, in trying to explain why lung cancer aggregates in families, it is crucial to collect information regarding cigarette smoking on each individual relative. This point is illustrated in a case-control study by Tokuhata and Lilienfeld (1963) in which relatives were classified according to their own smoking status in addition to the smoking status of the index cases and controls. Results from this analysis are summarized in Table 6–11. It is clear that the proportion of deaths from lung cancer in first-degree relatives depended both on the biologic relationship to a case or a control (a measure of familial "exposure"), as well as on the relatives' own smoking habits. From these data, the excess familial risk of lung cancer seems to be present among both smoker and nonsmoker relatives of lung cancer cases, but with different magnitudes. In other words, smoking did not seem to act only as a *confounding factor* in this instance. Recall, from Chapter 3, that a confounder is a variable associated with both the disease outcome and the risk factor (here being related to a case versus a control). The suggestion that smoking might be a confounder is reasonable, since (1) smoking is an important risk factor for lung cancer, and (2) relatives of lung cancer cases have a higher rate of smoking than relatives of controls (Tokuhata and Lilienfeld, 1963).

The study of Tokuhata and Lilienfeld illustrates the concept of *interaction* between familial and environmental factors. From Table 6–11, one can infer that the combined effect of smoking and being a relative of a case is more than the merely additive effect of each alone on the final risk of lung cancer. This suggests some biologic interaction between smoking and familial susceptibility factors (be they genetic or environmental). Nonetheless, this example underscores the need to measure any known risk factors for disease

Table 6–11. Percentage of lung cancer deaths in first-degree relatives of lung cancer cases and controls by own smoking status

		Among relatives	
Index	Smoking status of relative	% Lung cancer deaths	Relative risk
Control	Nonsmoker	0.28	1.0
Case	Nonsmoker	1.11	4.0
Control	Smoker	1.47	5.3
Case	Smoker	3.82	13.6

Adapted from Tokuhata and Lilienfeld (1963).

in a family study. The approach can be extended to other observable covariates in relatives such as age, sex, race, behavioral habits, and occupational exposures, if such information is available.

Can familial aggregation of an environmental risk factor account for familial aggregation of disease in the absence of any genetic susceptibility? Clearly, it is possible for environmental factors to produce familial clustering and the expected degree of familial aggregation will depend on the disease frequency, the exposure frequency, and the extent of familial aggregation of the risk factor. Familial clustering of infectious agents such as kuru and hepatitis B provides a good example of such nongenetic familial aggregation (Bennett et al., 1959; Blumberg et al., 1966). However, for etiologically heterogeneous diseases that manifest strong evidence of familial aggregation (e.g., certain birth defects), it can be shown, on theoretical grounds, that environmental risk factors alone are unlikely to account for such strong familial aggregation, unless the presumed environmental factors are associated with extreme relative risks (100 or more) and show extreme patterns of familial clustering (Khoury et al., 1988b). It has been difficult to document such environmental factors in birth defects studies to date.

Genetic Traits in Relatives

In addition to measuring environmental risk factors in relatives, investigators can also collect data on genetic markers that may be associated with the disease. If a genetic marker is associated with the disease, it may reflect a cause-effect relationship, an association due to linkage disequilibrium, or confounding (see Chapter 9). There are several reasons for routinely including genetic marker data in family studies.

First, such measured genetic markers could be partially responsible for the observed familial aggregation, especially if markers at or near candidate genes are selected. Because of the likely etiologic heterogeneity of most chronic diseases, however, one should not expect to attribute familial aggregation to one single mechanism. For example, in the case of the α-1 antitrypsin deficiency due to the PiZ phenotype, some familial aggregation in emphysema could be expected to be attributed to this simple genetic marker. However, due to its rarity, this deficiency genotype (i.e., *PiZ* homozygote) accounts for very little of all emphysema or other forms of COPD in the general population. Studies have shown that there is substantial familial aggregation in COPD even after taking into account effects of this genetic marker (Cohen, 1980; Khoury et al., 1985a). Methods of adjustment for measured genetic traits in case-control studies can be similar to adjustment procedures for other risk factors. Adjustment for measured genotypes in population studies can reveal important phenotypic effects directly attributable to alleles at the marker locus, either for risk of disease or quantitative traits associated with the disease. Such associations can point out areas for fruitful investigation.

Second, measured genetic markers can be extremely useful in extending genetic analyses. More explicit tests of association between markers and disease using either affected sibs or other relatives can be easily incorporated into family studies. These approaches test for association between marker alleles shared among affected relatives by comparing the observed distribution of shared markers to that expected under independence. The presence of a strong statistical association may indicate genetic linkage or a causal association. Finding cosegregation (i.e., genetic linkage) between a marker locus and a disease provides strong statistical evidence for genetic control of the disease in itself, as discussed in more detail in Chapter 9.

Third, measuring genetic markers in family studies gives an opportunity to test for specific genetic-environmental interactions that may be related to the disease. For example, the effects of cigarette smoking on the airways may be more deleterious in individuals who carry the α_1-antitrypsin deficiency allele. In this instance, one should expect to see distinct patterns reflecting statistical interaction between these genetic and environmental factors in either predicting the risk of airways obstruction both in families of affected individuals and in the population at large. From this, the effects of specific environmental factors on identifiable genotypes can clarify risk patterns in families and possibly provide a better understanding of pathogenetic mechanisms.

6.5.3. Adjusting for Covariates in Family Studies

Measures of familial aggregation summarize the increased risk of being affected given a relative is known to be affected. For most chronic diseases, however, there are usually other recognized risk factors that directly influence risk also. Whenever possible, information on such covariates must be collected on each individual relative and incorporated into the analysis. The example of lung cancer and smoking in Table 6–11 illustrates the importance of considering risk factors in relatives.

Extensions to Matched Case-Control Studies

For relatives of matched case and control pairs, observed risk factors can be incorporated by extending the traditional logistic regression model. Under this model, the log-odds of a relative's being affected is expressed as a linear function of his or her own covariates, while the status of the index (case versus control) serves as one additional independent variable, that is,

$$\ln \frac{P(Y_{ij} = 1)}{1 - P(Y_{ij} = 1)} = \alpha + \beta X_{ij} + \gamma\, \delta_{ij}, \tag{6-6}$$

where Y_{ij} is the outcome on the jth relative from the ith strata (the ith case-control pair), X_{ij} is the vector of covariates on this person, and δ_{ij} represents an indicator which is 1 if the ijth person is a relative of a case and 0 otherwise. This coefficient γ reflects the increase in risk associated with being ascertained through a case, and exp (γ) is the odds ratio comparing risk in relatives of cases to that in relatives of controls. Liang (1987) employed a pseudolikelihood approach that uses all possible pairs of relatives of cases and relatives of controls within each stratum to obtain estimators for β and γ that are statistically consistent and do not depend on assuming complete independence among relatives of cases and controls.

This approach of converting a test for the odds ratio in a 2×2 table into a logistic regression model allows simultaneous consideration of risk factors on family members and the status of the index (case or control) when testing for familial aggregation. It also makes prediction of risk somewhat more straightforward. Maestri and coworkers (1988) used this approach to show that some forms of congenital cardiovascular malformations do show significant familial aggregation (i.e., relatives of cases are at higher risk compared to relatives of controls), while other types of heart malformations do not. Thus, appropriate analysis of families ascertained through a case-control study can confirm the existence of familial aggregation and can also aid in identifying heterogeneous subgroups of disease.

Incorporating Covariate Effects into Tests for Pairwise Association

More explicit statistical models based first on log-linear and later on logistic regression models can incorporate observed risk factors (covariates), parameters measuring the degree of familial aggregation of risk. Hopper and colleagues (1984) suggested a restricted class of log-linear models might be more suitable for analysis of binary data from families because it requires relatively few assumptions about the exact underlying processes. By assuming no second-order or higher level interactions in a standard log-linear model, Hopper and Derrick (1986) demonstrated how data from families of different sizes and structure can be used to estimate both within class and among class "correlations" for binary data as functions of their odds ratios. Under the approach of Hopper and colleagues (1984), the first-order interaction term can be interpreted as a conditional log odds ratio measuring familial aggregation (conditional on the observed structure of the rest of the family). A similar application was developed by Connolly and Liang (1988), where the count of all affected relatives becomes an independent variable to predict risk to the jth member of the ith family (of size n_i), that is,

$$\ln \frac{P(Y_{ij}|X_{ij}, Y_{ij'})}{1 - P(Y_{ij}|X_{ij}, Y_{ij'})} = \alpha + \beta X_{ij} + \gamma \sum_{j' \neq j}^{n_i} Y_{ij'}, \tag{6-7}$$

where X_{ij} is a vector of observed covariates on the ijth individual and the last term represents the sum over all relatives other than this ijth individual. Under this model, exp (γ) has the interpretation of being the pairwise odds ratio reflecting the risk associated with having one affected relative, independent of effects of the individual's own covariates. Connolly and Liang (1988) developed a pseudolikelihood approach for estimating the parameters of this model $(\alpha, \beta, \text{ and } \gamma)$ which gives estimators that are almost as efficient as conventional maximum likelihood estimators. This pseudolikelihood approach involves modeling conditional probabilities of all possible pairs of relatives within a family, and therefore is less cumbersome than a true likelihood approach.

An alternative approach to modeling multivariate binary data in a conditional approach (as in Equation 6-7) is to specify fixed effects separately from the correlation structure, as is done for continuous data in Chapter 7. Here the log-odds of the expected value is written as

$$\ln \frac{P(Y_{ij}|X_{ij})}{1 - P(Y_{ij}|X_{ij})} = \alpha + \beta X_{ij} \qquad (6\text{-}8)$$

for the jth member of the ith family, just like in the usual logistic regression. The dependency among family members can be summarized by the odds ratio

$$OR(Y_{ij} = Y_{ik}) = \frac{P(Y_{ij} = Y_{ik} = 1)\, P(Y_{ij} = Y_{ik} = 0)}{P(Y_{ij} = 1,\, Y_{ik} = 0)\, P(Y_{ij} = 0,\, Y_{ik} = 1)} = \gamma, \qquad (6\text{-}9)$$

which can either be constant among all family members or can be specific to certain classes of relatives (Liang et al., 1991; Qaqish and Liang, 1992). The generalized estimating equation approach provides consistent and robust estimators for this model (Liang and Zeger, 1986). While these models have limitations that can be severe in situations where data are sparse, they do offer the opportunity to examine directly both familial aggregation of disease and the effects of observable risk factors. Liang and Beaty (1991) used family data on relatives of Chinese liver cancer patients to illustrate this approach. One advantage of this regression approach is that the odds ratio measuring familial aggregation is independent of family size, while it is not in the model proposed independently by Hopper and colleagues (1984) or Connolly and Liang (1988).

Regressive Logistic Models

An alternative approach for using logistic models on family data is described by Bonney (1986), where the observations within a family are ordered in some logical fashion (e.g., father, mother, sib 1, sib 2, . . .), and the risk to any individual is written as a function of the outcomes of all preceding relatives. The probability of any observed ($n \times 1$) vector of outcomes $\mathbf{Y}$ in a family, given the observed ($n \times p$) matrix of covariates $\mathbf{X}$ on all family members can be written as a product of a series of conditional probabilities, that is,

$$P(\mathbf{Y}|\mathbf{X}) = P(Y_1|\mathbf{X})\, P(Y_2|Y_1, \mathbf{X}) \cdots P(Y_n|Y_1, Y_2, \cdots, Y_{n-1}, \mathbf{X}). \qquad (6\text{-}10)$$

If one is also willing to assume that the covariates $\mathbf{X}_i$ for the ith individual influence only his or her own risk, any term of this series can be written

$$P(Y_i|Y_1, Y_2, \cdots, Y_{i-1}, \mathbf{X}) = P(Y_i|Y_1, Y_2, \cdots, Y_{i-1}, X_i). \qquad (6\text{-}11)$$

Under this sequential approach, a conventional logistic model can be written where the outcome on the ith individual is expressed as a function of their own observed covariates and some (but not necessarily all) relatives, although the set of independent variables would be different for every individual in a family. To avoid the complexity of a constantly changing set of independent variables, however, one can simply substitute a linear function of these Y_i's into a similar logistic regression while retaining the essential form of this regressive logistic model. Consider, for example, the simple linear function $Z(Y)$, which is defined as

$$Z_{ij} = \begin{cases} 2Y_{ij} - 1 & \text{if } j < i \\ 0 & \text{if } j \geq i \end{cases} \tag{6-12}$$

such that the independent variable Z_{ij} is 1 if the jth preceding relative for the ith individual was affected, -1 if this jth relative is not affected, and 0 if the jth relative does *not* precede the ith individual in the ordered vector of family members. Table 6–12 shows the relationship between the original observed outcome (i.e., the Y_i's) and the resulting Z_{ij}'s of this regressive logistic model. In essence, this approach forces family data into a univariate logistic regression model on n independent variables without the problem of a constantly changing set of independent variables, while retaining the interpretation of both the coefficients for the covariates and the observations on preceding relatives. This logistic regressive model can be written as

$$\ln \frac{P(Y_i|Y, X_i)}{1 - P(Y_i|Y, X_i)} = \alpha + \beta X_i + \gamma_1 Z_{i,1} + \cdots + \gamma_{i-1} Z_{i,j-1}$$
$$+ \gamma_i Z_{i,j} + \cdots + \gamma_{n-1} Z_{i,n-1} \tag{6-13}$$

where, as noted above, $Z_{ij} = 0$ for any $j \geq i$, that is, only the lower triangular portion of the $(n \times n - 1)$ matrix is nonzero.

Table 6–12. Expressing family data in the format of a logistic regressive model

Outcome	Covariate	Outcome on preceding relatives
		Independent variables
		Observed
Y_1	X_1	
Y_2	X_2	Y_1
Y_3	X_3	$Y_1 Y_2$
$\vdots$	$\vdots$	$\vdots$
Y_n	X_n	$Y_1 Y_2 Y_3, \ldots, Y_{n-1}$
		Transformed
Y_1	X_1	$Z_{11} Z_{12} Z_{13}, \ldots, Z_{1n-1}$
Y_2	X_2	$Z_{21} Z_{22} Z_{23}, \ldots, Z_{2n-2}$
Y_3	X_3	$Z_{31} Z_{32} Z_{33}, \ldots, Z_{3n-1}$
$\vdots$	$\vdots$	$\cdots$
Y_n	X_n	$Z_{n1} Z_{n2} Z_{n3}, \ldots, Z_{nn-1}$

Note that $Z_{ij} = 2Y_{ij} - 1$ if $j < 1$, and $= 0$ if $j \geq 1$. Therefore, the upper triangular portion of the $(n \times n - 1)$ matrix Z is composed entirely of zeros.
Adapted from Bonney (1986).

While this regressive approach has succeeded in converting a multivariate problem with dependent data into a univariate problem which can easily be handled by standard statistical packages, for data sets containing a few large families there will be a large number of parameters to be estimated with very little information for many of the parameters (specifically, the γ_j's). It is also important to realize that the ordering of individuals with the vector of family data is the basis for this model, and changing the ordering scheme will create a different statistical model on a single set of family data. Estimators for coefficients and their standard errors may not be similar if the ordering is changed.

Nonetheless, for nuclear family data, it is a reasonable approach to assume that parents are independent of one another and children in the family are dependent solely because of their common parentage. The corresponding logistic regressive model for fathers would then be

$$\ln \frac{P(Y_F|X_F)}{1 - P(Y_F|X_F)} = \alpha + \beta_F X_F, \tag{6-14}$$

for mothers, it would be

$$\ln \frac{P(Y_M|(X_M)}{1 - P(Y_M|X_M)} = \alpha + \beta_M X_M, \tag{6-15}$$

and for the ith child among n in the family, it would be

$$\ln \frac{P(Y_i|X_i)}{1 - P(Y_i|X_i)} = \alpha + \beta_i X_i + \gamma_F Z_F + \gamma_M Z_M \qquad i = 1, 2, \ldots, n. \tag{6-16}$$

Under this model, the estimated regression coefficient for any covariate will reflect its impact on risk, where e^β can serve as a measure of the relative risk per unit change in the covariate X. The coefficients γ_F and γ_M reflect the change in risk associated with having an affected father and mother, respectively. Negative values mean children of affected parents are less likely to be affected, while positive values mean children of affected parents are more likely to be affected compared to the baseline group. Recall that the Z values for parents are always zero in this regressive model; thus only information from children contribute to the estimators for γ_F and γ_M. The intercepts (the α's) may be varied among fathers, mothers, and children. Also, tests for possible interactions among the Z's and the vector of covariates $\mathbf{X}$ can be made by simple manipulations of the matrix of independent variables.

These regressive models are quite versatile and can be extended to formal genetic analysis (see Chapter 8). Hopper and colleagues (1990) compared the log-linear approach described above with a particular class of logistic regressive models, and noted regressive models were more computationally efficient and at times offered greater insight into the various patterns of familial aggregation.

6.6. CONCLUDING REMARKS

Epidemiologic approaches can be used to identify and quantitate familial aggregation of disease while considering the impact of observable risk factors.

Family data for such studies can be collected in a number of ways ranging from unconfirmed reports of disease among relatives to extensive and direct observation on all family members. Constraints of resources often determine how family data are actually collected. The statistical analysis of family data can likewise range in complexity from simple tests of the null hypothesis of independence in risk of disease among relatives to simultaneous estimation of the impact of observed covariates on an individual's risk and the impact on risk of having one or more affected relatives.

It is important to understand, however, that these epidemiologic approaches are not explicitly designed to test specific genetic models which may underlie familial aggregation. Once familial aggregation has been identified, further analysis is then needed to separate effects of genetic and environmental factors shared among family members. Subsequently, tests of specific genetic models of inheritance may be done, as described in the following three chapters.

7

Genetic Approaches to Familial Aggregation

I. Analysis of Heritability

7.1 INTRODUCTION

After documenting familial aggregation for a trait or disease, and showing that this aggregation cannot be explained completely by environmental risk factors, the next logical step is to ask how much of the familial aggregation can be attributed to genetic causes. *Heritability* is typically used to answer this question because it is defined as the proportion of variation directly attributable to genetic differences among individuals relative to the total variation in a population (which includes variation due to both genetic and nongenetic factors).

Historically, the concept of heritability was developed as part of quantitative genetics which focused exclusively on continuous traits (such as height, IQ, serum cholesterol). The statistical techniques used in quantitative genetics were largely derived from analysis of variance. As discussed in section 7.5, however, the concept of heritability can also be applied to qualitative traits by reframing the question to ask how much of the variation in *risk* of disease can be attributed to genetic differences among individuals. In either case, heritability serves to summarize the degree of potential genetic control over an observed phenotype. A high heritability constitutes circumstantial evidence for genetic control of a trait or disease, since it means a large proportion of the phenotypic variation among relatives follows patterns predicted by simple genetic factors. It must be noted, however, that nongenetic factors can conceivably give rise to such patterns of familial aggregation. Furthermore, as discussed below, heritability is, by its nature, a population-specific parameter and must always be used within the context of the sample at hand and its corresponding reference population.

7.2 THE CONCEPT OF HERITABILITY

In quantitative genetics, phenotypes are measured on a continuous scale, and the observed distribution in a sample is frequently unimodal giving little or no evidence for any finite number of distinct genotypes. Consequently, the terminology, summary statistics, and analytic methods used in quantitative genetics are quite different from those of traditional Mendelian genetics, and this is often misinterpreted as implying that quantitative genetics is intrinsically different and separate from Mendelian genetics. This is not true. It is important to remember that all of quantitative genetics implicitly assumes the underlying biologic mechanisms are strictly Mendelian. Furthermore, the goal of quantitative genetics is the same as traditional human genetics, that is, to identify possible genetic mechanisms controlling the distribution of phenotypes in both families and populations.

Because the phenotypes in quantitative genetics are continuous, summary statistics (means, variances, and correlations) must be used to describe a particular sample or population. Table 7–1 contains simple definitions and formulas for some summary statistics used in quantitative genetics. It is noteworthy that the actual value of the individual's phenotype may become extraneous to the analysis, and even the mean and variance of an entire sample may be effectively nuisance parameters, as they can and do vary from sample to sample. Genetic analysis frequently focuses only on correlations or covariances among relatives and attempts to partition these observed correlations (or covariances) into components attributable to shared genes and shared environments. From these components, heritability can be calculated.

7.2.1 Definitions

Heritability is defined as a ratio of variances, specifically, the ratio of the genetic variance (i.e., that attributable to genotypic or allelic differences among individuals) to the total phenotypic variance in the population. It is necessary to measure the degree of genetic control as such a ratio of variances because, when the trait is quantitative, it is not generally possible to distinguish among genotypes in order to estimate genotypic means. Thus, in the absence of extensive experimental or breeding control to isolate genotypes and/or sophisticated statistical analysis to compute genotypic probabilities, a simple summary of how much of the total phenotypic variation could be attributed to differences in unobserved genetic factors must suffice.

Two types of heritability should be distinguished. First, there is *heritability in the broad sense*, which is the ratio of variance attributed to *all* genetic differences among individuals to the total phenotypic variance; and second, there is *heritability in the narrow sense*, which is the ratio of variance contributed by the additive effects of alleles at one or more loci to the total phenotypic variance. Distinctions between these two measures of heritability are discussed later, but broad-sense heritability can be thought of as that proportion of variation attributable to all genotypic differences among indi-

Table 7–1. Common summary statistics used in quantitative genetics

Parameter (symbol)	Estimation formula	Interpretation
Mean (μ)	$$\overline{Y} = \frac{1}{n} \sum_{i=1}^{n} Y_i$$	The arithmetic mean or first central moment of a distribution
Variance (σ^2)	$$\mathrm{Var}\,(Y) = \frac{\frac{1}{n} \sum_{i=1}^{n} (Y_i - \overline{Y})^2}{n-1}$$ $$= \frac{\sum Y_i^2 - \frac{(\sum Y_i)^2}{n}}{n-1}$$	A measure of dispersion about the mean, also called the second central moment Computational formula
Standard deviation (σ)	$$\hat{\sigma} = \sqrt{\mathrm{Var}\,(Y)}$$	The square root of the variance which restores the original unit of scale
Covariance (σ_{xy})	$$\mathrm{cov}\,(XY) = \sum_{i=1}^{n} (X_i - \overline{X})(Y_i - \overline{Y})$$	A measure of similarity between two variables, ranging from $-\infty$ to $+\infty$
Interclass Correlation (ρ)	$$r = \frac{\Sigma(X_i - \overline{X})\,(Y_i - \overline{Y})}{\sigma_x \sigma_y}$$	A standardized covariance between paired observations X and Y. Ranges between -1 and 1
Intraclass Correlation* (ρ_I)	$$r_I = \frac{(\mathrm{MSA} - \mathrm{MSW})}{[\mathrm{MSA} + (n-1)\,\mathrm{MSW}]}$$	The common correlation in a trait shared by n members of a group. Ranges between $-1/(n-1)$ and 1

*Based on 1-way ANOVA where MSA = mean squared deviation among groups and MSW = mean squared deviation within groups

viduals, while narrow-sense heritability can be thought of as variation attributable to differences among alleles at one or more Mendelian loci.

It is important to remember that both these measures of heritability are ratios of a genetic component of variance to the total variance, and thus they must both lie between 0 and 1.0. The lower limit of zero heritability occurs when all of the observed phenotypic variation is attributable to nongenetic factors, while the upper limit of 100% heritability exists when there is no phenotypic variation *not* due to genetic differences. The use of such a ratio of variances to summarize the action of biologic entities (genes) has its disadvantages, of course, since the magnitude of this ratio is a function of both the genetic and nongenetic components. In principle, a given phenotypic trait could be under direct Mendelian control, and yet the heritability could be 0 (for example, if all individuals had the same genotype, there would be no genetic variation) or it could approach 1.0 (if there were very little differences in environmental factors influencing the trait, i.e., if there were no nongenetic sources variation).

When studying human populations, therefore, it is always important to consider the impact of small differences in these sources of variation that may well vary across populations. In general, greater diversity of environmental factors present in a population will lower the estimated heritability, while populations with more homogeneous environments will give higher estimates of heritability, even though the biologic mechanism underlying the trait may be identical. Similarly, it is unwise to compare directly populations that differ greatly in their degree of genetic variability. A population that is relatively genetically homogeneous will produce a lower estimate of heritability than will a genetically heterogeneous population. Of course, no human population is truly genetically homogeneous, but it is reasonable to assume small, closed human populations are more genetically homogeneous than larger populations composed of recent mixtures of diverse racial or ethnic groups. As a result, it is hazardous to apply an estimated heritability obtained from one population to another population for predictive purposes. Nonetheless, general patterns of familial aggregation are reflected in estimates of heritability, and these can indicate where genetic mechanisms are operating. The purpose of estimating the heritability of a trait or of risk of disease is to confirm and quantitate familial aggregation, and to identify phenotypes where a more detailed search for a genetic mechanism is warranted.

7.2.2 Estimation From a Simple Linear Model

Many widely used statistical techniques were first developed to measure the degree of family resemblance, and several early statisticians were often motivated by questions of genetic control. As discussed in Chapter 2, the concept of linear regression was first posed by Galton (1887) to summarize the relationship between parents and their adult offspring for a quantitative trait (height). This type of linear regression model is quite general and makes no assumptions about the biologic mechanisms underlying familial resemblance. The purpose of this approach is merely to describe and quantitate the resemblance between pairs of relatives.

A simple linear relationship between height in the offspring (Y_0) and height in one parent (Y_p) can be written as

$$Y_0 = \mu_0 + \beta(Y_p - \mu_p) + e, \tag{7-1}$$

where μ_0 is the mean height of offspring, μ_p is the mean height for parents, and e represents the deviation of observed from predicted offspring's height due to random factors. Here the regression coefficient β summarizes the effect of parent's height on predicting offspring's height. If β is positive, offspring of a tall parent will, on average, be tall (although not necessarily as tall as the parent). In other words, the expected value of height in an offspring conditional on his or her observed parent's height can be written

$$\mathbf{E}(Y_0|Y_p) = \mu_0 + \beta(Y_p - \mu_p), \tag{7-2}$$

merely from the definition of conditional probability (the expected value notation $\mathbf{E}$ is equivalent to finding the mean of a random variable; and here the random variable is the offspring height Y_0 conditional on the parent's height Y_p). The variance of this conditional mean for offspring given one parent's observed height is

$$\text{Var} \{\mathbf{E}(Y_0|Y_p)\} = \text{Var} \{\beta(Y_p - \mu_p)\} = \beta^2 \, \text{Var} \,(Y_p). \qquad (7\text{-}3)$$

Note that the variance of a constant is zero, so both the means (μ_0 and μ_p) drop out when computing this variance. Similarly, when a random variable, here Y_p, is multiplied by a constant, here β, the variance of the resulting product is increased by the square of that constant. This type of simple linear relationship alone would allow a certain degree of success in predicting height of offspring in the next generation, assuming conditions influencing the means and variances remain constant.

Looking at the total variation among offspring Var (Y_0), however, reveals that it too can be written as the sum of two components, one reflecting the expected values of offspring given observations on one parent, and the other component representing the remaining variation about these conditional means, that is,

$$\text{Var} \,(Y_0) = \text{Var} \{\mathbf{E}(Y_0|Y_p)\} + \mathbf{E}\{\text{Var} \,(Y_0|Y_p)\}. \qquad (7\text{-}4)$$

This decomposition of variance in offspring is a consequence of the linear model given in Equation 7-1 (Lindgren, 1976). In essence, the first component reflects the differences among all offspring attributable to differences among their parents, while the second component reflects residual variation in offspring not directly attributable to parental differences.

This partitioning of variance in the sample of offspring permits developing a relationship between the regression coefficient, β, and the coefficient of determination, D, which commonly serves as an assessment of the amount of information conveyed by any linear regression model. The coefficient of determination reflects the reduction in variation in the dependent variables (here Y_0) attributable to the linear relationship with the independent variable (Y_p), that is,

$$D = 1 - \frac{\mathbf{E}[\text{Var} \,(Y_0|Y_p)]}{\text{Var} \,(Y_0)}. \qquad (7\text{-}5)$$

Assuming the means and variances of parents and offspring were equal (i.e., $\mu_0 = \mu_p = \mu$ and Var $(Y_0) = $ Var $(Y_p) = $ Var (Y)) and substituting Equation 7-4 into this numerator, D becomes

$$
\begin{aligned}
D &= \frac{\text{Var} \,(Y_0) - \mathbf{E}[\text{Var} \,(Y_0|Y_p)]}{\text{Var} \,(Y_0)} \\[2ex]
&= \frac{\text{Var} \,\mathbf{E}[(Y_0|Y_p)] + \mathbf{E}[\text{Var} \,(Y_0|Y_p)] - \mathbf{E}[\text{Var} \,(Y_0|Y_p)]}{\text{Var} \,(Y_0)} \\[2ex]
&= \frac{\text{Var} \,[\mathbf{E}(Y_0|Y_p)]}{\text{Var} \,(Y_0)} = \frac{\beta^2 \text{Var} \,(Y_p)}{\text{Var} \,(Y_0)} = \beta^2.
\end{aligned}
\qquad (7\text{-}6)
$$

Thus, the regression coefficient β serves both as a predictive tool and a measure of the reduction in variance among offspring attributable to observing the height of one parent. If there were complete determination ($\beta = 1$), then offspring's height could be predicted without error; if there were no relationship between parent and offspring ($\beta = 0$) with regard to height, the conditional variance in offspring given the parent's value would be the same as its unconditional variance, that is, $D = 0$.

The coefficient of determination from a linear regression of offspring on one parent can therefore serve to measure the phenotypic resemblance between relatives. Specifically, twice this regression coefficient is termed the "empirical" heritability (Jacquard, 1983). Since only one parent was considered here, heritability itself is twice this regression coefficient, that is, $h^2 = 2\beta$. However, if the regression had been on the average of both parents simultaneously (and the two parents were phenotypically independent), a similar estimate of this empirical heritability would be obtained directly (that is, $h^2 = \beta$) from the regression model

$$Y_0 = \mu + \beta \frac{(Y_m + Y_f)}{2} + e \qquad (7\text{-}7)$$

where the $(Y_m + Y_f)/2$ is termed the *midparent value*. In this case again, the square of regression coefficient (β^2) will serve as a measure of the amount of variation in offspring height directly attributable to the observed height of the two parents.

It must be emphasized here that this "empirical heritability" makes *no* assumptions beyond the simple linear model listed in Equation 7-1 with its implied constant error variance along the range of observed parental values. No assumptions about biologic mechanisms are involved; and such mechanisms may involve genetic factors, environmental factors or both. This measure of empirical heritability (i.e., twice the regression coefficient of the child on one parent or the coefficient itself from a regression of the child's values on the average of both parents) can be used to predict offspring phenotype given parental phenotype. However, it is important to appreciate the limitations of such predictions.

Consider the following example from Jacquard (1983): If the empirical heritability were .80 (implying $\beta = .4 = h^2/2$) for a character Y that had a mean of 100 and variance Var $(Y) = 225$ (i.e., a standard deviation of 15, as is the case with standardized intelligence quotients [IQ]), one could predict that children of a parent with a value of 120 would follow a phenotypic distribution with a conditional mean of 108 ($\mathbf{E}(Y_0|Y_p) = 100 + 0.5(0.80)(120 - 100)$), and an expected conditional variance of 189, that is, $\mathbf{E}[\text{Var}\,(Y_0|Y_p)] = \text{Var}\,(Y_0)[1 - (\beta/2)^2] = 225\,(1 - [0.5(0.80)]^2) = 189$. This expected conditional standard deviation is thus 13.75, only 9% less than the standard deviation in the total population despite this seemingly high heritability. The reduction in the standard deviation among offspring due to observing one parent's value is approximately $(1 - h^4/4)^{1/2}$. Thus, while empirical heritability has some predictive value, the final variance among offspring changes relatively little except when the heritability is extremely close to 1, that is, those cases with almost complete determination.

7.3 VARIANCE COMPONENTS MODELS

Most of quantitative genetics involves more elaborate statistical models for estimating heritability. These techniques require additional assumptions about the underlying biologic mechanisms, but they do permit partitioning phenotypic variation into both genetic and nongenetic components, and they do allow greater predictions about the structure of populations under various conditions. The former feature provides estimates of the two types of heritability (narrow-sense and broad-sense heritability) to summarize familial aggregation, while the latter has great utility for designing selection and breeding schemes for domestic plants and animals.

The primary statistical tool for quantitative genetics is analysis of variance, where the observed phenotypic variance is partitioned into components reflecting differences in unobserved genetic factors and environmental factors, both of which must be estimated from covariances or correlations among relatives. This approach assumes an underlying linear model where the observed phenotype, Y, is a linear function of genetic and environmental factors, that is,

$$Y_{kl} = \mu + g_k + c_l + e_{kl},\qquad(7\text{-}8)$$

and where neither the effects of different genotypes (g_k, where $k = 1, \ldots,$ K) nor the various environmental factors (c_l, where $l = 1, \ldots, L$) are directly observable. The classic analysis of variance approach is termed a random-effects model because the parameters of interest are the variances attributable to differences in these genetic or environmental factors rather than the mean of any particular genotype or environment.

If the genotypes and environments are independent, the total variance of the trait, Y, can be written as

$$\text{Var}\,(Y) = \sigma^2 = \sigma_g^2 + \sigma_c^2 + \sigma_e^2\qquad(7\text{-}9)$$

and is merely a sum of these separate components of variance. From this breakdown, the "heritability in the broad sense" $h_B^2 = \sigma_g^2/\sigma^2$ can be obtained. This broad-sense heritability represents the proportion of variation attributable to *all* genetic differences, and would be directly analogous to the β^2, the regression coefficient from a regression of offspring on midparent value *if* there were no shared environmental factors affecting the phenotype of parents and offspring. This decomposition of the total variance is not strictly valid if there is any correlation among the unspecified genetic and environmental factors, nor is it valid if the observed phenotype is a nonlinear function of these two unobserved factors (i.e., the genetic and environmental factors). Since, in human studies, it is rarely possible to control for either correlation or interactions, it is important to understand how disregarding them can influence the final result of the analysis.

When there is a correlation between genotypic factors and environmental factors, the total variance is increased by twice this covariance, that is,

$$\sigma^2 = \sigma_g^2 + \sigma_c^2 + 2 \text{ cov } (gc) + \sigma_e^2. \tag{7-10}$$

In experimental situations, this correlation or covariance can be forced to zero by randomly assigning individuals of different genotypes to different environments. In observational studies of humans, however, it is impossible to force complete independence between genotypes influencing the trait and environmental factors influencing the trait. Ignoring such correlation when it does exist leads to an inflated estimate of the total genetic variance ($\hat{\sigma}_g^2$) and, therefore, an inflated estimate of broad-sense heritability.

When the relationship among different genotypic means is not constant over all environmental conditions, a statistical interaction between genotype and environments is created. This phenomenon is sometimes termed "genotypic instability across environments," and can be illustrated by data on growth of two inbred strains of mice shown in Table 7-2 (where strain serves as the definition of genotype) reared in two defined environments, good and poor nutrition (adapted from Falconer, 1960). While both strains obviously showed less growth under poor nutrition, their relative growth (the strain or genotypic effect) reversed itself across the two nutritional environments. Ideally, this instability across environments should be considered as a part of the total variance. Specifically, the total variance should be written as

$$\sigma^2 = \sigma_g^2 + \sigma_c^2 + 2 \text{ cov } (ge) + \sigma_{ge}^2 + \sigma_e^2, \tag{7-11}$$

and the analysis should attempt to estimate this additional component of variance (Falconer, 1981).

In experimental studies, it is sometimes possible to measure such a component due to genotype-environment interaction by incorporating a linear function measuring the "stability" of an observable genotype (e.g., a pure bred strain of plants or animals) over several observed environmental classes (Bulmer, 1985). However, human studies frequently involve both unobserved genotypes and environments, and it is extremely difficult, if not impossible, to estimate a separate component attributable to genotype-environment interaction. Ignoring such an interaction term leads to an inflated estimate of the environmental variance, and thus an underestimate of the total genetic component ($\hat{\sigma}_g^2$) and the broad-sense heritability. This is illustrated in Table 7-2 where the marginal growth differences between strains A and

Table 7-2. Mean weight gain between 3 and 6 weeks of age in two strains of inbred mice

	Nutrition		
	Good	*Poor*	*Marginal means*
Strain A	17.2	12.6	14.9
Strain B	16.6	13.3	15.0
Means	16.9	13.0	

Adapted from Falconer (1960).

B are effectively concealed by their reversal across the two nutritional environments.

7.3.1 Components of Genetic Variance

The genetic component of variance itself, σ_g^2, represents a sum of distinct components reflecting the different ways in which genes can act. Specifically, the genetic component can be partitioned as

$$\sigma_g^2 = \sigma_A^2 + \sigma_d^2 + \sigma_I^2, \tag{7-12}$$

where σ_A^2 represents the effects of individual alleles on the trait and is termed the *additive genetic variance*, σ_d^2 represents the nonlinear interaction effect between alleles at the same locus or *dominance variance*, and σ_I^2 represents the nonlinear interaction effects between alleles at different loci (termed *epistatic variance*). Most texts define these sources of variation in the context of a single-locus, two-allele model, where the additive effects of an allele represents the average deviation from the overall mean of all genotypes carrying a particular allele, and dominance deviations are computed as the deviation of a heterozygote from the mean of the two appropriate homozygotes (see Figure 7–1). However, it is important to realize that these genetic variance components themselves do not specify how many Mendelian loci may be involved; there may be a single locus with two alleles or there may be many independently segregating loci, each contributing equally to the phenotype (i.e., polygenes). Nonetheless, the interpretation of these genetic components is relatively straightforward.

The *additive genetic variance*, σ_A^2, represents variation in the phenotype which is transmissible from parents to offspring. As such, this component forms the basis for most of the observable covariance or correlation among relatives, and is used to compute heritability in the narrow sense ($h_N^2 = \sigma_A^2/\sigma^2$). This narrow-sense heritability dictates the response to selective pressures across generations, since it is this component that determines the correlation between parents and offspring (Hartl and Clark, 1989).

The *dominance variance* represents variation due to nonlinear interaction

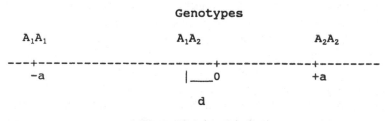

Figure 7–1 Additive effects of alleles and deviations due to dominance under a general multifactorial model. Here, the average effect of allele substitution is a and the deviation due to dominance is d. When $d = 0$, the heterozygote is exactly intermediate to the two homozygotes. When $d \neq 0$, there is allelic interaction and $\sigma_d^2 > 0$.

between these transmissible alleles at a single locus, and contributes only to covariance or correlation between relatives who can actually share a genotype identical by descent, most importantly full sibs and twins.

Epistatic variance is another form of nonadditive genetic variance and summarizes all nonlinear interaction among alleles at different loci. Epistatic interaction includes all effects of modifying loci and is not limited to situations of complete masking of the expression of one locus by another (the common definition of epistasis). The epistatic component encompasses nonlinear interactions both between pairs of loci and among trios (or even larger sets) of loci. As described in section 7.3.4, ignoring epistatic variance, when it in fact exists, will result in a predictable inflation of the additive genetic variance and possibly an inflation of the dominance genetic variance (if interaction between alleles at different loci can obliterate or alter the dominance relationship between alleles at one locus). However, it is very difficult to estimate all possible epistatic components separately from general family data. Studies of monozygotic twins provide some of the necessary contrasts for isolating epistatic components of variance (Bulmer, 1985); however, it is difficult to distinguish between epistatic components of variance and differences in the variances due to environmental factors shared between co-twins.

7.3.2 Components of Environmental Variance

Just as genetic variance can be further partitioned into distinct components, the total environmental component can also be divided into distinct components. Of course, both the σ_c^2 and σ_e^2 in Equation 7-9 are environmental components, with the former reflecting variation due to environmental factors possibly shared among relatives, and the latter reflecting factors unique to each individual (including simple measurement error for the phenotype in question). However, there is no general conceptual framework on which to build definitions of all possible levels of shared environments. As discussed later, some simple definitions of shared environments lead to near complete confounding between environmental and genetic components. Frequently, definitions of environmental components are designed as crude alternatives for genetic factors. If, for example, all the observed familial resemblance in a trait can be attributed to some household environment shared among relatives living together, there would be little point in further genetic analysis. However, if a genetic component remained statistically significant in the presence of such simple models of shared environment, further genetic analysis is warranted.

7.3.3 Estimating Variance Components From Data on Relatives

The linear model in Equation 7-8 can be generalized to include separate additive and dominance effects by writing

$$Y_{kk'l} = \mu + (a_k^m + a_{k'}^p) + d_{kk'} + c_l + e_{kk'l}, \qquad (7\text{-}13)$$

where the average effect of the kth allele inherited from the mother (a_k^m) (or $a_{k'}^g$ the k'th allele inherited from the father) represents the additive effects of alleles at any autosomal locus; $d_{kk'}$ represents possible interactions between these alleles ($d_{kk'}$ can be greater than zero only when $k \neq k'$); the impact of the lth environment is represented by c_l; and the error term $e_{kk'l}$ represents independent factors not shared among relatives. Note that here epistatic interaction among loci, as well as correlation between genotypes and environments are not considered.

Since the focus is on the components of variance associated with these four types of factors (i.e., σ_A^2, σ_d^2, σ_c^2 and σ_e^2), it is more useful to look at the covariance between pairs of relatives predicted under this linear model rather than the predicted phenotypes of single individuals. Recall from Table 7–1 that the covariance measures how two traits are jointly distributed, and the correlation is merely a standardized covariance. Under this linear model, the expected covariance between any two relatives I and J can be written as

$$\text{Cov}(Y_i Y_j) = 2\phi_{ij}\sigma_A^2 + \Delta_{ij}\sigma_d^2 + \gamma_{ij}\sigma_c^2 + \delta_{ij}\sigma_e^2 \qquad (7\text{-}14)$$

where ϕ_{ij} is the *kinship coefficient* between individuals I and J defined as the probability of randomly drawing an allele in individual J that is identical by descent (*ibd*) to an allele at the same locus randomly drawn from individual I; Δ_{ij} is the probability that both alleles at an autosomal locus are *ibd* in individuals I and J and is identical to Jacquard's (1974) Δ_7 coefficient; γ_{ij} is the probability that two relatives share a particular environmental factor, and this may be defined in several ways, as discussed later; the coefficient for the residual component δ_{ij} is 1 if I = J, and zero for all other cases. This definition preserves the decomposition of total variance into separate and independent components, that is, the overall variance can still be written as

$$\sigma^2 = \sigma_A^2 + \sigma_d^2 + \sigma_c^2 + \sigma_e^2. \qquad (7\text{-}15)$$

Table 7–3 gives the expected phenotypic covariances for a number of types of relatives where some environment shared among persons living in the same household also affects the observed phenotype. From simple comparisons of observed covariances or correlations on pairs of relatives, crude inferences about the degree of genetic control can be made. For example, if a trait shows a correlation near .5 between sibs, dizygotic twins, and parent-offspring pairs while monozygotic twins have a correlation near 1.0; one could infer that there was little evidence for any substantial nonadditive genetic component (i.e., σ_d^2 is likely zero), while the additive genetic component may be important and the narrow-sense heritability may be high.

Although estimating covariances or correlations for various types of relatives is instructive, when these pairs are drawn from families in a single study, these estimated correlations are not statistically independent since the same individual may contribute to more than one type of correlation. For example, a parent contributes to both the spouse correlation and the parent-offspring correlation. Calculating standard errors for these correlations using conventional pairwise approaches rarely takes this dependence into account,

Table 7–3. Expected covariances for pairs of relatives

Types of relatives	Coefficient for		
	σ_A^2	σ_d^2	σ_C^2
Spouse-spouse	0	0	1
Parent-offspring (living together)	1/2	0	1
Full sibs (living together)	1/2	1/4	1
Full sibs (living apart)	1/2	1/4	0
Half sibs (living together)	1/4	0	1
Half sibs (living apart)	1/4	0	0
Aunt/uncle–niece/nephew	1/4	0	0
First cousins (living apart)	1/8	0	0
Double first cousins (living apart)	1/4	1/16	0
Dizygotic twins (living together)	1/2	1/4	1
Monozygotic twins (living together)	1	1	1

In general, the coefficient for the additive genetic variance (σ_A^2) is $2\phi_{ij}$, and for dominance variance (σ_d^2) is Δ_7 (Jacquard, 1983). Shared environment is denoted by a simple binary variable indicating living together (yes, no) and this is the coefficient for common environmental variance (σ_C^2).

although it is possible to simultaneously estimate most common familial correlations (and the correlations among them) using general maximum likelihood techniques (Donner and Koval, 1981).

Analysis of Fixed Sets of Relatives

Family studies always involve intrinsic differences in the age and sex of relatives, and age and sex are themselves frequently important covariates for quantitative traits associated with chronic diseases. One epidemiologic approach to address this problem has been the "family set" approach (described in Chapter 6) where fixed sets of relatives all within a specified age range are sampled and stratified by major covariates of interest. Relatives in a family set typically include an index, his/her spouse, a sib of the same sex as the index, a first cousin also sex matched to the index, and an unrelated control also matched to the index for age, sex, and possibly other demographic characteristics. Specialized least squares regression models to obtain estimators for the narrow-sense heritability have been developed explicitly for such family sets (Schull et al., 1977), and general maximum likelihood estimators have also been used to estimate components of variance from family sets (Moll et al., 1983).

The major advantage of the family set method lies in the deliberate matching for age, sex, and certain observable risk factors while retaining both genetic and environmental contrasts among members of the set. For example, the index-sib and index-cousin supply contrasts on genetic relationships, while the index-spouse and index-control provide contrasts over observable environmental risk factors. Moll and colleagues (1983) in a reanalysis of blood pressure data from a stratified sample of family sets matched for race and neighborhood environment estimated both genetic and environmental components of variance.

Twin Studies

Another fixed sample design provided by nature is twins, which are uniquely matched for age and many environmental factors. Twins have been used to study the role of genetic factors for a large number of different phenotypes. The goal of twin studies is to compare similarities (correlations) and/or differences (within-pair variances) in monozygotic and dizygotic twins to infer and measure genetic control. While greater concordance in MZ twins compared to DZ twins can argue in favor of genetic factors, any discordance in MZ twins underscores a role for environmental factors. The classic twin study involves several key assumptions, however: (1) monozygotic twins are completely identical for all genetic factors; (2) dizygotic twins are no more alike genetically than full sibs and share, on average, half their genes; (3) both types of twins are samples from the same gene pool; and (4) the environmental components of variance of both types of twins are similar. While the first three assumptions are fairly reasonable, the fourth may be quite weak, especially for behavioral traits. Nonetheless, under these assumptions, a simple comparison of within-pair variances using the F-statistic provides a quick and easy test for a possible genetic component of variance on any quantitative trait.

Table 7–4 shows how a one-way analysis of variance table can be used for twin studies. A sequential approach for analysis of twin data is used. First, the total variance in both types of twins is compared, and then the null hypothesis of no additive genetic variance is tested. Lastly, estimates of the different genetic components can be obtained and used to compute broad sense heritabilities, if desired (Christian et al., 1974). However, there is still debate over the ability to generalize results of twin studies to the broader population of nontwins, because twins share environmental factors to a unique degree (Vogel and Motulsky, 1986). In general, classic analysis of twins provides an upper estimate of heritability, which may not accurately measure the degree of genetic control in the nontwin population.

In addition to obtaining estimators of heritability from twin studies, twins and their families can be used to test for genotype-environment interactions and other components of variation not usually addressable in family studies. Note that for MZ twins, the offspring of co-twins are biologically half-sibs. Extending the standard twin design to include the spouses and offspring of twins allows direct testing for sex effects on the expression of genetic components, longitudinal differences in these same components, and tests for possible genotype by environment interaction (Nance, 1984). Using the twin family design and the techniques of path analysis to partition correlation in MZ twin families, Nance and coworkers (1983) suggested that some of the maternal influence on birthweight could be genetic in origin. Despite the fact that analysis of twin data alone is restricted both in terms of the underlying assumptions and inferences to the general population that can be made, much information can still be gained about the degree of genetic control over a trait from using this natural fixed sampling design.

Table 7–4. Analyses of twin data usually involves a one-way analysis of variance (ANOVA) computed on monozygotic (MZ) and dizygotic (DZ) twins separately

From a sample of n twins, the ANOVA table is constructed as

Source of variation	df	Sum of squares	Mean squares	E(MS)
Among pair	$n - 1$	SS_{Am}	$MSA = SS_{Am}/(n - 1)$	$\sigma_W^2 + 2\sigma_{Am}^2$
Within pair	n	SS_W	$MSW = SS_W/n$	σ_W^2

Assuming the total variance, σ^2, is the sum of genetic components (σ_A^2 & σ_d^2) and environmental components (σ_c^2 & σ_e^2), i.e.,

$$\sigma^2 = \sigma_{Am}^2 + \sigma_W^2 = \sigma_A^2 + \sigma_d^2 + \sigma_c^2 + \sigma_e^2$$

the expected values for these within and among mean squares can be written for MZ and DZ twins.

For MZ twins $E(MS \text{ among}) = \sigma_A^2 + \sigma_d^2 + \sigma_c^2$
$E(MS \text{ within}) = \sigma_e^2$

For DZ twins $E(MS \text{ among}) = \frac{1}{2}\sigma_A^2 + \frac{1}{4}\sigma_d^2 + \sigma_c^2$
$E(MS \text{ within}) = \frac{1}{2}\sigma_A^2 + \frac{3}{4}\sigma_d^2 + \sigma_e^2$

Note that the among and within mean squares are constrained to sum to the total variance ($\sigma^2 = \sigma_{Am}^2 + \sigma_W^2$).

In classic twin analysis, *first* test for equal variances in MZ and DZ twins using the F test.

$$H_0: \sigma_{MZ}^2 = \sigma_{DZ}^2 \qquad F' = \frac{(MSA_{MZ} + MSW_{MZ})}{(MSA_{DZ} + MSW_{DZ})} \quad \text{or} \quad \frac{(MSA_{DZ} + MSW_{DZ})}{(MSA_{MZ} + MSW_{MZ})}$$

depending on which ratio is greater than one. Degrees of freedom for each zygosity class are computed as

$$df = \frac{(MSA + MSW)^2}{MSA^2/(n - 1) + MSW^2/n}$$

Second, test the null hypothesis that $\sigma_A^2 = 0$. If there was no difference in the total variance between zygosity classes, the within pair approach is preferred

$$F = \frac{MSW_{DZ}}{MSW_{MZ}} \qquad df = (n_{DZ} - 1, n_{MZ} - 1)$$

If there was a significant difference in total variance, it is most likely due to unequal environmental covariances between MZ and DZ twins. Therefore, the preferred test is based on the among components approach,

$$F = \frac{(MSA_{MZ} + MSW_{DZ})}{(MSA_{DZ} + MSW_{MZ})} \quad \text{with } (df_1, df_2)$$

(Continued)

Table 7-4. (Continued)

where

$$df_1 = \frac{(MSA_{MZ} + MSW_{DZ})^2}{MSA_{MZ}^2/(n_{MZ} - 1) + MSW_{DZ}^2/n_{DZ}}$$

$$df_2 = \frac{(MSA_{DZ} + MSW_{MZ})^2}{MSA_{DZ}^2/(n_{DZ} - 1) + MSW_{MZ}^2/n_{MZ}}$$

Third, each of these methods can provide estimates of broad sense heritability. Based on the "within pair" approach,

$$\hat{h}_B^2 = \frac{2(MSW_{DZ} - MSW_{MZ})}{\frac{1}{2}(MSA_{MZ} + MSW_{MZ} + MSA_{DZ} + MSW_{DZ})}$$

Based on the among component approach

$$\hat{h}_B^2 = \frac{(MSW_{DZ} - MSW_{MZ}) + (MSA_{MZ} - MSA_{DZ})}{\frac{1}{2}(MSA_{MZ} + MSW_{MZ} + MSA_{DZ} + MSW_{DZ})}$$

Both of these estimates are slightly inflated estimators of broad sense heritability with expectation of $(\sigma_A^2 + \frac{3}{2}\sigma_d^2)/\sigma^2$.

7.3.4 General Approaches to Variance Components

From the general model shown in Equation 7-14, the $(n \times n)$ expected covariance matrix for an entire family of n individuals can be written as:

$$\Omega = 2\Phi\sigma_A^2 + \Delta\sigma_d^2 + \Gamma\sigma_c^2 + I\sigma_e^2, \tag{7-16}$$

where each $(n \times n)$ matrix of coefficients (Φ, Δ, Γ, and I) dictates the contribution of their respective components of variance to the overall covariance between relatives. Both the matrix of kinship coefficients and the matrix of Δ coefficients are familiar to geneticists. Note, however that aside from monozygotic twins, Jacquard's Δ_7 coefficient is nonzero only for full sibs ($\Delta_7 = \frac{1}{4}$) and double first cousins ($\Delta_7 = \frac{1}{16}$).

It is possible to incorporate epistatic genetic components into the general model using functions of these two matrices of genetic coefficients. If only two locus interactions were considered, for example, the appropriate matrix of coefficients for epistatic variance contains squared values from the term-by-term product $(2\Phi) \otimes (2\Phi)'$. An analogous matrix for further epistatic components may be constructed as term-by-term products of the kinship matrix and the Δ matrix (i.e., $2\Phi \otimes \Delta$), if the model must include epistatic effects on the relationship between alleles at a single locus (i.e., if the modifier locus alters the dominance relationship between alleles).

The common environmental matrix (Γ) can be constructed in any number of ways within the constraint that it remains symmetric and nonnegative definite. For example, a simple sibship environment could be defined by computing a matrix product based on the relationship matrix (R) of Marayuma and Yasuda (1970). This nonsymmetric R matrix is an $(n \times n)$ matrix whose (i, j)th element is 1 if I is an offspring of J, and zero otherwise. The matrix of coefficients for a simple sibship common environment is then given by RR' +

I which is symmetric and nonnegative definite, but still needs appropriate scaling to force diagonal elements to 1 (Astemborski et al., 1985). However, it is sometimes difficult to distinguish between such simplistic, fixed shared environments and certain genetic components. For example, the dominance genetic component (σ_d^2) contributes to the covariance only among sibs and double first cousins, so it is difficult to disentangle this genetic component from that of a simple unobserved environment shared only among full sibs.

The matrices of coefficients for such simplistic shared environments are set by the data (i.e., two individuals are observed to live together or not, they are sibs or not, etc.), and do not require estimation of any additional parameters. However, it is also possible to reconstruct the general linear model in Equation 7-13 so that parameters reflecting the degree of sharing are estimated along with the environmental component of variance (i.e., σ_c^2). Exponential functions that allow the sharing of environmental factors to increase with time spent together or decrease with time spent apart have been proposed (Hopper and Mathews, 1983); and these may be most appropriate for certain phenotypic traits where learned behavior or cumulative exposures are critical. The parameters of these exponential functions may then be estimated along with the components of variance.

Maximum Likelihood Methods of Estimation

From the linear model in Equation 7-13 and the resulting partitioning of the covariance matrix given in Equation 7-14, it is possible to use maximum likelihood techniques to estimate components of variance (both genetic and nongenetic), *if* one can reasonably assume a particular form for the distribution of the phenotype within a family. In all such maximum likelihood procedures, the goal is to obtain those values of the parameters which maximize the probability of the observed data (Edwards, 1978). The resulting maximum likelihood estimators (MLE) for the parameters of the model (here, $\hat{\sigma}_A^2$, $\hat{\sigma}_d^2$, etc.) have desirable statistical properties of efficiency and consistency, but to employ such maximum likelihood methods one must specify the underlying distribution for the phenotype in families (which is the sampling unit). For reasons of convenience more than anything else, the multivariate normal distribution was chosen to represent quantitative traits within families. This choice is not without theoretical justification (Lange, 1978), but it must nonetheless be recognized as arbitrary.

The assumption of multivariate normality permits the likelihood function for the ($n \times 1$) vector of observations $\mathbf{Y}$ to be written as

$$\mathbf{L} = -\frac{1}{2} |\Omega|^{-1/2} \exp\left[(\mathbf{Y} - \mathbf{E(Y)})'\Omega^{-1}(\mathbf{Y} - \mathbf{E(Y)})\right], \quad (7\text{-}17)$$

where the expected value of ($\mathbf{E(Y)}$) may be a constant mean (μ) or may reflect fixed effects of observed covariates (e.g., $\mathbf{E(Y)} = \beta'(X)$), and the covariance matrix Ω is given in Equation 7-16. From this, the ln-likelihood function is written as

$$\ln \mathbf{L} = -\frac{1}{2} \ln |\Omega| - \frac{1}{2}\left[(\mathbf{Y} - \mathbf{E(Y)})'\Omega^{-1}(\mathbf{Y} - \mathbf{E(Y)})\right]. \quad (7\text{-}18)$$

Without too much difficulty, first and second derivatives of this ln-likelihood function can be obtained, and these turn out to be functions of the coefficients given in Equation 7-14 (Lange et al., 1976). Using these derivatives in either Fisher's scoring or in a classic Newton-Raphson algorithm, MLEs can be obtained for the different components of variance from a sample of families of varying size and structure. The resulting MLEs for both genetic and environmental components of variance reflect the relative importance of each in determining variation in the observed phenotype, and these MLEs for the genetic components can be used to compute heritabilities, if desired.

Another benefit of this likelihood approach is that a series of hierarchical models can be compared using the likelihood ratio test (LRT) to select the most parsimonious model for any given set of data. The LRT statistic is computed as twice the difference in ln-likelihoods of a reduced model (where one or more parameters are fixed at some null hypothesis value) and a complete model (where these parameters are estimated), that is, the test statistic is

$$\text{LRT} = -2[\ln L(\text{reduced model}) - \ln L(\text{complete model})]. \quad (7\text{-}19)$$

In general, this LRT statistic asymptotically follows a chi-square distribution with degrees of freedom equal to the number of parameters fixed in the reduced model (Edwards, 1978). Since the individual components of variance are constrained to be nonnegative under the classic random effects model, however, this LRT statistic does not actually follow a simple chi-square distribution for the null hypothesis that a given component is zero because this point is on the boundary of the parameter space (Self and Liang, 1987). Nonetheless, it is relatively straightforward to calculate the true distribution of this test statistic when testing the null hypothesis that any single component is zero. In this case, the LRT statistic asymptotically follows an equal mixture of the usual chi-square distribution with 1 df and a degenerate chi-square distribution with 0 df, so the 5% critical value of the LRT is equal to the 10% value for a chi-square with 1 df (Beaty et al., 1985). Similarly, the true distribution of the LRT for a test that two components are both zero is also a mixture of chi-squares, but the formula is somewhat more complicated.

The assumption of multivariate normality within pedigrees is an important one, since it allows implementation of this entire likelihood procedure, although it is also quite difficult to test its validity. For pedigrees of fixed size and structure, it would be possible to test explicitly for multivariate normality in most situations (Box and Cox, 1964). However, when pedigrees in the sample vary in both size and structure, it is not possible to test this critical assumption. Furthermore, it is important to realize that any deviations from normality in the observed phenotype may result from the fixed effects of covariates (such as age or gender). The critical assumption of the model is that the residual phenotype, after adjusting for all such covariates, follows a multivariate normal distribution.

One strategy to relax this assumption is to rely on a less restrictive method for calculating variances about the final estimators and for testing hypotheses. By modifying slightly the usual variance covariance matrix for the MLEs (which is based on the second derivatives of Equation 7-18), a more robust estimate of standard errors for estimated components of variance can be computed. This same robust estimate of variation about the MLEs can be used in an alternative test statistic, the score test, to test the null hypothesis that a given component of variance is zero. It is interesting, however, in the special case of testing the null hypothesis that a single component is zero against its alternative hypothesis that there is one variance component plus residual variation, both the LRT and this score test are equally robust (Beaty et al., 1985).

Another approach for dealing with nonnormality is to estimate parameters of a generalized transformation function that will assure multivariate normality after transformation, while simultaneously estimating the variance components themselves. Most nonnormal quantitative data can be forced to follow a multivariate normal distribution by using the appropriate power transformation (Clifford et al., 1984). One problem in relying on such power transformations, however, is that the relationship between the observed phenotype, Y, and covariates can be altered if Y is transformed. It must be remembered that the assumption of multivariate normality applies to the residual term after considering possible covariates. More general transformation techniques have been proposed to consider covariate effects while assuring full adherence to the assumption of multivariate normality (George and Elston, 1987). However, such transformation functions must be used with extreme caution because (1) transforming quantitative phenotypes obscures or obliterates the original scale of measurement and complicates final interpretation, and (2) transformations can, in the extreme, conceal important facts about the original phenotype and its distribution. For example, using the generalized modulus transformation function described by George and Elston (1987), it is possible to convert a bimodal distribution into a unimodal normal distribution. Thus, arbitrary transformation to meet one assumption of variance components analysis can obscure information critical to later genetic analysis.

Extensions to Variance Components Models

The purpose of variance components models is to partition variation which *could* be attributed to unobserved Mendelian factors. If the genetic component of variance represents a substantial proportion of the total variation in a trait, there is clearly a need for further genetic analysis. However, it is important to realize that the random effects model described here does not specify the number of Mendelian loci or their exact mode of action. Recent extensions to the classic variance components models permit further inquiry into mode of action of unobserved Mendelian factors and also allow corrections for nonrandom sampling of families.

Multivariate Phenotypes. The general linear models upon which variance components analysis is based can also be extended to bivariate and higher order phenotypes (Lange and Boehnke, 1983). The usual ($n \times n$) covariance matrix for a family of n individuals now becomes a $(2n \times 2n)$ matrix Ω^* which can be written as

$$\Omega^* = \begin{bmatrix} \Omega_{11} & \Omega_{12} \\ \Omega_{21} & \Omega_{22} \end{bmatrix}, \tag{7-20}$$

where the submatrices Ω_{11} and Ω_{22} are linear functions of components affecting trait 1 and 2, respectively, and are equivalent to that seen in Equation 7-16. The $(n \times n)$ off-diagonal submatrix Ω_{12} ($=\Omega_{21}$) is also a linear function of genetic and nongenetic components of variance, but now these reflect the role of shared genes and shared environments in determining the covariance between two phenotypes. The genetic covariance term can be interpreted as a measure of *pleiotropic effects* of genes influencing both traits simultaneously. If this genetic component were sufficiently large, it would suggest a single genetic mechanism may be operating (Boehnke et al., 1986). Similarly, the nongenetic component of covariation represents unobserved environmental factors that can be shared among relatives and that contribute to the covariance of the two traits both within and between individuals. Boehnke and colleagues (1986) used this bivariate model to estimate the degree of genetic correlation in total cholesterol and triglyceride levels in a sample of families ascertained through schoolchildren. This analysis showed that both genetic and environmental factors contributed to the observed correlation between these lipid phenotypes.

Incorporating Information on Genetic Markers. The influence of observable covariates (such as age and gender) on the phenotype can be incorporated as fixed effects in the linear model given in Equation 7-13; and appropriate regression coefficients can be estimated along with the variance components. When such observed covariates include genetic markers, it is also possible to partition out a distinct component of the total variance that represents fixed effects of alleles at the marker locus on the phenotype. This approach, when applied to samples of unrelated individuals, is completely analogous to the traditional one-way ANOVA; and the average effect of each marker allele may be estimated directly (Falconer, 1981). This average effect of an allele is merely the weighted phenotypic mean of all genotypes carrying that allele, and the sum of the weighted squared deviations for each genotype at the marker locus serves as a measure of phenotypic variation attributable to the marker locus (Boerwinkle et al., 1986). However, a significant marker effect does not necessarily imply genetic linkage. Rather it could reflect a direct biologic effect of the allele at the marker locus on the quantitative phenotype.

One example of this approach in humans is the apolipoprotein E locus which carries three polymorphic alleles in most populations. Surveys of unrelated individuals show that the e_4 allele is associated with an increase in serum total cholesterol levels while the e_2 allele is associated with a decrease in total cholesterol levels (Boerwinkle and Sing, 1987). This allelic effect is likely due to decreased binding of the apolipoprotein molecule coded for by the e_4 allele to its receptor (Mahley, 1988). Analysis of family data where the means were estimated for the different *apoE* genotypes along with the genetic and nongenetic variance components revealed that 7% of the total variance in adjusted total cholesterol could be attributed to this marker locus alone (Sing et al., 1988). While this component of variance attributable to the marker locus is small compared to the total genetic component (i.e., it represents just 11% of all genetic variation), it clearly points out that multiple loci are involved in the control of total cholesterol levels.

When applied to family data, it is necessary to incorporate the probability of observing marker genotypes in family members into the likelihood function and to estimate genotypic means at the marker locus along with the usual variance components (Boerwinkle et al., 1986). Further partitioning of the genetic variation into components attributable to marker loci (be they candidate genes or unrelated genetic markers) opens the door to further genetic analysis. Identification of a genetic marker accounting for a significant fraction of the total genetic variation serves to flag actual chromosomal segments for further genetic and biochemical investigation. Variations on this approach of testing for genetic markers that account for substantial fractions of variance can be used within fixed sample designs (e.g., pairs of sibs) to screen for marker loci which are closely linked to unobservable Mendelian loci exerting a major impact on the phenotype, that is, previously unknown "major genes" controlling a quantitative trait (Haseman and Elston, 1972; Elston, 1990).

Correcting for Ascertainment. The usual presentation of variance component analysis is correct for families randomly sampled from the general population. Frequently, however, families are ascertained through a proband with an extreme phenotypic value. The proband may have a value above (or below) an arbitrary cutoff value, say above the 95th percentile for a well-defined reference population, or may have a clinical disease associated with extreme values of the quantitative trait (as diabetes is associated with high blood glucose values). When the proband is identified as being beyond a defined cut-point, the likelihood function in Equation 7-17 can be replaced with a conditional likelihood function representing the joint distribution of all non-proband relatives and a proband known to have been drawn from a specified tail of the distribution (Rao and Wette, 1987). Alternatively, the original likelihood function in Equation 7-17 can be conditioned on the observed phenotype of the proband, and this conditional likelihood function could then be used to estimate components of variance. This latter approach is slightly less efficient (in the statistical sense of having larger standard errors about the final estimators) than using the joint likelihood function itself, but it has several important advantages. First, only rarely is the exact cut-point known for probands; and second, in some situations the proband may be recognizably different on other grounds. Consider the case of families ascertained through non-insulin-dependent diabetics: at the time of sampling a known diabetic proband may not be hyperglycemic due to clinical control of his or her disease, yet some adjustment for the nonrandom selection of these families must still be made.

The likelihood function conditioned on the proband's value can be used either under the strict assumption of multivariate normality (Hopper and Mathews, 1982) or with this assumption relaxed (Beaty and Liang, 1987). It must be noted, however, that implicit in this conditioning process is the assumption that ascertainment of probands is such that there is only one per family (Ewens and Shute, 1986). This is termed *single ascertainment* and is discussed in more detail in Chapter 8.

7.3.5 Interpreting Variance Components Models

The main purpose of conducting variance components analysis in family studies is to quantitate the potential degree of genetic control, and to test whether simple nongenetic mechanisms could possibly account for the observed distribution of a phenotype and its pattern of familial aggregation. If a quantitative trait showed significant familial correlation, variance components analysis can identify that proportion of variation which could be attributed to genetic differences, and could systematically test for the effects of a limited range of nongenetic explanations for such observed correlations. If a substantial proportion of the variance can be attributed to genetic factors even in the presence of arbitrary shared environmental factors, more explicit genetic models should then be examined. These explicit Mendelian models, which require formal segregation analysis, are discussed in detail in Chapter 8.

In variance components analysis, it also is possible to conduct a preliminary screening of all families to identify families or individuals who do not fit the overall pattern for one reason or another. Hopper and Mathews (1982) proposed two types of goodness-of-fit statistics (one computed for each family, and one computed for all individuals in a family), which are useful for screening samples of families. The first goodness-of-fit statistic is merely the squared deviation for a family from its expected mean, weighted by its expected covariance matrix (i.e., this goodness-of-fit statistic is merely the Mahalanobis distance of the observed phenotypic vector for a family from that predicted by the overall MLEs). Families poorly fit by the overall model may simply contain outlier individuals or may reflect distinctive patterns of familial aggregation arising from different etiologic mechanisms. These goodness-of-fit statistics can be used to select for families which may be segregating for a Mendelian locus influencing the quantitative phenotype under consideration (Boehnke and Lange, 1984). Frequently outliers have relatively modest effects on final estimators of the variance components (perhaps underscoring the robustness of analysis of variance techniques), nonetheless it is important to identify such individuals or families when analyzing large samples.

7.4 PATH ANALYSIS

Path analysis represents an alternative approach to classic variance components models for partitioning genetic and nongenetic components. It is important to recognize, however, that both approaches are based on the same linear model (shown in Equation 7-8) where unobserved genetic and nongenetic factors contribute to the observed phenotype (i.e., the classic random effects models). The goal of variance components analysis is to estimate components of total variance or covariance that result from shared unobserved factors (genes or environments). Path analysis, on the other hand, was developed to partition observed *correlations* into components reflecting such shared causal factors. Path analysis evolved from linear regression, and it is designed to reflect relationships between one or more observed phenotypes when there are linear combinations of causal factors.

Path analysis uses exclusively standardized phenotypes where the sample mean is subtracted from each individual's phenotypic value and then divided by the sample standard deviation. Using Equation 7-8 to write an appropriate linear model for such a standardized phenotype gives

$$
\begin{aligned}
Y_{kl} - \frac{\mu}{\sigma} &= \frac{g_k + c_l + e_{kl}}{\sigma} \\
&= \left(\frac{\sigma_g}{\sigma}\right)\left(\frac{g_k}{\sigma_g}\right) + \left(\frac{\sigma_c}{\sigma}\right)\left(\frac{c_l}{\sigma_c}\right) + \left(\frac{\sigma_r}{\sigma}\right)\left(\frac{e_{kl}}{\sigma_r}\right) \qquad (7\text{-}21) \\
&= \mathbf{h}\left(\frac{g_k}{\sigma_g}\right) + \mathbf{c}\left(\frac{c_l}{\sigma_c}\right) + \mathbf{e}\left(\frac{e_{kl}}{\sigma_r}\right).
\end{aligned}
$$

Thus, it can be seen that the path coefficients (**h**, **c**, and **e**) are merely standardized regression coefficients on the unobserved genetic and environmental factors. Note that assumptions about the independence of genetic and environmental factors in the underlying linear model are still in effect when using path analysis, unless otherwise explicitly indicated in the path model.

Because the variance of the standardized phenotype is fixed at 1, there is a constraint on the sum of these path coefficients, specifically,

$$
\mathrm{Var}\ \frac{Y - \mu}{\sigma} = 1 = \mathbf{h}^2 + \mathbf{c}^2 + \mathbf{e}^2. \qquad (7\text{-}22)
$$

Indeed the use of h^2 as the standard notation for heritability originated when Sewall Wright (1934) pointed out that the square of the path coefficient describing the relative impact of genes on a phenotype was equivalent to the ratio of genetic variance to the total phenotypic variance.

7.4.1 Constructing Path Models

Although based on the same underlying linear model, path analysis enjoys a flexibility that classic variance components models do not have. Given a path diagram detailing the causal relationship between observable and unobservable factors, it is relatively simple to obtain expected values for all possible correlations following a minimum number of tracing rules (Li, 1975). These rules, summarized in Table 7–5, guarantee a set of consistent equations for the expected correlations for a phenotype between two individuals, correlations between one phenotype and another within individuals, and correlations

Table 7−5. Rules for constructing equations for expected correlations and variances using path models

I. *Notational rules*:
   1. Observed variables are enclosed by squares, unobserved variables by circles.
   2. Causal pathways between two variables are denoted by single-headed arrows.
   3. Correlations are denoted by double-headed arrows.

II. *Rules for writing equations:*
   1. The variance of any observed variable is the sum of the squared path coefficients for each arrow leading into it. Note: All observed variables must have a variance of 1.0.
   2. The correlations from a causal variable to an effected variable is the respective path coefficient, if there are no intermediate variables.
   3. The correlation between two variables is the sum of all connecting pathways.
   4. No connecting pathway may contain more than one change in direction.
   5. A compound pathway through one or more intermediate variables is the product of all elementary paths along the connecting route.
   6. No connecting pathway should contain more than one correlation (double-headed arrow).
   7. No connecting pathway should contain "forward then backward" movement.

Adapted from Li (1975).

between different phenotypes across individuals as linear functions of these path coefficients. It is up to the user to construct a biologically meaningful path model, of course. Thus, while path analysis is extremely flexible, it does not offer much guidance in constructing causal models.

The equations for the expected correlations, along with constraints on the total variance, constitute a system of simultaneous equations relating the observed correlations to the parameters of the path model itself. If there are fewer equations than unknown parameters (path coefficients), then it is not possible to obtain unique estimators; if the number of equations is equal to the number of unknown parameters, then a single unique solution exists, and therefore there will be no variation in the resulting estimators; if the number of equations is larger than the number of path coefficients in the model, the system is "overdetermined" and it becomes possible to use maximum likelihood techniques to estimate the path coefficients. Consider a simplistic path diagram shown in Figure 7−2 where a single phenotype (Y) is a linear function of genetic factors, a single environment shared among parents and offspring, and independent residual factors (not shown). By convention, observed traits are enclosed by squares, while unobserved traits are enclosed by circles. Causal pathways are denoted by single-headed arrows and correlations by double-headed arrows. There are three path coefficients (h, c, and r), as well as the unknown correlation in the shared environments (a) in the simple model shown here. From nuclear family data, only three correlations can be estimated if sex is ignored (parent-offspring, parent-parent, and the correlation among offspring); however, it is not possible to estimate all four parameters because two of these correlations have identical expectations (i.e., two equations are not linearly independent). In this simple model, one is then left with three independent equations and four unknowns, so it is not generally

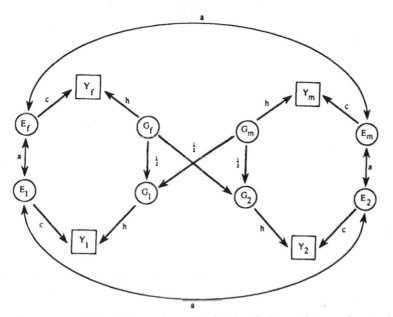

Figure 7–2. Simplistic path model for familial correlation of a single phenotype. Expected correlations are as follows:

$$E\,[\mathrm{cor}\,(Y_f,\,Y_m)] = c^2 a$$
$$E\,[\mathrm{cor}\,(Y_f,\,Y_i)] = E\,[\mathrm{cor}(Y_m,\,Y_i)] = \tfrac{1}{2}h^2 + c^2 a \quad \text{for } i = 1, 2$$
$$E\,[\mathrm{cor}\,(Y_1,\,Y_2)] = \tfrac{1}{2}h^2 + c^2 a$$

possible to separate effects of shared genes from shared environments and residual variation using a single observed phenotype for each individual in nuclear families.

The addition of a second observation on each family member makes it possible to obtain more observed correlations, and so construct an overdetermined system of equations where there are more independent equations available than parameters to be estimated. The exact nature of the path model and therefore the equations depend on question at hand, of course, but Figure 7–3 offers one simple example. Here an observed trait X is modeled as having a direct effect on the phenotype Y, which has some genetic basis. This path model predicts the observed correlations in terms of four path coefficients, and was applied to family data on smoking and pulmonary function in adults by Cotch and coworkers (1990).

Rao (1985) proposed another path model for nuclear family data where one observation on each individual is simply that person's predicted value based on a regression of the phenotype on relevant covariates, and the residual value from this same regression model serves as the second observed phenotype. In this standardized model, 16 independent equations for expected correlations and 6 additional constraints on variances are used to iteratively estimate 10 path coefficients. This particular path model separates genetic components from nongenetic culturally transmitted components, while allow-

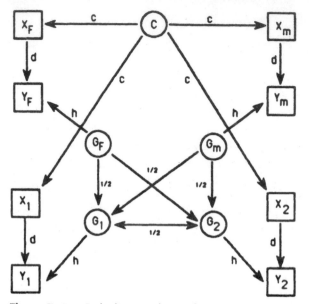

Figure 7–3. Path diagram for analysis of two phenotypic traits where one (X) exerts a direct effect on the other (Y).

Expected correlations are as follows:

$r(X_iY_i) = d$ for $i = F, M, 1, 2$
$r(X_iX_j) = c^2$ for all $i \neq j$
$r(Y_iX_j) = dc^2$ for all $i \neq j$
$r(Y_FY_M) = d^2c^2$
$r(Y_FY_1) = r(Y_FY_2) = \frac{1}{2}h^2 + d^2c^2$
$r(Y_MY_1) = r(Y_MY_2) = \frac{1}{2}h^2 + d^2c^2$
$r(Y_1Y_2) = \frac{1}{2}h^2 + d^2c^2$

ing for parental correlation and shared sibship environments. Since this particular model allows for one of the main comparisons of interest (i.e., estimating genetic heritability and testing for a generalized, nongenetic basis for familial correlation), it has been applied to a number of diverse phenotypic traits (Rao et al., 1983). These path models have also been adapted to adjust for certain ascertainment schemes (Rice et al., 1991).

7.4.2 Estimating Path Coefficients

The estimation procedure for any path model typically involves an algorithm which minimizes the squared deviations between the observed correlations and their expectations in the system of m equations. The original phenotypic data on individuals is not used directly in this type of path analysis, as all analysis is done on the estimated correlations (r_i, $i = 1 \cdots m$). These m estimated correlations are transformed, using Fisher's z transformation, to obtain normalized correlation statistics

$$z_i = \frac{1}{2} \ln \frac{1 + r_i}{1 - r_i} \tag{7-23}$$

that asymptotically follow a normal distribution with expectation

$$\mathbf{E}(z_i) = \frac{1}{2} \ln \frac{1 + \rho_i}{1 - \rho_i},$$

where ρ_i is the true value of the ith correlation, and a variance of $1/n_i$ where n is the number of pairs used to estimate this correlation. These expectations for the z values are linear functions of the path coefficients used in the path model, and the overall chi-square value

$$\chi^2 = \sum_{i=1}^{m} n_i[z_i - \mathbf{E}(z_i)]^2 \tag{7-24}$$

serves as a measure of the fit of the data to the model. As these z_i statistics are asymptotically normally distributed (if the original data are themselves multivariate normal), this same chi-square value is proportional to the ln-likelihood of the model itself. Thus, the minimum chi-square approach is effectively a maximum likelihood approach. This series of assumptions about the underlying data and the distribution of the normalized correlations allows the likelihood ratio test to be used to compare submodels where one or more path coefficients are set to zero.

The assumptions about the distribution of the original phenotype or the transformed correlation coefficients computed from them are relatively mild, if the different observed correlations in each of the m equations are indeed independent of one another. However, in family studies, observed correlations are rarely truly independent because individuals contribute to more than one correlation (Elston, 1975). For example, the same data on parents are used when estimating a parent-parent correlation and a parent-offspring correlation. This double counting induces a dependence or correlation among the observed correlations coefficients which are to be used in fitting the path model. Simulation studies of standard path models suggest that this dependence among correlations has relatively little impact on the final estimators for the path coefficients themselves, but test statistics are more sensitive to this violation of the underlying assumptions (McGue et al. 1984; Rao et al., 1987).

Solutions for dealing with these correlations among correlations involve more assumptions about the distributional forms for either the observed correlations, the phenotype itself, or both (Rao, 1985). Furthermore, the direct approach proposed by Rao (1985) for estimation of path coefficients from family data is, in itself, a likelihood method where the usual likelihood ratio tests are available for testing hierarchical models, but the goodness-of-fit statistics for families under any particular model are no longer available (Hopper, 1986). Using a strict maximum likelihood approach for path analysis blurs the distinction between variance components models and path models for nuclear family data, since there are only minor differences in the parameterizations of the two underlying statistical models.

7.4.3 Interpreting Path Models

The main advantage of path analysis lies in its flexible approach to constructing causal models for observable phenotypes. It is relatively simple to specify path models for traits where one phenotype has a direct effect on another and often this is biologically appropriate. For example, studies of both weight and blood pressure in sibs using path analysis have shown that approximately 30% of the sib correlation in blood pressure can be attributed to an underlying correlation in weight (Hanis et al., 1983). The main disadvantage in path analysis is its lack of a clearly specified mathematical form for the wide scope of possible path models. Not only does this impair the testing of hypotheses and statistical inference in general, but it creates a degree of ambiguity which makes many uneasy. The construction of path models is, by its nature, subjective and it is almost always possible to construct more than one path model that will fit any given set of data. Therefore, the investigator must exercise an appropriate degree of caution when proposing path models, and the criterion should always be the biologic relevance of the model to the question at hand.

Given a biologically reasonable path model, the currently available methods for estimating path coefficients allow the observed correlations to be partitioned into components reflecting the relative importance of genetic and a limited range of nongenetic factors. Specific hypotheses can easily be tested about parameters within the general model, for example, it is relatively easy to test whether a given path coefficient is different from zero. However, the validity of such test statistics rely heavily on the assumptions of normality of either the correlation coefficients or the raw data underlying them. These assumptions are both difficult to test and to avoid. Path analysis should be viewed as a flexible alternative to the traditional variance components models, but one where the ability to test hypotheses is, at least slightly, lessened. In those situations where partitioning of familial correlations is more important than testing hypotheses, however, path analysis may be the more appropriate analytic tool for family studies in genetic epidemiology.

7.5 MEASURING HERITABILITY FOR DISCRETE TRAITS

When the phenotype of interest is qualitative or discrete, rather than quantitative, the approach to measuring the possible role of genetic factors takes on a slightly different form. It is still possible to think in terms of the general model given in Equation 7-8, where unobserved genetic and environmental factors contribute additively to a continuous phenotype Y, but now Y itself is also unobserved and only a binary indicator function of it can be directly observed (i.e., an individual either has a disease or does not). Traditionally, this has been modeled where the phenotype Y, now termed "liability," is the sole determinant of disease, and family data on prevalence of disease in various classes of relatives is used to estimate the correlation in liability among relatives. From such correlations in liability, estimates of genetic heritability can be obtained (Falconer, 1965; Curnow and Smith, 1975).

It is important to realize, however, that the multifactorial model for liability is constructed by layering several assumptions upon one another, which individually are not very restrictive, but collectively can be difficult to defend. A clear perspective of the purpose of using this multifactorial model for liability must be maintained. Its utility comes from the ability to quantitate the degree of familial aggregation of disease and the assessment it provides of the role genetic factors *may* play in the etiology of disease, rather than any definitive description of the actual mode of inheritance.

As with the multifactorial model for a quantitative trait, the multifactorial model for liability assumes that genetic and environmental factors are independent and uncorrelated, and that there is no interaction between them. Therefore, the total variance in liability is simply the sum of the variance due to genetic differences (σ_g^2) and the variance due to environmental factors (σ_e^2). The model further assumes that liability is normally distributed among individuals in the population and follows a multivariate normal distribution among relatives. This assumption is without biological justification, but is mathematically convenient. One could argue that it is not critical that liability actually be multivariate normal, since it is possible to transform any distribution to fit normality. However, since liability is unobservable, tests of this assumption or transformation to meet this assumption are not feasible. Only the end results of predicted risks to relatives provide information on the final efficacy of the model, and it is possible to obtain very similar estimates of risk assuming either multivariate normality for liability or entirely different distributional forms (T. P. Hutchinson, 1980).

7.5.1 Defining the Risk Function

Given that liability controls risk of disease, it is logical to assume that individuals with higher liability values (either from genetic or environmental causes) are at higher risk of disease. Some risk function must then be defined to determine whether or not a particular individual is actually affected. Graphically, it is easier to think of a simple threshold point (T) on the liability scale beyond which an individual is affected, as shown in Figure 7–4; however, such a simple step function (Φ) may not be biologically realistic. A more mathematically attractive, continuous risk function is given by the cumulative normal function where risk for a particular genotypic value, g, is a function of the environmental variance (σ_e^2) and the threshold value (T), that is,

$$
\begin{aligned}
P(\text{affected}|g) &= \Phi\left[\frac{g - T}{\sigma_e}\right] \\
&= \int_{-\infty}^{(g-T)/\sigma_e} (2\pi)^{-1/2} \exp\frac{-\mu^2}{2} \, d\mu \\
&= \int_{-\infty}^{g} (2\pi)^{-1/2} \exp\left(-\frac{1}{2}\frac{(x - T)^2}{\sigma_e}\right) dx
\end{aligned}
\tag{7-25}
$$

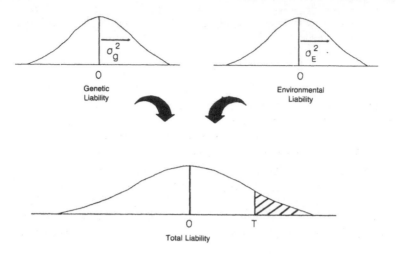

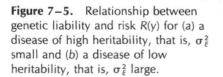

Figure 7–4 Multifactorial model for liability with a threshold-determining discrete phenotype.

(Elston, 1981). This sigmoidal risk function for the genetically determined component of liability is mathematically equivalent to the concept of a simple threshold for the total liability (diagrammed in Figure 7–4), but its exact form reflects the impact of the nongenetic variance in liability. Specifically the risk function will rise more steeply as g increases when σ_e^2 is small, and less steeply when σ_e^2 is large (see Figure 7–5). Again, the choice of this particular risk function is arbitrary and is based on mathematical convenience rather than any biologic mechanism.

Given a risk function to relate the unobserved liability value to the probability of being affected, the assumed normality of liability permits data on disease prevalence, in either the general population or in classes of relatives ascertained through an affected individual, to be used to estimate parameters of the multifactorial model for liability. Initially, risk of disease in the general population is used to determine the mean and variance of liability in affected individuals. First, note that the risk in the general population is simply the

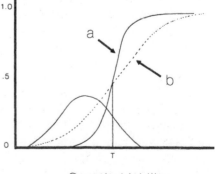

Figure 7–5. Relationship between genetic liability and risk $R(y)$ for (a) a disease of high heritability, that is, σ_E^2 small and (b) a disease of low heritability, that is, σ_E^2 large.

product of the risk function, $R(y)$, and the density function for total liability integrated over the full range of its possible values, that is,

$$P_1 = P(\text{affected}) = \int_{-\infty}^{\infty} R(y)\phi(y) \, dy, \qquad (7\text{-}26)$$

which is interpreted graphically as the area under the curve beyond the threshold T seen in Figure 7–4. From this, the mean liability among affected individuals can be computed as μ_A:

$$\mu_A = \frac{\phi(T)}{P_1}, \qquad (7\text{-}27)$$

with variance given by

$$1 - \mu_A(\mu_A - T) \qquad (7\text{-}28)$$

(Rice, 1986). Similarly, information on risk in relatives of affected individuals can be used to estimate the mean and variance in liability in this group. The displacement in the liability distribution among relatives reflects the degree of resemblance in liability between affected individuals and their relatives (i.e., it is a measure of the correlation in liability). This idea of using the proportion of individuals beyond a given point in a bivariate distribution to estimate the underlying correlation dates back to the early part of the twentieth century, when Pearson (1901) introduced the concept of a tetrachoric correlation. In short, the higher the risk of disease among relatives of cases, the greater must be the correlation in underlying liability.

7.5.2 Analogy With Variance Components Models

By adhering to the concept of a multivariate normal distribution for liability among relatives, data from the general population and in various classes of relatives (1°, 2° relatives, etc.) can be used to estimate an overall correlation in liability. Exact estimation of this correlation involves numerical integration of the multivariate normal distribution which can be cumbersome, if special situations do not apply (Curnow and Smith, 1975). If all correlation in liability were due to shared genes acting in a strictly additive fashion, it would be simple to generalize and predict the correlation for various types of relationships. It must be remembered, however, that any correlation in nongenetic factors controlling liability inflates the estimated heritability of liability. Also, when dealing with a discrete trait, it is not possible to estimate the actual components of variance for liability (σ_g^2, σ_e^2, etc.), but only their relative magnitude ($\sigma_g^2/(\sigma_g^2 + \sigma_e^2) = h^2$) (Elston, 1981).

It should be noted that the multifactorial model for liability can be extended to consider observable covariates, although this is at times awkward. First, consider the case of a fixed effect of gender on risk, for example, where males are uniformly at higher risk than females. This is best incorporated into the multifactorial model for liability as separate thresholds for males and females or, equivalently, as a simple displacement of the distribution of liability in males and females. In the former situation, affected females represent a more extreme tail of the normal distribution than do affected males and, as a result, their relatives will have a liability distribution that is shifted further to the right than do relatives of affected males. In the latter situation of shifted distributions, the higher risk to males may be partially offset by sex-specific correlations in liability. Statistically, these two alternative parameterizations are practically indistinguishable. Pyloric stenosis, which uniformly shows a higher prevalence in males, appears to be quite compatible with this simple displacement of the distribution of liability in males, and this leads to different predictions for recurrence risks in families ascertained through affected males and those ascertained through affected females (Chakraborty, 1986). In general, multiple threshold models (or their equivalent) should provide more statistical power to discriminate among polygenic multifactorial models and single-locus multifactorial models, if only because there are more observations available (i.e., male relatives of male probands, female relatives of male probands, male relatives of female probands, etc.).

Information on quantitative covariates can also be incorporated into the general multifactorial model for liability by assuming an observed covariate follows a bivariate normal distribution with the still unobserved, normally distributed liability (Smith and Mendell, 1974). Approximate methods for estimating the correlation between liability and the observed covariate, the correlation for the covariate in different relatives, and the correlation in liability have been proposed and these can be used to predict risk to a relative. Recent generalizations of this concept suggest covariate information can improve its predictive ability, even if there is only a moderate correlation between liability and covariate (Moldin et al., 1990). However, the incorporation of an observed covariate into the general multifactorial model creates a paradox. Specifically, when the correlation between the covariate and liability is modest, the covariate contributes little information about risk, while when this correlation is large, information on the disease status in a relative is minor compared to observing the covariate in the individual directly. In cases where the individual cannot be observed either because he/she is not yet born or because he or she is currently at low risk (perhaps below the age of risk), this approach may be most worthwhile.

7.5.3 Analogy With Path Models

In any situation where estimates of familial correlations can be obtained, it is possible to use path analysis to partition such correlations into components representing the effects of different unobserved, underlying factors. Therefore, it is possible to use the estimated correlations in liability obtained from a multifactorial model for a discrete trait to estimate genetic components of correlation (heritability) and nongenetic components (Rice and Reich, 1985). However, without data on risk in a variety of relatives (1° and 2° relatives, possibly stratified by gender) and without additional information on some measure of shared environment, it is still quite difficult to discriminate between genetic and nongenetic components contributing to the correlation in liability to disease. It may be more appropriate to use the tools of path analysis simply to partition familial correlations in liability (preferably considering sex-specific transmission) without attempting to disentangle genetic and environmental causal factors underlying such correlations. Rice and colleagues (1981) have developed a general path model for estimating sex-specific transmission of a discrete trait from family data.

7.5.4 Predicting Recurrence Risks From the Multifactorial Model

Beyond quantitating familial correlation in liability or risk, the primary application of the multifactorial model for liability is in calculating recurrence risks for individuals at risk for any of the many diseases that can be described by this general model. Many chronic diseases and congenital malformations are typically classified as multifactorial, in that they show consistent familial aggregation, but are not clearly Mendelian. Thus it is necessary to offer some estimate of recurrence risk for counseling purposes even in the absence of any defined mechanism of inheritance. To this end, the multifactorial model for liability can be quite useful because, given an estimate of the correlation in liability, risk of individuals with different configurations of affected and nonaffected relatives can be calculated under the multivariate normal distribution. Essentially, recurrence risks are computed as a series of joint and marginal probabilities, which can then be used under Bayes' theorem to give the probability of having a liability beyond the threshold, given one or more affected relatives. In general, for fixed heritability (i.e., a fixed correlation in liability) these recurrence risks are approximately linear functions of prevalence when plotted on a logarithmic scale. Beyond this, the addition of an affected relative uniformly increases the risk while the addition of nonaffected relatives uniformly decreases the risk (although by smaller increments).

It is important to realize, however, that such risk calculations are invalidated by violations of the underlying assumptions of the multifactorial model. In particular, the classic multifactorial model for liability assumes that liability determines risk and that all correlation in risk among relatives is due to genetic factors. If this assumption is false because environmental factors shared among relatives also contribute to risk, the estimated correlation in liability could still be used to predict risk (although it is an inflated estimate of genetic heritability), as long as only relationships represented in original data set are considered. For example, if data on sibs is used to estimate the total correlation in liability, this estimator could still be used to calculate recurrence risks to sibs but should not be extended to 2° relatives.

Nonetheless, it is quite possible for more than one distributional form to give very similar estimated recurrence risks. T. P. Hutchinson (1980) showed how the Pareto distribution, commonly used in survival analysis, can be used to estimate the equivalent of a correlation in risk from prevalence data; and then used to predict recurrence risks for individuals with various configurations of affected relatives. These estimates are surprisingly close to those calculated under the assumption of a multivariate normal distribution for liability, underscoring the generality of the multifactorial model for liability.

One must remember that the original motivation for developing and applying the multifactorial model for liability was to quantitate the degree of familial aggregation of disease in the context of possible genetic transmission. Heritability estimates for liability obtained from this model are invariably crude indicators of whether a genetic mechanism might be controlling the disease, and are subject to substantial biases.

7.6 CONCLUDING REMARKS

One of the primary goals of quantitative genetics is to confirm that a phenotype shows familial aggregation, and assess the relative importance of genetic control while explicitly considering nongenetic alternatives that might lead to similar patterns of familial clustering. The available statistical tools in quantitative genetics reflect an essential imbalance between models for genetic and environmental factors jointly controlling the phenotype. The expected effects of shared genetic components of variance are well-defined consequences of Mendelian genetics, although not all can be estimated from observational studies. The expected effects of shared environmental components lack a solid foundation, however, and there are many more opportunities to create arbitrary models of cultural inheritance. Problems arise, however, in that it may not always be possible to discriminate among the various sources of variation with studies of small families where there is no control over either genotypic or environmental factors (as is always the situation in studies of humans). Nonetheless, analysis of multifactorial models is a critical intermediate step in genetic epidemiology, and this route ultimately holds the promise of defining the interactions between genes and environments.

Genetic Approaches to Familial Aggregation

II. Segregation Analysis

8.1 INTRODUCTION

Mendel first proposed for each phenotype that individuals receive two distinct "factors" from their parents and that these may be different forms (or alleles) of a given gene. He further proposed that these two factors would separate or segregate from one another in the process of forming gametes that determine the genetic makeup of the next generation. The segregation of these alleles in any particular mating type gives rise to fixed ratios of genotypes (and of phenotypes) among offspring. Thus, *segregation analysis* was originally designed to test whether or not an observed mixture of phenotypes among offspring is compatible with Mendelian inheritance. In medical genetics, classic segregation analysis has focused almost exclusively on estimating the proportion of affected and nonaffected offspring in sibships, and the hypotheses of interest were whether or not this proportion was compatible with the expectations of simple Mendelian models. Over the years, segregation analysis has broadened to encompass fitting more general models of inheritance to pedigrees of arbitrary structure, but the ultimate goal is the same: to test for compatibility with Mendelian expectations by estimating parameters of a given model of inheritance.

Segregation analysis tests explicit models of inheritance on family data. The analytic strategy relies heavily on fitting genetic models, along with a few arbitrary nongenetic models, and selecting the model that best explains the data. While showing an adequate fit to a genetic model of inheritance in a single data set does not constitute proof that a trait or disease is in truth under genetic control, it may be considered strong statistical evidence. Even though segregation analysis has its limitations, as will be discussed below, it remains a powerful tool for identifying genetic mechanisms that may control traits associated with disease or contribute to disease risk.

8.2 COMPARING SEGREGATION ANALYSIS WITH EPIDEMIOLOGIC APPROACHES

The general approaches and limitations of segregation analysis can be compared with traditional epidemiologic analysis of risk factor-disease associations, for example, from case-control studies (see Table 8–1). Both types of studies are usually observational in nature, and both can offer only circumstantial evidence either for or against their null hypotheses, never proof. Case-

Table 8–1. Comparison of the approaches and limitations of segregation analysis of family data with epidemiologic analysis for associations between risk factors and outcomes

Characteristic	Epidemiologic methods	Segregation analysis
Approach	Observational	Observational
Null hypothesis	No association exists between factor and outcome (e.g., odds ratio = 1)	A specific genetic model can explain family data (e.g., autosomal dominant)
Statistical evaluation	To reject the null hypothesis	To identify the best fitting model
Type II errors (lack of power)	Even if an association exists, small sample size may limit the ability to reject the null hypothesis	Even if the genetic model is incorrect, small sample size may limit the ability to reject it
Type I errors	Spurious associations can occur due to chance and other biases	Even if the model is correct, the analysis may still reject it in favor of alternative models
Selection bias	If persons with certain outcome-factor combinations are more likely to be in the study sample, bias can distort odds ratios	When families with certain genotypic/phenotypic characteristics are more (or less) likely to be in the study sample, ascertainment bias can distort the final inference
Misclassification bias	When outcome or risk factors are incorrectly classified (e.g., recall bias), estimates of odds ratio can be altered	When outcome is incorrectly identified (e.g., recall bias), final statistical inference can be altered
Confounding	Associations may be due to unmeasured confounder associated with both risk factor and outcome	Consistency with a genetic model may be due to measured or unmeasured environmental factors
Representativeness	Inference is applicable to the cases evaluated, and may preclude generalization to populations	Inference is applicable to the families evaluated, and may preclude generalization to other populations

control studies can never prove that a statistical association between an exposure and a disease is causal in nature. Similarly, segregation analysis alone can never prove that a particular genetic model is correct. Other biologic data are required, such as biochemically identified gene products. Statistical analyses can be used only to determine whether observed familial patterns of a trait or disease are consistent with a specific model of inheritance when compared with more generalized models.

There is, however, a fundamental difference between statistical tests carried out in epidemiology and those in segregation analyses. In the usual epidemiologic studies, the null hypothesis states that no relationship exists between a factor and an outcome; while in segregation analysis, the null hypothesis is that the data do fit with some model of inheritance (genetic or nongenetic). Thus in the epidemiologic setting, statistical tests are based on "badness-of-fit," while in genetic analysis, tests are typically based on "goodness-of-fit" measures (Murphy, 1989). In both situations, type I and type II errors can and do occur, but they have different implications. In epidemiologic studies, a type II error occurs when a true underlying association between a risk factor and a disease is not detected statistically, frequently due to a small sample size. On the other hand, in segregation analysis, a type II error occurs when the genetic model is incorrect, but statistical testing fails to reject it, again frequently because of a small sample size. Thus, in genetic analysis, small sample sizes may lead to the inability to reject an incorrect model in favor of the true model.

In epidemiologic studies, type I errors occur when the analysis incorrectly rejects the null hypothesis and suggests an association between the risk factor and the disease. Spurious associations can occur by chance alone, and become more likely when multiple statistical tests are done on a single data set or when there are underlying biases in study design. On the other hand, type I errors occur in segregation analysis when the investigators reject a true underlying genetic model in favor of some alternative model; and sampling or ascertainment biases can be implicated here too. Selection or ascertainment bias can occur in both types of studies. While in epidemiologic studies, selection bias involves the differential sampling of individuals with different combinations of disease and risk factors; in segregation analysis, it involves the differential sampling of certain configurations of families. Ascertainment bias in segregation analysis is discussed in section 8.3.2.

Misclassification bias can also occur in both types of studies, and generally refers to the situation when the phenotypic information on individuals is incorrect (e.g., the reported disease status is not correct). In epidemiologic studies, this leads to either dilution or distortion in the magnitude of any associations. One example of misclassification bias in segregation analysis is the possible bias in reported disease status among relatives not directly contacted but classified from interviews with probands or their family members. Another source of misclassification bias occurs when relatives of cases are misclassified as unaffected because they are below the age of risk for a late-onset disease. Incorrectly classifying relatives' phenotype will compromise any statistical analysis. A unique problem in genetic analysis is the misclassification of biologic relationships among relatives. While seldom a widespread problem, it does demand diligence in data collection and interviewing techniques and can be tested for, if appropriate marker data are available.

Confounding is a problem that plagues all observational studies. In segregation analysis, in particular, environmental risk factors can be confounders, and they may mimic genetic patterns within families. Therefore, care must be exercised in collecting and analyzing risk-factor information on relatives. General approaches to considering covariate effects in segregation analysis are discussed in section 8.4.6.

Finally, the issue of representativeness needs to be addressed. In any case-control study, inferences regarding the association of disease with a particular exposure is limited to the sample at hand. Generalization to other populations and samples depends on how the cases were collected, and replication is essential before intervention or other public health policies can be initiated. The ideal design for an epidemiologic study calls for ascertainment of all new cases in a well-defined population (e.g., population-based registries). This approach maximizes the opportunities for making general inferences. The problem of generalizing to a reference population is certainly applicable to segregation analysis, although often overlooked in genetic studies. Frequently, investigators analyze a highly select group of pedigrees with multiple affected individuals for evidence of genetic mechanisms. Such pedigrees may not be ascertained from any defined population or in any systemic way, and medical genetics is replete with rare Mendelian diseases identified in one or a few families. If investigators find strong statistical evidence for a single-gene mechanism in such pedigrees, it may indeed represent a rare Mendelian disease or a rare genetic form of a common disease, but it remains unclear as to the contribution of this gene to the etiology of the disease in the population at large. Thus, while substantial progress in human genetics has been built upon analysis of isolated pedigrees, genetic epidemiology must work to place these findings into the general context of public health by assessing their applicability to the overall population. Again, the ideal design for segregation analysis calls for ascertainment of families through probands that are themselves chosen for the ideal design of an epidemiologic study, namely, incident cases from population-based registries.

8.3 SEGREGATION ANALYSIS IN SIBSHIPS

In this section, the basic approaches for performing segregation analysis in the simplest family structure (sibships) under the simplest parameterization of Mendelian models are presented. In addition to considering questions of statistical power, the issue of ascertainment bias is developed.

8.3.1 Fundamentals

When analyzing a simple discrete phenotype (e.g., affected versus nonaffected) in sibships from a single mating type, the probability of any given offspring being affected (p) is unknown, and the goal of the analysis is to estimate this probability and to test for departure from Mendelian expectations. Assuming children within a sibship are independent observations, the binomial distribution describes the probability of observing r affected offspring from a total of s sibs, as

$$P(r;s,p) = \binom{s}{r} p^r (1 - p)^{s-r},$$
(8-1)

where the coefficient "s choose r" is $s!/\{r!(s - r)!\}$ and represents the number of different combinations in which r affected offspring can occur among a total of s sibs. This binomial distribution serves as the likelihood function for a single sibship and, for a sample of n independent sibships of this same mating type, the likelihood of the total sample is simply the product of this binomial function taken over all sibships, that is,

$$\prod_{i=1}^{n} \binom{s_i}{r_i} p^{r_i} (1 - p)^{s_i - r_i}.$$
(8-2)

Whenever a single mating type among parents can be identified, therefore, it is relatively simple to estimate p and to test whether or not it is compatible with a given Mendelian expectation. For example, for a rare autosomal dominant disease (with complete penetrance and no etiologic heterogeneity), it is reasonable to assume that all matings between an affected individual and a nonaffected individual (i.e., $A \times N$ matings) represent a mutant heterozygote by normal homozygote mating type (Aa $\times$ aa) with the expected $p = .5$. Thus, the overall proportion of affected children serves as the estimator, that is,

$$\hat{p} = \frac{R}{S} = \frac{\sum_{i=1}^{n} r_i}{\sum_{i=1}^{n} s_i}.$$
(8-3)

The variance of this estimated proportion is

$$\text{Var}(\hat{p}) = \frac{\hat{p}(1 - \hat{p})}{S},$$
(8-4)

which makes it easy to test the null hypothesis of interest (i.e., that $\hat{p}$ is not significantly different from .5). For example, if one had 100 offspring from 20 sibships ascertained though a single affected parent, an observed proportion of 0.42 would have a 95% confidence interval (CI) of $[.32, .52]$ which encompasses the null hypothesis value of 0.5, and so could not be taken as evidence *against* the autosomal dominant model. Similarly an observed $\hat{p}$ of .58 has 95% CI $[.48, .68]$, which also spans the null hypothesis value. An observed value of .35 from this same sample, however, has confidence limits of $[.26, .45]$, which do not span the null hypothesis value and would lead to rejecting the autosomal dominant model. Similarly, an observed value of .65 with 95% CI of [.55, .74] would constitute evidence of non-Mendelian segregation in the sample. Note that the number of sibships does not enter into these calculations directly, due to the assumption of a single mating type (i.e., the 100 offspring could come from any number of sibships).

More often, however, the mating types of parents are *not* known with certainty. For example, a particular sample could give an apparently non-Mendelian estimate for the segregation proportion (even if the disease were in truth autosomal dominant) if the mating type $(A \times N)$ were not genetically homogeneous. For example, if $A \times N$ matings included some homozygous affected parents (e.g., $AA \times aa$ matings), the expected proportion of affected children is 1.0 for a subset of families. This is not a serious problem for rare diseases, but can be a real concern for more common traits. Consider that, if the frequency of the mutant allele is .01, 99.5% of affected individuals are expected to be heterozygous, but if the frequency of the mutant allele is .4, only 75% of all affected individuals are expected to be heterozygous. Alternatively, some of the affected parents might not carry the mutant allele at all (i.e., some affected individuals may be phenocopies), thus the expected proportion of affected offspring is effectively zero for these matings. In either situation, the ability of segregation analysis based on a single binomial distribution is severely compromised, unless a more complex likelihood function is used to reflect such mixtures of mating types among parents.

8.3.2 Ascertainment Bias and Estimating the Segregation Proportion

A fundamental problem arises in segregation analysis because families are commonly ascertained through affected offspring rather than through the parental mating types. Sampling through affected offspring considerably alters the expected ratio of affected to unaffected offspring, and induces a substantial bias in the estimate of the segregation proportion if the simplistic approach described above is adopted. For example, matings between two heterozygotes $(Aa \times Aa)$ give the familiar 1:2:1 ratio of AA, Aa, and aa genotypes among offspring and will result in a segregation proportion of .25 for strictly autosomal recessive diseases. However, if only families with one or more affected offspring are sampled, then a certain percentage of all $Aa \times Aa$ matings will never be identified because, by chance alone, they did not have an affected offspring. Specifically, 75% of all sibships of size 1 will not be sampled ($= 1 - 0.25$), 56.3% ($= 0.75^2$) of all sibships of size 2 will be missed, 42.2% ($= 0.75^3$) of all sibships of size 3 will have no affected offspring and will be missed, and so on. In effect, therefore, the binomial distribution is truncated by sampling through an affected offspring. Specifically, the proportion $(1 - p)^s$ of all sibships of size s are no longer eligible to enter the sample. Thus, the distribution of affected offspring among those sibships eligible to enter the sample is better described by the conditional probability

$$P(r > 0;s,p) = \frac{P(r;s,p)}{P(r > 0)}$$

(8-5)

$$= \frac{\binom{s}{r}p^r(1 - p)^{s-r}}{1 - (1 - p)^s}.$$

From this truncated binomial distribution, it is possible to use maximum likelihood methods to estimate the segregation proportion, although the formulas are somewhat cumbersome (Elandt-Johnson, 1971). In 1912, Weinberg used this truncated binomial distribution to obtain an estimator of the segregation proportion, $\hat{p}$, which is equivalent to the conventional maximum likelihood estimator (MLE), although it has a larger variance. An even simpler approximation for the segregation proportion in this situation of sampling from a truncated binomial distribution was developed by Li and Mantel (1968). Here, the estimator for the segregation proportion is computed as

$$\hat{p} = \frac{R - J_1}{S - J_1},$$

(8-6)

where R is the total number of affected offspring in a sample of S offspring, and J_1 represents the number of simplex sibships, that is, the number of sibships with only one affected member. The variance of this approximate estimator is generally greater than that of the regular maximum likelihood estimator, but less than that of Weinberg's original estimator. For large samples, the variance of this estimator is

$$\text{Var}\,(\hat{p}) = \frac{(R - J_1)(S - R)}{(S - J_1)^3} + \frac{2J_2(S - R)^2}{(S - J_1)^4},$$

(8-7)

where J_2 is the number of sibships with two affected individuals (Davie, 1979).

The truncated binomial distribution given in Equation 8-4 represents only the distribution of affected and unaffected offspring in *eligible* sibships. This will be an adequate description of the data present in a given study if, and only if, there is no further distortion created by the sampling process, that is, if all eligible sibships are identified with the same probability as they occur in the population. However, often sibships with two or more affected individuals (multiplex sibships) are more likely to enter the sample than simplex sibships (sibships with only one affected), and this will obviously distort the distribution of affected and nonaffected offspring and therefore bias the estimator of p. To address this problem, the concept of a *proband* was developed. Traditionally, a proband is defined as an affected individual who serves to bring a family (or sibship) into the sample and who has been ascertained *independently* of all other probands (either in the family or outside it). Families may have more than one proband (e.g., a search of a statewide registry of birth defects might ascertain two members of the same sibship); they may have affected members who are not probands (e.g., such a registry would not contain an affected sib born out of state); but no family in the sample may have zero probands (i.e., the family with only one affected sib born out of state would not be identified by the study). In comparing epidemiologic and genetic studies, an index case is effectively a proband.

By specifying the probability of an affected individual's becoming a proband, it should be possible to obtain an unbiased estimator for p, the segregation proportion; however, some assumptions are required. The simplest model assumes that all affected individuals have some constant probability of being ascertained as a proband, say π. Under the assumption that all probands are truly independently ascertained, the same binomial distribution seen in Equation 8-1 can be used to describe the distribution of c probands among r affected sibs in a family, that is,

$$P(c;r,\pi) = \binom{r}{c}\pi^c(1 - \pi)^{r-c}. \tag{8-8}$$

Because families with $c = 0$ will not be identified, the distribution of probands among r affected individuals in *sampled* sibships is itself a truncated binomial distribution:

$$P(c > 0;r,\pi) = 1 - (1 - \pi)^r. \tag{8-9}$$

In other words, sibships where all r affected individuals are missed by the sampling procedure will be lost to the study. The probability distribution for probands among the affected individuals must be combined with the distribution of affected individuals among all sibs to obtain the probability of ascertaining a sibship (Elandt-Johnson, 1971). For this, one writes

$$P(c>0;s,p,\pi) = \sum_{r=1}^{s} \binom{s}{r} p^r(1-p)^{s-r}[1 - (1 - \pi)^r]$$

$$= \sum_{r=1}^{s} \binom{s}{r} p^r(1-p)^{s-r} - \sum_{r=1}^{s} \binom{s}{r} p^r(1-p)^{s-r}(1 - \pi)^r \tag{8-10}$$

(Note the first term merely represents the loss of sibships where r is zero, while the second can itself be written as a binomial with terms $(1 - \pi)p$ and $(1 - p)$.) We may continue

$$= 1 - (1 - p)^s - \sum_{r=1}^{s} \binom{s}{r} [(1 - \pi)p]^r(1 - p)^{s-r}$$

$$= 1 - (1 - p)^s - \{(1 - p)^s + [(1 - \pi)p + (1 - p)]^s\} \tag{8-11}$$

$$= 1 - (1 - \pi p)^s.$$

This result can be understood by noting that πp represents the *joint* probability of being affected and being ascertained as a proband. Therefore, the only families not represented in the sample are those where all s offspring are *not* both affected and a proband (Morton, 1982). This probability of at least one proband in each sibship can then be used to condition the original distribution of affected offspring in sibships (given in Equation 8-1) on the fact that they were ascertained through an affected proband. The conditional distribution of r affected individuals in sibships of size s *in the sample* is then computed from the joint probability distribution for affected individuals in a sibship and the distribution of probands in ascertained sibships (Equation 8-8) divided by the probability of ascertaining the sibship (Equation 8-9), that is,

$$P(r|c>0; s, p, \pi) = \frac{P(r; s, p) \cap P(c>0; r, \pi)}{P(c>0; s, p, \pi)}$$

$$= \frac{\binom{s}{r} p^r (1-p)^{s-r} [1 - (1-\pi)^r]}{1 - (1-p\pi)^s}.$$

(8-12)

This conditional probability distribution can then serve as the likelihood function to estimate the main parameter of interest (p, the segregation ratio) as well as the secondary parameter (π, the probability of an affected individual becoming a proband).

While maximum likelihood estimators obtained from Equation 8-12 represent the most efficient way to estimate both p and π, in most situations, the segregation ratio p is of primary interest, and often the ascertainment probability π is little more than a nuisance parameter. Therefore, it is convenient to note that the simple approximation given in Equation 8-6 is valid as long as the distinction between probands and affected nonprobands is carefully maintained. While this estimator was originally developed for situations of *complete ascertainment* (i.e., where π in Equation 8-7 is fixed at 1.0), later workers have shown this method of subtracting off the number of sibships with only one proband (simplex sibships with respect to proband status) is also valid for situations where π is less than 1.0 (Davie, 1979; Li et al., 1987). The key to using this simple estimator is to note consistently the proband versus nonproband status of all affected sibs within a family. The generalization of Equation 8-6 results if J_1 is the number of sibships with only one proband, although there may be other affected nonprobands in the sibship. Similarly Equation 8-7 can be generalized by letting J_2 be the number of sibships with exactly two probands, regardless of whether or not there are affected nonprobands in the sibship.

An interesting result occurs if one considers π to be fixed at some very small value in this model, that is, if very few affected individuals are identified as probands. Specifically, because $(1 - x)^y = 1 - yx$ when x is near 0, Equation 8-12 reduces to

$$P(r|c>0; s, p, \pi=0) = \frac{\binom{s}{r} p^r (1-p)^{s-r} [1 - (1-r\pi)]}{1 - (1-sp\pi)}$$

$$= \frac{\binom{s}{r} p^r (1-p)^{s-r} r\pi}{sp\pi}$$

(8-13)

$$= \binom{s-1}{r-1} p^{r-1} (1-p)^{s-r}$$

Note that this is merely the binomial distribution for affected *nonprobands* in the sibship. This situation of very inefficient sampling, where the probability of an affected individual's becoming a proband (π) is quite small, is frequently referred to as *single ascertainment* because no sibship is likely to have more than one proband. If the assumption of strict independence among probands holds so that Equation 8-8 remains valid, then the distribution of affected individuals among sibs of affected probands follows a simple binomial form after excluding the proband (Morton, 1982). This allows estimation of the segregation parameter as

$$\hat{p} = \frac{R - N}{S - N},$$
(8-14)

where, as before, R is the total number of affecteds, S is the total number of offspring, and N is the total number of sibships (which here is equivalent to the number of sibships with a single proband since there can be only one proband per sibship, that is, $N = J_1$). Despite the similarity with Equation 8-6, one must return to the binomial distribution in Equation 8-11 to compute the variance about the MLE in this situation of single ascertainment, that is,

$$\text{Var}\ (\hat{p}) = \frac{\hat{p}(1 - \hat{p})}{S - N}.$$
(8-15)

In this situation of single ascertainment (i.e., where π is very small), the distortion of the distribution of affected and nonaffected offspring is at its greatest under the binomial model given in Equation 8-8. When the ascertainment probability (π) is one under this model, it is often presented as implying all affected offspring are ascertained as probands (hence the term "complete ascertainment"). In truth, however, there is merely no distortion in favor of multiplex sibships during the sampling process. Thus, the sample distribution is merely truncated by loss of sibships where $r = 0$, but not distorted from its natural form. Under single ascertainment, however, sibships with two affected individuals will be represented in the sample at twice their population rate, sibships with three affected individuals will be represented at three times their population rate, and so on. While this linear distortion in the distribution of multiplex sibships is the worst case possible under this binomial model of ascertainment, other models with greater levels of distortion are conceivable, as discussed in section 8.3.4.

8.3.3 Statistical Power in Segregation Analysis of Sibships

Using the binomial distribution to calculate the probability of observing various numbers of affected children, the minimum sample size needed to reject a wrong null hypothesis value (H_0) at the 5% significance level (in a one-sided test) can be computed for any specific value of the alternative hypothesis (H_A). Table 8-2 shows such minimal sample sizes along with value expected under the null hypothesis, the critical value for the test, and the actual attained power at that critical value. Since the critical value (i.e., the number of

Table 8–2. Minimum samples needed in segregation analysis of sibships (without ascertainment bias)

H_A	H_0: $p = 0.5$				H_0: $p = 0.25$			
	Minimum sample size	Expected	Critical value	Attained power (%)	Minimum sample size	Expected	Critical value	Attained power (%)
0.01	5	2.5	0	95.1	11	2.8	0	89.6
0.10	11	5.5	2	91.0	50	12.5	7	87.8
0.20	18	9.0	5	86.7	463	115.8	100	82.2
0.25	28	14.0	9	86.2	—	—	—	—
0.30	42	21.0	15	88.6	522	130.5	148	80.8
0.40	169	84.5	73	82.3	68	17.0	24	82.8
0.50	—	—	—	—	28	7.0	12	82.8
0.60	169	84.5	96	82.3	16	4.0	8	85.8
0.70	42	21.0	27	83.6	8	2.0	5	80.6

Two values of the null hypothesis were considered, $p = 0.5$ corresponding to an autosomal dominant model and $p = 0.25$ corresponding to an autosomal recessive model. Minimum sample sizes needed to reject a false null hypothesis at the $\alpha = 0.05$ level (one-sided test) with 80% power under binomial model.

affected offspring at which H_0 will be rejected) must be an integer, often the attained power is greater than 80%. Consider the example where the true proportion of affected offspring from a series of $A \times N$ matings were 0.1 (and thus clearly non-Mendelian), one would need only observe 11 offspring to reject the erroneous null hypothesis of $p = 0.5$ with at least 80% power, that is, 80 times out of 100. More specifically, the erroneous null hypothesis would have predicted 5.5 affected offspring, but observing 2 or fewer affected offspring in a sample of 11 would lead to rejecting the null hypothesis 91% of the time.

Note that these minimum sample sizes represent the total number of sibs over all sibships, regardless of the size of individual sibships, because it was assumed sibs are independent of one another, given the mating type of the parents (this implies there is no environmental component to risk that varies across families). Clearly relatively modest sample sizes are quite adequate when the true segregation proportion is far from the Mendelian expectation, but, as the difference between the true value and the Mendelian value decreases, much larger sample sizes are required to detect non-Mendelian segregation.

Also shown in Table 8–2 are minimum sample sizes required to reject the null hypothesis that the proportion of affected children is 0.25, as would occur when analyzing offspring of matings between two heterozygous carriers of a recessive disease (again assuming complete penetrance, no variability in the age of onset, and no etiologic heterogeneity). Whenever the mating types of the parents are known, such that the outcomes among offspring are essentially drawn from a binomial distribution with some constant parameter p, such simple tables are sufficient guides to selecting the sample sizes necessary to rigorously test Mendelian models.

When there is the potential for ascertainment bias, that is, when families are sampled through an affected offspring, the likelihood function given in Equation 8-12 is used to obtain MLEs for p which will be asymptotically normally distributed with a variance that reflects the sibship size, the number of sibships observed, the true values of the ascertainment probability (π) and the true value of segregation parameter (p) (Elandt-Johnson, 1971). By taking advantage of this asymptotic normality of the MLEs, approximate minimum sample sizes needed to test the two simplest Mendelian null hypotheses (autosomal recessive and autosomal dominant) can be computed for a range of alternative values (Wong and Rotter, 1984). Such information is critical when designing family studies to ensure a final sample size large enough to reject a false null hypothesis most of the time (typically a power of 80% or more is the minimal acceptable). The sample size needed to achieve this level of statistical power is always a function of the difference between the true value of the parameter being tested (here p) and the null hypothesis value, but the specification of other parameters also influence these minimum sample sizes. Table 8–3 shows some estimated minimum sample sizes needed to test for autosomal recessive and dominant segregation in sibships. For example, only 36 sibships of size 2 are needed to reject a false null hypothesis ($p = .25$) with probability 0.8 when the true value is $p = .5$; however, vastly larger sample sizes are required when the true value is quite close to the null hy-

Table 8–3. Minimum samples needed in segregation analysis of sibships (with ascertainment bias)

	π = 1.0 (complete)			π = 0.5			π = 0.05			π → 0 (single)		
True p	S = 2	S = 3	S = 4	S = 2	S = 3	S = 4	S = 2	S = 3	S = 4	S = 2	S = 3	S = 4
Null hypothesis: p = 0.25 [autosomal recessive model]												
0.10	86	40	25	64	16	21	55	27	18	54	27	18
0.30	916	425	266	708	350	231	616	308	205	609	305	204
0.50	36	17	10	29	14	9	26	13	9	26	13	9
Null hypothesis: p = 0.50 [autosomal dominant model]												
0.10	12	5	3	10	5	3	9	5	3	9	5	3
0.25	36	16	10	31	15	10	29	15	10	29	14	10
0.40	227	103	64	201	99	66	194	97	65	194	97	65

Two values of the null hypothesis were considered, p = 0.5 corresponding to an autosomal dominant model and p = 0.25 corresponding to an autosomal recessive model. Minimum number of sibships required to reject a false null hypothesis at the α = 0.05 level with power of 80% under the binomial model.

Adapted from Wong and Rotter (1984).

245

pothesis value (e.g., 916 sib pairs would be needed to achieve this same level of statistical power when the true $p = .3$).

Furthermore, larger sibships bring more information per individual than smaller sibships. Table 8–3 shows that 10 sibships of size 4 (40 individuals) carry as much information for distinguishing between an autosomal recessive null hypothesis and an autosomal dominant alternative hypothesis, as do 36 sibships of size 2 (72 individuals) under complete ascertainment. In general, it is more cost-effective to sample larger sibships, because fewer total people need to be examined to distinguish between competing genetic models. This possible gain in efficiency is constrained by the availability of larger sibships, of course. When it becomes more expensive and/or difficult to identify or recruit large sibships, the preferred strategy would be to take the more common smaller sibships. One must also consider whether large sibships are representative of the general population or a select subset. It is important to realize that these minimum sample sizes are only approximate, however, primarily because the methods used to compute variances about the parameter values assume samples of only one sibship size at a time. Nonetheless, they do serve as a useful guide in designing family studies.

8.3.4 Alternative Models for Correcting for Ascertainment Bias

As stated earlier, the use of the binomial distribution to describe the distribution of probands among affected individuals (given in Equation 8-7) requires two key assumptions. Specifically, first, one must assume there is some constant probability that an affected individual will be ascertained as a proband, and, second, one must assume all probands are truly independent of one another. Neither of these assumptions is easily testable in family studies, however, and it is difficult to support either assumption. It is reasonable to suppose that certain groups of affected individuals may have different probabilities of being ascertained depending on their access to medical care, the severity and age of onset of their disease, and so on. Furthermore, several sources of ascertainment are often used by any one study: clinic referrals, disease registries, vital records, population surveys, etc. Each source is likely to have a different probability of identifying affected individuals as probands, and these may not be constant among all groups in the population. For example, vital records could provide more complete coverage of a defined population but may underreport the true disease frequency, while hospital or clinic referral sources may accurately report all affected patients but may only draw from selected subsets of the population. Some information on the probability of ascertaining an affected individual as a proband (π) can be gained by noting the number of overlapping ascertainments for each proband, that is, how many probands were ascertained by only one source, by two sources, and so on (Morton, 1982). Frequently, however, the sources of ascertainment are not independent (i.e., ascertainment through death records may preclude ascertainment through clinic referral), and this will lead to an underestimate of π.

While it is difficult to give a simple definition of the "best" ascertainment scheme for any disease, some criteria can be given. First, every effort should be made to attain complete ascertainment where there is no distortion in the underlying distribution of sibships with 1, 2, and so on affected members. This does not necessarily imply that *all* affected individuals be identified as probands (although that certainly removes any distortion), but rather multiplex sibships should not be overrepresented in the sample. Reliance on disease registries is recommended, although, for severe diseases requiring medical treatment, clinic-based studies can achieve nearly complete ascertainment. Second, the ascertainment scheme should specify the population of reference in terms of geography and time covered, as well as in terms of the genetic composition of the subjects (i.e., membership in ethnic group). In some populations with high levels of inbreeding, it may be necessary to consider individual inbreeding levels and thus collect genealogical data on all probands. Wherever appropriate, information on environmental covariates should be incorporated into the segregation analysis. Reliance on population-based samples provides the opportunity for broad inferences about the public health impact of genetic factors.

The second assumption of complete independence among probands is also difficult to justify, especially within a sibship or pedigree. A second affected child in a family may be brought to attention more readily than the first affected child because the parents are more informed about the disease. This dependence may also extend beyond the sibship, such that a cousin of a proband may have a greater chance of being ascertained through a single clinic because the extended family is more informed about the disease. Alternatively, a negative effect within sibship is also possible if medical treatment is ineffective or the "disease" is relatively minor. For example, parents may judge it not worthwhile to bring a second affected child into a study if no benefit resulted from enrolling the first. Similarly, if the disease or trait is judged as "normal" by the family, a second affected child may be less likely to enter the study. Greenberg (1986) has shown that such dependence among potential probands can result in severe biases in the estimated segregation ratio and compromise tests of genetic mechanisms.

One unfortunate consequence of relying exclusively on Equation 8-7 is that many mistakenly consider single ascertainment ($\pi \rightarrow 0$) to be the limiting case of the distortion possible when ascertaining sibships through an affected offspring. As described above, under the binomial assumption, when π approaches 0, the probability of a sibship entering the study is a strict linear function of the number of affected offspring (r). Sibships with two affected offspring are represented in the sample twice as frequently as they occur in the population, sibships with three affected offspring are represented at three times their population rate, and so on. Since simple estimators have been worked out for this situation of single ascertainment and for the case of complete ascertainment (where $\pi \rightarrow 1.0$), a common strategy is to estimate the segregation parameter (p) under both complete and under single ascertainment, assuming these two situations represent the limits of all possible biases. If the resulting estimate of p under both single and complete ascertainment are compatible with Mendelian inheritance, this is often taken as strong evidence in favor of a genetic mechanism.

However, distortions beyond the linear pattern may well occur. For example, the probability of ascertaining a family may increase exponentially with the number of affected individuals. Thus, multiplex sibships can be vastly overrepresented in the sample, for example, sibships with two affected offspring occur in the sample at four times their population frequency, sibships with three affected offspring occur at nine times their true rate, and so on. Ewens and Shute (1986) point out that some sets of family data appear to fit such a quadratic function where the probability of the family's being ascertained increases with the square of the number of affected individuals. This quadratic pattern of bias could easily result from two layers of single ascertainment, where the first layer of bias might occur at the clinic level and the second at the level of a collaborative study among clinics.

A nonparametric approach for adjusting for ascertainment has been proposed by Ewens and Shute (1986), where no specific form of the probability of ascertaining a family is assumed. Rather, the likelihood function of the genetic model is conditioned first on that subset of the data that is relevant to ascertainment. In the case of nuclear families ascertained through affected children, this subset would constitute the number of affected children and possibly the status of their parents; in the case of larger pedigrees, it might be sibships or families, which could have been ascertained through a single source (e.g., only those residing in the geographic region served by a given clinic). Only after this first step of conditioning, are the parameters of the genetic model estimated in a second stage of analysis, and thus this approach is more computationally intensive (Hopper et al., 1990). It has been demonstrated that misspecifying the ascertainment function for family data can lead to biases in estimates of genetic parameters (Shute and Ewens 1988a, 1988b). The cost of this conditioning on subsets of the data is an unavoidable loss of precision in the final estimators, that is, because the conditioning process removes information contained in part of the data, the standard errors about the final estimators will be larger than those obtained if an unconditional process were adopted (Shute and Ewens, 1988a). It can be shown, however, that this conditioning on an unknown ascertainment process will not invariably result in a "conditioning out" of all information in the sample at hand, but will give the same MLEs for genetic parameters as would the correct choice of ascertainment model (Hodge, 1988).

8.4 SEGREGATION ANALYSIS IN PEDIGREES

The use of sibship data alone to estimate the proportion of affected offspring represents a limited form of segregation analysis. Not only is it limited by the assumption about the form of ascertainment, but it does not offer an opportunity to disentangle the underlying causal factors that could produce non-Mendelian ratios. For example, a segregation proportion of 40% in a sample of sibships could result from non-Mendelian transmission of the causal factor, from a reduced penetrance of the mutant allele for an autosomal dominant disease, or from the presence of some percentage of phenocopies among families. When estimating the single summary parameter (p, the proportion of affected offspring), it is not possible to distinguish among these explanations. By explicitly defining the parameters of a more complete model of inheritance, however, it is possible to use maximum likelihood techniques to test hypotheses representing these separate and distinct biologic mechanisms that might account for a non-Mendelian distribution of phenotypes among sibs.

8.4.1 Defining a General Model of Inheritance

The extension to a general model of inheritance requires explicit definition of all the basic parameters involved. First among these parameters is the number of different types of individuals possible. These essential "types," termed *ousiotypes* by Cannings and colleagues (1978) from the Greek word *oussos* for essence, are required to construct any model of inheritance. Since single-locus, diallelic models represent the simplest Mendelian model, general models of inheritance usually permit three such ousiotypes, and these may actually correspond to the three genotypes of a single-locus trait with two alleles. While one can think of these essential "types" as genotypes, it must be understood that until there is evidence of Mendelian transmission they must be treated in a more general manner.

Beyond this implicit assumption of the number of relevant "types" of individuals, three general classes of parameters are required to construct the likelihood function for a general model of inheritance. The first two classes specify the frequency with which these different "types" of individuals may occur. In pedigree data, there are two kinds of individuals: *founders* (or originals) whose parents are unknown, and *nonfounders* (or nonoriginals) who are the offspring or descendants of founders. *Frequency parameters* specify the probability of any founder having each of the essential "types" (i.e., each ousiotype). These frequency parameters may be simple products of a binomial proportion (which is the underpinning of Hardy-Weinberg equilibrium in a population), or they may be more general multinomial frequencies.

While frequency parameters determine the probability of a founder having each possible "type" or ousiotype, the probability of a nonfounder having each "type" is a function of the actual transmission of alleles from parent to offspring (be they true alleles at a genetic locus or more general, nongenetic "factors"). Therefore *transmission parameters* must be defined to represent the probability of each parental "type" transmitting an underlying "factor" or allele to an offspring. One subset of all possible transmission probabilities corresponds exactly to Mendelian inheritance, but non-Mendelian inheritance must also be considered.

The third and final class of parameters in any general model of inheritance defines the relationship between the unobserved, essential "type" (or ousiotype) and the observed phenotype. These parameters are termed *penetrance parameters* because they reflect the conditional probability of observing the phenotype given the individual's "type" or ousiotype. These penetrance functions can be probability functions for discrete phenotypes (either simple probabilities or cumulative incidence functions, depending on age) or density functions describing the distribution of a quantitative phenotype.

8.4.2 Likelihood Functions on Pedigrees

The likelihood function of any statistical model evaluated on a set of data is proportional to the probability of the observed data under the model at hand (Edwards, 1978). In segregation analysis, a likelihood function is constructed by considering the genotypic probabilities of all individuals in the pedigree (or more generally, the probability of each individual's having each possible "type" or ousiotype) and the probability of each observed phenotype occurring under each possible ousiotype. Conceptually, this likelihood can be visualized as a series of joint probabilities summed over all possible combinations of essential "types" or ousiotypes. For example, if there are $m = 1 \cdots M$ "types" possible under the model, let $f(m)$ represent the frequency of the mth "type" and $P(Y|m)$ be the penetrance function of this "type" or ousiotype (where either $P(Y_I|m)$ is a conditional probability that person I has an observed discrete phenotype Y_I given ousiotype m; or an analogous conditional density function for ousiotype m, if the observed phenotype Y_I is continuous). Then any founder individual I in a pedigree contributes

$$\sum_{m=1}^{M} P(Y_I|m)f(m) \tag{8-16}$$

to the likelihood function. In other words, the likelihood function is merely the product of the prior probability of having a given essential "type" or ousiotype times the conditional probability of having the observed phenotype given this "type," summed over all possible "types." If matings are independent of such "types" or ousiotypes, the joint probability of pair of founder parents I and J can be written as

$$\sum_{i=1}^{M} P(Y_I|i)f(i) \sum_{j=1}^{M} P(Y_J|j)f(j)$$
$$= \sum_i \sum_j P(Y_I|i)P(Y_J|j)f(i)f(j). \tag{8-17}$$

Furthermore, letting the transmission parameters $t(k|ij)$ describe the probability of the kth "type" in offspring K of parents I and J, allows the likelihood of such a parent-offspring trio to be written as

$$\sum_{i=1}^{M} P(Y_I|i)f(i) \sum_{j=1}^{M} P(Y_J|j)f(j) \sum_{k=1}^{M} P(Y_K|k)t(k|i,j)$$
$$= \sum_i \sum_j \sum_k P(Y_I|i)P(Y_J|j)P(Y_K|k)f(i)f(j)t(k|i,j). \tag{8-18}$$

Note that the sequential summations over all possible "types" or ousiotypes for this parent-offspring trio are in effect computing a nonnormalized conditional probability (or likelihood) of the observed data on parents I and J and their offspring K (each with the observed phenotypes Y_I, Y_J, and Y_K, respectively), weighted by the appropriate prior probabilities (Smith, 1976). In general, if a pedigree contains N individuals, N_1 of whom are founders (and N_2 of whom are nonfounders with both parents contained in the pedigree), the likelihood function of the entire pedigree can be written as

$$\sum_{i_1} \sum_{i_2} \cdots \sum_{i_N} \prod_{j=1}^{N} P(Y_j|i_j) \prod_{k=1}^{N_1} f(i_k) \prod_{m=1}^{N_2} t(i_m|i_{m_1},i_{m_2}). \qquad (8\text{-}19)$$

Note the first product (that for the penetrance parameters) is over all N members of the pedigrees, while the middle product (for frequency parameters) is over the N_1 founders, and the last product (for transmission parameters) is over the $N_2(=N-N_1)$ nonfounders in the pedigree (Hasstedt, 1982).

From this formulation, the likelihood function can be visualized as a complete enumeration of all possible combinations of the essential "types" or ousiotypes that can occur in the pedigree considering both their prior probabilities (either in terms of frequencies for founders, or transmission probabilities for nonfounders) and the conditional probability of their observed phenotypes given each ousiotype. To compute the likelihood as it is written here, however, would be impractical, since it requires summing products of probabilities for $(M)^N$ combinations of ousiotypes. Even for moderate-sized pedigrees, this becomes computationally intractable. For example, the minimal Mendelian model requires $M = 3$, so a simple parent-offspring trio represents 27 genotypic combinations, while a pedigree of size 10 represents 59,049 distinct genotypic combinations. Computing the likelihood function on larger pedigrees would be technically difficult for fixed values of the parameters (i.e., frequency, penetrance, and transmission parameters), and iterative procedures for estimating these parameters would be generally prohibitive, using this approach of complete enumeration.

The repetitive internal structure of pedigrees, however, permits recursive methods to be used that sequentially accumulate the components of this overall likelihood function (Lange and Elston, 1975; Cannings et al., 1976; Cannings et al., 1978). These recursive methods originally employed graph theory to note that any pedigree, regardless of its structure and complexity, can be represented as a series of interconnected units involving a limited variety of connections. For example, a member of a large pedigree may have an impressive array of relatives (first cousins, great-uncles, second cousins once removed, etc.), but all such relationships can be expressed as repeated parent-offspring, spouse, or sib relationships. In other words, a first cousin is merely the offspring of a parent's sib; a great-uncle is the sib of a parent's parent; a second cousin once removed is the grandchild (= offspring's offspring) of a parent's parent's sib's offspring.

The nuclear family, which is a combination of the essential parent-offspring, spouse, and sib relationship, serves as the basic unit for this sequential conditioning process. In simple pedigrees, that is, those without marriage or inbreeding loops, the likelihood is constructed by sequentially "peeling" information from a nuclear family either "up" onto a parent connecting two nuclear families or "down" onto an offspring connecting two nuclear families. Such connecting individuals, termed "pivots" by Cannings and colleagues (1978), are the connections between nuclear families in any extended pedigree. This permits all information to be separated into mutually exclusive subsets—that "above" the pivot (connected through his or her parents) and that "below" the pivot (connected through his or her spouse and offspring). By sequentially calculating the conditional probabilities through a series of such pivots, the likelihood for an entire extended pedigree can be obtained (Thompson, 1986). In other words, a series of single individuals (pivots) connect all nuclear families in the pedigree into a "peeling" sequence for sequentially conditioning one nuclear family subunit onto another. The conditional likelihood obtained at the end of this peeling sequence is exactly proportional to the probability of the observed data under the model at hand, that is, it *is* the likelihood of the model.

In terms of the graph theory behind the "peeling" process, a simple pedigree is one where each pivot divides the remaining pedigree into mutually exclusive subsets. When there are inbreeding or marriage loops, however, the subset of the pedigree "above" a pivot and that "below" the pivot are no longer mutually exclusive, that is, one or more individuals may be connected to the pivot both through his or her parents *and* through his or her spouse or offspring. For example, in a mating between first cousins, the spouse of a pivot is related to the parents of the pivot. In these situations, it becomes necessary to consider the joint probability of more than one individual when following the peeling sequence through the pedigree. The computation of the necessary conditional probabilities becomes more cumbersome and increases exponentially with the number of individuals that must be jointly considered. However, because the number of individuals who must be considered jointly is generally small even for quite complex pedigrees, it is still possible to use this sequential approach to compute likelihood functions on complex pedigrees. Thompson (1986) has shown how this sequential process for accumulating the likelihood function can be used on pedigrees that represent the entire genealogy over many generations of an isolated population.

Defining the Parameters for Mendelian and Polygenic Models

An important goal of segregation analysis is to distinguish between competing genetic models. The primary competitors are the single-locus Mendelian model and the more amorphous "polygenic" model. While the polygenic model is built upon the principles of Mendelian inheritance, it does not attempt to identify individual loci exerting large effects on the phenotype (e.g., genotypic effects or allele frequencies), rather it relies on the summary statistic of heritability to quantitate the degree of genetic control. Under the general multifactorial model described in Chapter 7, the expected covariances among relatives are identical under a single Mendelian locus and under the traditional additive polygenic model. Therefore it is of prime interest to distinguish between these two competing genetic models. To accomplish this, a complete notation for these two models of inheritance is presented.

Frequency Parameters. For a single locus, the number of frequency parameters needed is one less than the number of alleles (assuming the population of inference is in Hardy-Weinberg equilibrium), and otherwise is at a maximum of one less than the number of possible genotypes. For example, for a single-locus model (with alleles A_1 and A_2), the frequency parameters would be

$$f(A_1A_1) = p^2,$$

$$f(A_1A_2) = 2pq, \tag{8-20}$$

$$f(A_2A_2) = q^2,$$

if Hardy-Weinberg equilibrium exists (where $q = 1 - p$). For multiple loci, the number of distinct genotypes increases geometrically, but again the assumption of multilocus Hardy-Weinberg equilibrium minimizes the number of frequency parameters. It is worth noting that, in general, multilocus models require specification of the degree of disequilibrium present between linked loci when defining the corresponding frequency of genotypes. This disequilibrium component is distinct from the recombination fraction between loci specified as part of the transmission parameters.

The other model of inheritance commonly considered is the additive *polygenic model* where the individual genotypes are no longer of interest, but only the variation induced by them is estimated. Under the strict additive polygenic model, a given "polygenotype" G can be treated as an unobserved random variable that follows a normal distribution with a population mean of zero and variance σ_A^2 (Elston, 1981). Under this polygenic model, therefore, the frequency parameter is written as

$$f(G) = (2\pi\sigma_A^2)^{-1/2} \exp \frac{1}{2}\frac{G}{\sigma_A^2} = \phi(G, \sigma_A^2). \tag{8-21}$$

Under the polygenic model, no attempt is made to estimate the actual expected frequency of any given "polygenotype," but only the phenotypic variance associated with all such genotypes. Thus, the polygenic model is quite close to the classic random effects model used in analysis of variance.

If mating is random with respect to genotype (be it a genotype at a single locus or a "polygenotype"), the frequency of a pair of parents can be computed simply as the product of their individual frequencies. If there is assortative mating (either negative or positive), however, the conditional probability of the genotype in one parent given the genotype of the other parent must be used instead. This is only a minor problem for Mendelian models as long as there is some reasonable structure for specifying these conditional probabilities. For example, if founders were drawn from a population with average inbreeding coefficient F, the appropriate genotypic frequencies would be

$$f(A_1A_1) = p^2(1 - F) + pF$$

$$f(A_1A_2) = 2pq(1 - F) \tag{8-22}$$

$$f(A_1A_2) = q^2(1 - F) + qF$$

rather than those given in Equation 8-20. No other changes in the parameterization of the model are necessary.

For polygenic models, however, assortative mating has effects beyond simple changes in frequency parameters. Assortative mating must be based on phenotypic similarities, and, to the extent that "polygenes" control the phenotype, a phenotypic correlation in general leads to a correlation in the underlying genetic factors. In the presence of positive assortative mating, the additive genetic variance is increased (and therefore heritability also increases) because the differences between families are greater. In other words, because parents are more similar to one another, there are greater differences among families. At equilibrium, if there were a correlation r between parental phenotypes, the additive genetic variance (σ_A^2) would be

$$\sigma_A^2 = \frac{\sigma_A^{2*}}{(1 - rh^2)}, \tag{8-23}$$

where σ_A^{2*} represents the additive genetic variance which would exist if mating were truly random and h^2 is the narrow-sense heritability at equilibrium (i.e., $h^2 = \sigma_A^2/\sigma^2$, where σ^2 is the total phenotypic variance at equilibrium) (Falconer, 1981; Bulmer, 1985). In addition to this increase in the additive genetic component created by assortative mating, however, the expected correlation between parents and offspring is also inflated. Thus, not only do the frequency parameters change, but the actual transmission parameters are influenced by assortative mating for traits strictly controlled by polygenes (Thompson, 1986).

It is important to remember that this inflation due to assortative mating generally has a modest effect on the final estimate of heritability. If, for example, a trait had a narrow-sense heritability of .5 under random mating, the introduction of a positive correlation of $r = .5$ between mates would only inflate the equilibrium heritability to .58 (Bulmer, 1985). Also, it is important to note that an observed phenotypic correlation of r may not always induce the same level of correlation in additive genetic factors between parents. Specifically, in Equation 8-23 it was implicitly assumed the phenotypic correlation between spouses (r) translated in a straightforward manner into a correlation in breeding values of rh^2. It is conceivable, however, that the phenotypic correlation between spouses could originate primarily from common environmental factors and remain unrelated to genetic factors influencing the phenotype. For example, if environmental factors influencing performance on IQ tests (e.g., schools attended) were truly independent of genetic factors influencing IQ but played a strong role in mate selection, there would be a phenotypic correlation between spouses but no carryover correlation in the genes influencing the trait, and thus no effect on $\hat{\sigma}_A^2$ or on heritability (Falconer, 1981).

Transmission Parameters. The transmission parameters for simple Mendelian models define the probabilities of each mating type transmitting a specified genotype to an offspring. Elston and Stewart (1971) showed that three basic transmission parameters are sufficient to specify the genotypic probabilities of offspring under a single-locus, two-allele Mendelian model. The probability of a parent's transmitting the A_1 allele to an offspring can be written as a (3×1) vector $\boldsymbol{\tau}$, where each element reflects the three possible parental genotypes

Parental genotype P (transmitting allele A_1)

$$\begin{array}{cc} A_1A_1 \\ A_1A_2 \\ A_2A_2 \end{array} \qquad \begin{bmatrix} 1 \\ 1/2 \\ 0 \end{bmatrix} = \boldsymbol{\tau}$$

Note that from this, it is easy to obtain the probability of receiving the alternate allele (i.e., the probability of transmitting the A_2 alleles is $\boldsymbol{\tau}^* = 1 - \boldsymbol{\tau}$). Using this vector notation, the probability of an offspring K having each genotype can be represented as a series of direct products of these (3×1) transmission vectors for parents I and J (the direct product $\otimes$ involves multiplying each element of the first vector by the entire second vector). The resulting product matrix, **T**, is

$$\tau(k|i,j) = \mathbf{T} = [\tau_i \otimes \tau_j \{(\tau_i \otimes \tau_j^*) + (\tau_i \otimes \tau_j^*)\} \tau_i^* \otimes \tau_j^*] \qquad (8\text{-}24)$$

This product matrix has dimensions of (9×3) since taking a direct product of a $(r_1 \times c_1)$ matrix and a $(r_2 \times c_2)$ matrix results in a $(r_1r_2 \times c_1c_2)$ matrix. Table 8–4 shows the full (9×3) matrix of transmission probabilities for a single Mendelian locus with two alleles, in the absence of mutation or segregation distortion. Each column of this matrix corresponds to one of the three possible genotypes in an offspring.

Similar vectors of probabilities can be written for X-linked loci. The number of genotypes differs between males and females, however, and the transmission parameters depend on the sex of the offspring. Specifically, the 3×1 vector $\boldsymbol{\tau}$ for mothers is identical to that listed above, but, for fathers, $\boldsymbol{\tau}$ is a (2×1) vector for the two possible paternal genotypes (i.e., $\boldsymbol{\tau}' = (1,0)$). For daughters, this leads to a (6×3) transmission matrix computed as in Equation 8-24, which is also shown in Table 8-4. For sons, however, the corresponding matrix is

$$\tau(k|i,j) = [\tau_i \otimes \mathbf{1}, (1 - \tau_i) \otimes \mathbf{1}], \qquad (8\text{-}25)$$

where **1** is the (2×1) unit vector $(1,1)$. This results in transmission probabilities for sons that are functions of only the mother's genotype (see Table 8–4).

Similar matrices of genotypic probabilities can be constructed for multiple alleles at a single locus and for multiple loci. For any multiallelic system, the number of basic transmission parameters is one less than the number of alleles. These parameters define the probability of transmitting alleles from each possible genotype, with the probability of transmitting the remaining allele computed by subtraction.

For multiple-locus systems, not only is the number of genotypes increased,

Table 8–4. Transmission probabilities for single-locus models with two alleles (A_1 and A_2)

Parental mating type	For a single autosomal locus		
	Offspring genotype		
	A_1A_1	A_1A_2	A_2A_2
$A_1A_1 \times A_1A_1$	1	0	0
$A_1A_1 \times A_1A_2$	1/2	1/2	0
$A_1A_1 \times A_2A_2$	0	1	0
$A_1A_2 \times A_1A_1$	1/2	1/2	0
$A_1A_2 \times A_1A_2$	1/4	1/2	1/4
$A_1A_2 \times A_2A_2$	0	1/2	1/2
$A_2A_2 \times A_1A_1$	0	1	0
$A_2A_2 \times A_1A_2$	0	1/2	1/2
$A_2A_2 \times A_2A_2$	0	0	1

For a single X-linked locus, the analogous transmission probabilities depend on the sex of the offspring

Parental mating type	Daughter's genotype			Son's genotype	
	A_1A_1	A_1A_2	A_2A_2	A_1Y	A_2Y
$A_1A_1 \times A_1Y$	1	0	0	1	0
$A_1A_1 \times A_2Y$	0	1	0	1	0
$A_1A_2 \times A_1Y$	1/2	1/2	0	1/2	1/2
$A_1A_2 \times A_2Y$	0	1/2	1/2	1/2	1/2
$A_2A_2 \times A_1Y$	0	1	0	0	1
$A_2A_2 \times A_2Y$	0	0	1	0	1

but the transmission parameters must specify the probability of transmitting each unique gametic combination. In the simplest possible situation of two loci with two alleles each (locus 1 with alleles A_1 and A_2; locus 2 with alleles B_1 and B_2), this means there are four unique gametes (A_1B_1, A_1B_2, A_2B_1, and A_2A_2). Therefore, just as the (3 × 1) vector τ' ($= [1, \frac{1}{2}, 0]$) was defined for the single-locus case, four (10 × 1) transmission vectors can be defined for the two-locus situation (τ_1 for gametes A_1B_1, τ_2 for A_1B_2, τ_3 for A_2B_1, and τ_4 for A_2B_2). These transmission vectors contain the probability of each of the 10 possible genotypes donating a particular gamete to an offspring. Table 8–5 shows both the frequency and transition parameters for a simple two-locus model. It is a simple (though cumbersome) matter to construct the transmission matrix for this genetic model.

$$T = [\tau_1 \otimes \tau_1, (\tau_1 \otimes \tau_2 + \tau_2 \otimes \tau_1), \tau_2 \otimes \tau_2, (\tau_1 \otimes \tau_3 + \tau_3 \otimes \tau_1),$$

$$(\tau_1 \otimes \tau_4 + \tau_4 \otimes \tau_1), (\tau_2 \otimes \tau_3 + \tau_3 \otimes \tau_2), (\tau_2 \otimes \tau_4 + \tau_4 \otimes \tau_2), \quad (8\text{-}26)$$

$$\tau_3 \otimes \tau_3, (\tau_3 \otimes \tau_4 + \tau_4 \otimes \tau_3), \tau_4 \otimes \tau_4].$$

Note that in the absence of linkage disequilibrium (where $D = 0$ and the frequency of double heterozygotes in coupling and repulsion are equal), this (100 × 10) transmission matrix can be collapsed to a (81 × 9) matrix cor-

Table 8–5. Frequency and transmission parameters for a simple two-locus Mendelian model

Genotype	Frequency		Transmission			
	$D = 0$	General	τ_1	τ_2	τ_3	τ_4
$A_1A_1B_1B_1$	p^2r^2	$(pr + D)^2$	1	0	0	0
$A_1A_1B_1B_2$	p^22rs	$2(pr + D)(ps - D)$	1/2	1/2	0	0
$A_1A_1B_2B_2$	p^2s^2	$(ps - D)^2$	0	1	0	0
$A_1A_2B_1B_1$	$2pqr^2$	$2(pr + D)(qr - D)$	1/2	1/2	0	0
$A_1A_2B_1B_2^c$	$4pqrs$	$2(pr + D)(qs + D)$	$1/2(1 - \Theta)$	$1/2\,\Theta$	$1/2\,\Theta$	$1/2(1 - \Theta)$
$A_1A_2B_1B_2^R$	$4pqrs$	$2(ps - D)(qr - D)$	$1/2\,\Theta$	$1/2(1 - \Theta)$	$1/2(1 - \Theta)$	$1/2\,\Theta$
$A_1A_2B_2B_2$	$2pqs^2$	$2(ps - D)(qs + D)$	0	1/2	1/2	0
$A_2A_2B_1B_1$	q^2r^2	$(qr - D)^2$	0	0	1	0
$A_2A_2B_1B_2$	q^22rs	$2(qr - D)(qs + D)$	0	0	1/2	1/2
$A_2A_2B_2B_2$	q^2s^2	$(qs + D)^2$	0	0	0	1

p = frequency of A_1 allele, $q = 1 - p$; r = frequency of B_1 allele, $s = 1 - r$.
D is a measure of linkage disequilibrium given by $P(A_1B_1)P(A_2B_2) - P(A_1B_2)P(A_2B_1)$.
[c] Double heterozygote in coupling
[R] Double heterozygote in repulsion
Θ is the recombination fraction between loci A and B.

responding to the 81 mating types and 9 genotypes possible. If there are no sex differences in either frequencies or transmission parameters, these 81 mating types represent 45 unique pairs of parents.

Under simple additive polygenic models, on the other hand, the "polygenotype" of an offspring becomes an unobserved random variable, which is assumed to be normally distributed about the midparent value with a variance equal to one-half the additive genetic variance. Thus, the transmission probability for any offspring K of parents I and J is a random variable distributed as

$$\tau(k|i,j) \sim N\left(\frac{I + J}{2}, \frac{1}{2}\sigma_A^2\right). \tag{8-27}$$

Recalling the earlier discussion of assortative mating under polygenic inheritance, it has been shown that the expected parent-offspring covariance becomes

$$\text{Cov}\,(Y_p, Y_0) = \frac{1}{2}\sigma_A^2(1 + r) \tag{8-28}$$

in the presence of assortative mating (Bulmer, 1985). Given this new parent-offspring covariance, the distribution of the transmission parameters becomes

$$\tau(k|ij) \sim N\left(\frac{I + J}{2}, \frac{1}{2}\sigma_A^2(1 + r)\right) \tag{8-29}$$

when there is a correlation r between the phenotype of parents. Since the polygenic model is in essence a random effects model for analysis of variance, the mean values of neither the offspring (K) nor the parents $(I$ and $J)$ are directly estimated; rather the observed covariance is partitioned into components of variance as discussed in Chapter 7.

Penetrance Parameters. The final class of parameters that must be defined specifies the relationship between the genotype (a discrete Mendelian genotype, an unobserved continuous "polygenotype," or a truly general "ousiotype") and the observed phenotype. Obviously, if the phenotype is discrete and falls into two or more mutually exclusive categories, the penetrance parameter must specify the probability of each genotype having one or the other outcome. This is quite simple for discrete Mendelian genotypes, and penetrance parameters alone distinguish between recessive and dominant Mendelian models. If the probability of the A_1A_1 genotype's displaying the trait is equal to that of the heterozygote (A_1A_2), A_1 is dominant to A_2. Table 8–6 lists the penetrance parameters for the simplest single-locus models. Note that when there are more than two phenotypic classes (e.g., a mild and severe form of the disease), separate penetrance parameters are needed for each class. In general, there must be $k - 1$ parameters to define the probability of falling into k phenotypic classes.

Under the polygenic model, however, the "polygenotype" is treated as a

Table 8-6. Penetrance parameters for simple Mendelian models

	Single-locus models where the A_1 allele produces disease $P(\text{affected}|\text{genotype})$			$P(\text{severe})$	$P(\text{mild})$
	Dominant	Recessive	50% Penetrant	Codominant	
A_1A_1	1.0	1.0	1.0	1.0	0.0
A_1A_2	1.0	0.0	0.5	0.0	1.0
A_2A_2	0.0	0.0	0.0	0.0	0.0

	Two-locus models where the A_1 allele produces disease, while the B_2 masks the disease			
	Recessive recessive	Recessive dominant	Dominant recessive	Dominant dominant
$A_1A_1B_1B_1$	1.0	1.0	1.0	1.0
$A_1A_1B_1B_2$	1.0	0.0	1.0	0.0
$A_1A_1B_2B_2$	0.0	0.0	0.0	0.0
$A_1A_2B_1B_1$	0.0	0.0	1.0	1.0
$A_1A_2B_1B_2$	0.0	0.0	1.0	0.0
$A_1A_2B_2B_2$	0.0	0.0	0.0	0.0
$A_2A_2B_1B_1$	0.0	0.0	0.0	0.0
$A_2A_2B_1B_2$	0.0	0.0	0.0	0.0
$A_2A_2B_2B_2$	0.0	0.0	0.0	0.0

random variable that follows a normal distribution in the population. Therefore, it becomes necessary to define a *risk function* to specify the probability of being affected as a function of this unobserved "polygenotype." Conventionally, this risk function assumes that the probability of being affected is an increasing function of the "polygenotype." As discussed in Chapter 7, the risk function was originally a simple and arbitrary cut-point along the scale of liability. A more mathematically appealing risk function is the cumulative normal function whose midpoint is identical to the cut-point or threshold of the original risk function (Elston, 1981). One important advantage to using the cumulative normal distribution as a continuous risk function is that it becomes relatively simple to make risk (a function of the "polygenotype") also dependent on the genotype at a "major" Mendelian locus. This point will be discussed in more detail when the "mixed model" is described in section 8.4.3.

For any continuous phenotype, the penetrance parameters must specify the distribution (mean and variance) for each "type" allowed. The normal distribution is one reasonable and well-recognized choice, such that the conditional density function for the ith "type" is

$$P(Y_i|i) = \frac{1}{\sqrt{2\pi\sigma^2}} \exp\left[-\frac{(Y_i - \mu_i)^2}{2\sigma^2}\right]. \tag{8-30}$$

In principle, this involves estimating up to three genotypic means and three variances for a general single-locus model, although it is common to assume a common variance to minimize the number of parameters. Under polygenic models, only a single mean would be fit, and the phenotypic variance about that mean (σ^2) would be partitioned into genetic and environmental components as described in Chapter 7.

The use of the normal distribution is the result of choice rather than any biologic imperative, and it is very difficult to test the validity of this assumption. In essence, fitting a major gene model with genotype-specific penetrance functions reduces to a mixtures problem, where two or more underlying distributions are fit to a single observed phenotypic distribution. The limitations on inferring genetic control from this approach are discussed in section 8.4.4.

An Example

To illustrate how a likelihood function is actually computed on a given pedigree, consider the pedigree in Figure 8–1. The model of inheritance considered is a single autosomal locus with two alleles A_1 (frequency p) and A_2 (with frequency $q = 1 - p$), where A_1 is responsible for the disease. If the mutant A_1A_1 homozygote has a 100% probability of having the disease, while the A_1A_2 heterozygote has only 50% risk, the penetrance parameters are given in the following table.

Genotype	P(affected)	P(unaffected)
A_1A_1	1.0	0.0
A_1A_2	0.5	0.5
A_2A_2	0.0	1.0

The transmission parameters are given in Table 8–4.

Following the matrix notation developed by Smith (1976), the sequential conditioning process (equivalent to the "peeling" process of Cannings and colleagues [1978]) can be thought of as a serial application of Bayesian prin-

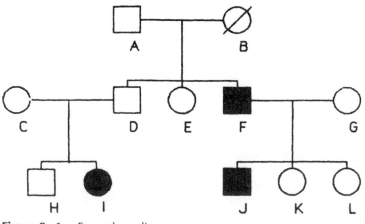

Figure 8–1. Example pedigree.

ciples where at each step a prior probability is multiplied by a conditional likelihood to give a posterior probability. It is important to note, however, that no normalization is done until the end of the "peeling" process on a single pedigree. At this point, the sum of these nonnormalized likelihoods over all possible genotypes (or more general "types" or ousiotypes for non-Mendelian models) serves as the likelihood function for the model. Table 8–7 lists each step for the conditioning process for the pedigree given in Figure 8–1.

The likelihood function obtained is a complex polynomial in terms of the underlying allele frequencies p and q. The coefficients of this polynomial are functions of the penetrance and transmission parameters that are fixed in this example. It is important to realize that other peeling sequences applied to this same pedigree will yield identical likelihoods, if the conditioning steps are done correctly and all available information is used. In other words, if the reverse pathway for this pedigree were used (where the G, J, K, and L were "peeled" onto F; then A, B, E and F were "peeled" onto D; and, lastly, C, D, and I were "peeled" onto the unaffected child H), the likelihood function would have the same value as shown in Table 8–7. For any pedigree, several valid peeling sequences exist, although some are computationally more efficient than others.

Beyond evaluating the total likelihood function for this particular genetic model as a function of allele frequencies, this conditional sequencing approach is useful for computing the probability of any individual's having a particular genotype. In the example given here, the final (3×1) vector of nonnormalized genotypic probabilities obtained at the end of this peeling process can be converted into a proper probability for that person by merely dividing each element by the likelihood itself. Thus, if L's phenotype were unknown because he was not yet born (or even conceived), the risk to some future child of F and G could be easily computed for any given value of the allele frequency or over a range of frequencies.

Clearly, this process is too cumbersome for routine hand calculation, but it is instructive at several levels. First, this matrix notation allows one to see the contribution of each individual to the total likelihood and at what points certain genotypes are excluded for certain individuals. Second, by systematically going through the pedigree in this manner, one can assure that even less likely genotypic combinations are not overlooked. For example, if the trait were a rare and easily diagnosed genetic disease, it is reasonable to assume F is a heterozygote and G is homozygous for the normal allele, which means the risk to L is 0.5, ignoring the possibility of new mutation. However, if the trait is common and/or imperfectly identified, the contribution of the terms representing other genotypes for F and G may play a bigger role in determining the risk to L. For the sake of completeness, the probability that G is a heterozygote or F is homozygous for the mutant allele should be considered. Computing risks in this systematic manner will account for all possible genotypic combinations.

Table 8–7. Calculation of the likelihood function of an autosomal model with 50% risk to the heterozygote on pedigree in Figure 8-1

Step I: Peel C, H, and I onto D

1.   Condition C and D on child I: $(cd)_I = Ti$

$$
= \begin{bmatrix}
1.0 & 0.0 & 0.0 \\
0.5 & 0.5 & 0.0 \\
0.0 & 1.0 & 0.0 \\
0.5 & 0.5 & 0.0 \\
0.25 & 0.5 & 0.25 \\
0.0 & 0.5 & 0.5 \\
0.0 & 1.0 & 0.0 \\
0.0 & 0.5 & 0.5 \\
0.0 & 0.0 & 1.0
\end{bmatrix}
\begin{bmatrix}
1.0 \\
0.5 \\
0.0
\end{bmatrix}
=
\begin{bmatrix}
1.0 \\
0.75 \\
0.5 \\
0.75 \\
0.5 \\
0.25 \\
0.5 \\
0.25 \\
0
\end{bmatrix}
$$

2.   Condition C and D on child H: $(cd)_H = Th$

$$
= \begin{bmatrix}
0.0 \\
0.25 \\
0.5 \\
0.25 \\
0.5 \\
0.75 \\
0.5 \\
0.75 \\
1.0
\end{bmatrix}
$$

3.   Combine these conditional vectors on C and D

$$
(cd)_{HI} = (cd)_I \wedge (cd)_H =
\begin{bmatrix}
0 \\
.19 \\
.25 \\
.19 \\
.25 \\
.19 \\
.25 \\
.19 \\
0
\end{bmatrix}
$$

Table 8–7. (Continued)

4. Condition D on C

$$\mathbf{d}_{\text{CHI}} = (I \otimes \mathbf{c}^*)' \, (\mathbf{cd})_{\text{HI}} = \left(\begin{bmatrix} 100 \\ 010 \\ 001 \end{bmatrix} \otimes \begin{bmatrix} 0 \\ pq \\ q^2 \end{bmatrix} \right)' (\mathbf{cd})_{\text{HI}}$$

$$= \begin{bmatrix} 0 & pq & q^2 & 0 & 0 & 0 & 0 & 0 & 0 \\ 0 & 0 & 0 & 0 & pq & q^2 & 0 & 0 & 0 \\ 0 & 0 & 0 & 0 & 0 & 0 & 0 & pq & q^2 \end{bmatrix} \begin{bmatrix} 0 \\ .19 \\ .25 \\ .19 \\ .25 \\ .19 \\ .25 \\ .19 \\ .25 \\ .19 \\ 0 \end{bmatrix}$$

$$= \begin{bmatrix} .19 \, pq + .25 \, q^2 \\ .25 \, pq + .19 \, q^2 \\ .19 \, pq \end{bmatrix}$$

NOTE: The prior probability vector for any original is $(p^2 \ 2pq \ q^2)'$.

Considering C is unaffected, $\mathbf{c}^* = \begin{bmatrix} p^2 \\ 2pq \\ q^2 \end{bmatrix} \wedge \begin{bmatrix} 0 \\ 0.5 \\ 1.0 \end{bmatrix} = \begin{bmatrix} 0 \\ pq \\ q^2 \end{bmatrix}$

5. Condition D on his phenotype

$$\mathbf{d}^* = \mathbf{d}_{\text{CHI}} \wedge \begin{bmatrix} 0 \\ 0.5 \\ 1.0 \end{bmatrix} = \begin{bmatrix} 0 \\ .13 \, pq + .09 \, q^2 \\ .19 \, pq \end{bmatrix}$$

Step II: Peel A, B, D, E onto F:

1. Condition A & B on D:

$$(\mathbf{ab})_{\text{D}} = \mathbf{T} \, \mathbf{d}^* = \begin{bmatrix} 0 \\ .06 \, pq + .05 \, q^2 \\ .13 \, pq + .09 \, q^2 \\ .06 \, pq + .05 \, q^2 \\ .11 \, pq + .05 \, q^2 \\ .16 \, pq + .05 \, q^2 \\ .13 \, pq + .09 \, q^2 \\ .16 \, pq + .05 \, q^2 \\ .19 \, pq \end{bmatrix}$$

Table 8–7. (Continued)

2. Condition A & B on E:

$$(\mathbf{ab})_E = \mathbf{T}\,\mathbf{e} = \begin{bmatrix} 0 \\ 0.25 \\ 1.0 \\ 0.25 \\ 0.5 \\ 0.75 \\ 0.5 \\ 0.75 \\ 1 \end{bmatrix}$$

3. Combine these conditional vectors

$$(\mathbf{ab})_{DE} = (\mathbf{ab})_D \,^\wedge\, (\mathbf{ab})_E = \begin{bmatrix} 0 \\ .016\,pq + .012\,q^2 \\ .125\,pq + .094\,q^2 \\ .016\,pq + .012\,q^2 \\ .055\,pq + .023\,q^2 \\ .117\,pq + .035\,q^2 \\ .063\,pq + .047\,q^2 \\ .117\,pq + .035\,q^2 \\ .188\,q^2 \end{bmatrix}$$

4. Incorporate phenotype on A

$$(\mathbf{ab})^* = (\mathbf{a}\otimes\mathbf{b}) \,^\wedge\, (\mathbf{ab})_{DE} = \left(\begin{bmatrix} 0 \\ pq \\ q^2 \end{bmatrix} \otimes \begin{bmatrix} p^2 \\ 2pq \\ q^2 \end{bmatrix} \right) \,^\wedge\, (\mathbf{ab})_{DE}$$

$$= \begin{bmatrix} 0 \\ 0 \\ 0 \\ .016\,p^4q^2 + .012\,p^3q^3 \\ .109\,p^3q^3 + .047\,p^2q^4 \\ .117\,p^2q^4 + .035\,pq^5 \\ .063\,p^3q^3 + .047\,p^2q^4 \\ .234\,p^2q^4 + .070\,pq^5 \\ .188\,q^6 \end{bmatrix}$$

NOTE: Because B has an unknown phenotype, the vector of priors is $\mathbf{b}' = (p^2\ \ 2pq\ \ q^2)$. Since A is unaffected,

$$\mathbf{a} = \begin{bmatrix} p^2 \\ 2pq \\ q^2 \end{bmatrix} \,^\wedge\, \begin{bmatrix} 0 \\ 0.5 \\ 1.0 \end{bmatrix} = \begin{bmatrix} 0 \\ pq \\ q^2 \end{bmatrix}$$

Table 8–7. (Continued)

5. Condition F on A and B: $\mathbf{f}_{AB} = \mathbf{T}'\,(\mathbf{ab})^*$

$$= \begin{bmatrix} .008\,p^4q^2 + .033\,p^3q^3 + .012\,p^2q^4 \\ .008\,p^4q^2 + .096\,p^3q^3 + .246\,p^2q^4 + .105\,pq^5 \\ .027\,p^3q^3 + .188\,p^2q^4 + .053\,pq^5 + .188\,q^6 \end{bmatrix}$$

6. Incorporate phenotype on F:

$$\mathbf{f}^* = \mathbf{f}_{AB} \mathbin{\char`\^} \begin{bmatrix} 1 \\ 0.5 \\ 0 \end{bmatrix} = \begin{bmatrix} .008\,p^4q^2 + .033\,p^3q^3 + .012\,p^2q^4 \\ .004\,p^4q^2 + .048\,p^3q^3 + .123\,p^2q^4 + .053\,pq^5 \\ 0 \end{bmatrix}$$

Step III: Peel F, G, J, K onto L:
1. Condition F and G on J and K:

$$(\mathbf{fg})_J = \mathbf{Tj} = \begin{bmatrix} 1 \\ 0.75 \\ 0.5 \\ 0.75 \\ 0.5 \\ 0.25 \\ 0.5 \\ 0.25 \\ 0 \end{bmatrix} \qquad (\mathbf{fg})_K = \mathbf{Tk} = \begin{bmatrix} 0 \\ 0.25 \\ 0.5 \\ 0.25 \\ 0.5 \\ 0.75 \\ 0.5 \\ 0.75 \\ 1 \end{bmatrix}$$

2. Compute prior vector on F and G:

$$\mathbf{f}^* \otimes \mathbf{g} = \mathbf{f}^* \otimes \begin{bmatrix} 0 \\ pq \\ q^2 \end{bmatrix} = \begin{bmatrix} 0 \\ .008\,p^5q^3 + .033\,p^4q^4 + .012\,p^3q^5 \\ .008\,p^4q^4 + .033\,p^3q^5 + .012\,p^2q^6 \\ 0 \\ .004\,p^5q^3 + .048\,p^4q^4 + .123\,p^3q^5 + .053\,p^2q^6 \\ .004\,p^4q^4 + .048\,p^3q^5 + .123\,p^2q^6 + .053\,pq^7 \\ 0 \\ 0 \\ 0 \end{bmatrix}$$

3. Combine prior and conditional

$$(\mathbf{fg})^*_{JK} = (\mathbf{fg}) \mathbin{\char`\^} (\mathbf{fg})_J \mathbin{\char`\^} (\mathbf{fg})_K$$

$$= \begin{bmatrix} 0 \\ .001\,p^5q^3 + .006\,p^4q^4 + .002\,p^3q^5 \\ .002\,p^4q^4 + .008\,p^3q^5 + .003\,p^2q^6 \\ 0 \\ .001\,p^5q^3 + .012\,p^4q^4 + .031\,p^3q^5 + .013\,p^2q^6 \\ .001\,p^4q^4 + .009\,p^3q^5 + .023\,p^2q^6 + .010\,pq^7 \\ 0 \\ 0 \\ 0 \end{bmatrix}$$

Table 8–7. (Continued)

4. Compute prior vector on L:

$$\mathbf{l}_{\text{FGJK}} = \mathbf{T}'(\mathbf{fg})^*_{\text{JK}}$$

$$= \begin{array}{l} .001\ p^5q^3 + .006\ p^4q^4 + .009\ p^3q^5 + .003\ p^2q^6 \\ .001\ p^5q^3 + .011\ p^4q^4 + .024\ p^3q^5 + .021\ p^2q^6 + .005\ pq^7 \\ .0002\ p^5q^3 + .003\ p^4q^4 + .012\ p^3q^5 + .015\ p^2q^6 + .005\ pq^7 \end{array}$$

At this point, since no additional information is available on L, the likelihood is the sum of all elements of this last vector, i.e.,

$$L(\text{model} \mid A - K) = .002\ p^5q^3 + .021\ p^4q^4$$

$$+ .045\ p^3q^5 + .039\ p^2q^6 + .010\ pq^7$$

To further compute the probability of individual L having any of the three possible genotypes, merely divide the appropriate element of the (3 × 1) vector given above by this likelihood.

8.4.3 Comparing Models in Segregation Analysis

As mentioned before, the likelihood of a model evaluated on a set of data (e.g., a pedigree) is proportional to the probability of observing that particular data under that particular model (Edwards, 1978). This is always true for binary phenotypes, where each component of the likelihood (penetrance, frequency, and transmission) is itself a probability. For quantitative traits, the penetrance functions used in this same procedure become the height of a normal distribution evaluated at a single point, so the likelihood itself is no longer constructed directly as a product of probabilities. Nonetheless, it does remain proportional to a true probability and can be treated as such.

This permits several approaches for comparing the likelihoods of different models of inheritance and selecting the best model among those examined for a given pedigree or for set of pedigrees. The first and most obvious situation is that when the likelihood function is zero, the model of inheritance is incompatible with the data. For example, if a set of pedigrees contains one affected individual with unaffected parents, then a strict autosomal dominant model will have a zero likelihood, unless some allowance is made for either new mutations or incomplete penetrance. Similarly, the occurrence of a single instance of father-son transmission will give a zero likelihood for an X-linked model of a rare disease.

Because the likelihood function on a set of pedigrees is computed as the product of individual likelihoods over all independent pedigrees (or equivalently as the sum of the log-likelihoods over all independent pedigrees), care must be taken to assure that a particular model is not excluded due to a single pedigree. Conversely, it is wise to estimate the appropriate penetrance or transmission parameters for a set of data when assessing the fit to a particular model of inheritance. As in all maximum likelihood procedures, estimation of parameters is achieved by iteratively searching the likelihood surface to find those parameter values that maximize the total likelihood on the entire sample. Minor deviations from the expectations of simple models may represent etiologic heterogeneity in only a few pedigrees among the entire data set.

Likelihood Ratio Tests

One major advantage of using the maximum likelihood approach rises from the availability of the likelihood ratio test (LRT) for evaluating specific hypotheses. This commonly used test statistic is based on the ratio of the maximum likelihood value of the null hypothesis (H_0) to that of a larger parameter space which encompasses both the null and the alternative hypothesis (H_A), that is,

$$\lambda = \frac{\max\limits_{H_0} L(\text{model}|\text{data})}{\max\limits_{H_0 + H_A} L(\text{model}|\text{data})},$$ (8-31)

where the numerator represents the maximum value of the likelihood function of the null hypothesis (i.e., the "reduced" model) and the denominator represents the corresponding maximum likelihood value of the "complete" model (where any constraints on parameters specified by H_0 are relaxed). This ratio has the advantage of ranging between 0 and 1.0. A likelihood of 0 means the data are incompatible with the null or "reduced" model, while a value of 1.0 implies the null hypothesis does *not* place any relevant constraints on the model. Since the "reduced" model generally restricts some parameter value, the likelihood of the "complete" model should always be greater than that of the "reduced" model.

Wilks' theorem states that, as the sample size gets large, -2 times the log of this ratio approaches a chi-square distribution, that is,

$$\begin{aligned} \text{LRT} &= -2 \ln \lambda \\ &= -2 \left[\ln L(\text{"reduced" model}|\text{data}) \right. \\ &\quad \left. - \ln L(\text{"complete model"}|\text{data})\right] \\ &\sim \chi^2_{m-n} \end{aligned}$$ (8-32)

where the degrees of freedom for this test statistic (i.e., $(m - n)$) represent the difference in the parameter space for the "complete" and "reduced" models. For example, if the likelihood of the complete model represented the maximum over an m-dimensional space, while the reduced model fixed one parameter at some value, the LRT would asymptotically approach a chi-square distribution with 1 degree of freedom.

Therefore, maximum likelihood methods can be used to iteratively estimate parameters of various models of inheritance from pedigree data, and the likelihood values themselves (or more commonly the ln-likelihood values) can be used to compare hierarchical models based on this widely recognized test statistic. It is important to understand, however, the limitations of this test statistic.

First, because the LRT is based on a comparison of strictly hierarchical models (i.e., the "reduced" or null model must be a subset of the "complete"), several models of prime interest cannot be directly compared. For example, a simple recessive model cannot be tested against a simple dominant model, rather these two fixed penetrance models must be tested against a more general model where the penetrance parameters are estimated from the data. Similarly, a single-locus model cannot be directly tested against a polygenic model of inheritance because these two models do not represent hierarchical parameter spaces. Again, each of these models must be compared to a more general alternative model of inheritance which encompasses both Mendelian and polygenic inheritance. Such a general model, termed the "mixed model," is discussed in greater detail in section 8.4.4.

Second, while the asymptotic distribution of the LRT approaches some form of a chi-square as the sample size increases, this theoretical finding is based on the assumption that the sampling units are independently and identically distributed. The sampling unit for segregation analysis is the pedigree, which varies in both size and structure and therefore cannot be considered identically distributed. By their nature, pedigrees must also vary in information content. Furthermore, in many instances the sample consists of a single large pedigree containing many individuals. Technically, in such situations, the sample size is 1; and, therefore, the LRT should not be viewed strictly as a chi-square statistic. Nevertheless, it can still serve as an indication of the relative fit of one model versus another.

It must also be remembered that even in samples of many families, a small number of families may be informative for certain parameters; thus dominating the likelihood function and, through it, both the estimation procedure and the LRT. This inequality in the information content of a pedigree depends on the size and structure of families, and on the models being considered. For example, if the question at hand is whether a trait is X-linked versus autosomal, nuclear families ascertained through an affected mother carry absolutely no information, regardless of the number of offspring, while nuclear families ascertained through an affected father are informative, regardless of the sex distribution of the offspring (daughters are informative for estimating penetrance, sons are informative for estimating transmission parameters). In general, it is difficult to predict which families will be most informative for a given comparison. Therefore, it becomes important to evaluate the "support" each family gives to a particular model of inheritance. Some methods for doing this are discussed in section 8.5.2.

Third, the distribution of the LRT is not a simple chi-square if the value of a parameter under the null hypothesis is at the boundary of the parameter space. As was the case in variance components models (discussed in Chapter 7), when the null value of a parameter is itself a boundary point, the LRT takes on the distribution of a mixture of chi-squares. For a single parameter, the LRT asymptotically follows an equal mixture of a chi-square with 1 degree of freedom (df) and a degenerate chi-square distribution with 0 df. In this simple case, the true critical value for the 5% significance level is the 10% value of a regular chi-square with 1 df. When testing the null hypothesis that two parameters are at boundary values, the LRT follows a more complex mixture that is $\frac{1}{4}$ a chi-square with 2 df, $\frac{1}{2}$ a chi-square with 1 df, and $\frac{1}{4}$ a chi-square with 0 df (Self and Liang, 1987).

In addition to causing problems with test statistics, however, having a critical parameter at a boundary value leads to problems in obtaining meaningful estimators. Frequently, there is not enough information to estimate all transmission parameters (especially for the rarer genotypes), and the final MLEs may or may not be close to the expected. The ideal situation is for the MLEs from a generalized single-locus model to be close to the Mendelian expectation of $\tau = (1, \frac{1}{2}, 0)$, with a nonsignificant difference in ln-likelihoods compared to a strict Mendelian model. Frequently the MLEs from a general model appear far from the expected, but the difference in ln-likelihoods may be small and nonsignificant (i.e., the likelihood surface is relatively flat) or standard errors for the MLEs cannot be computed due to boundary problems (e.g., the searching algorithm may lead to values outside the permissible range and prevent calculation of second derivatives). In these latter situations, the evidence for a Mendelian mechanism is less compelling, although the overall results may still suggest single-locus inheritance.

Comparing Nonhierarchical Models

Often the LRT cannot be used because the competing models of most interest do not represent a hierarchical parameter space where one model is a strict subset of the other. Even here, however, one can adapt a "model choice" approach to select the most likely model. Edwards (1978) treats the topic of relative likelihoods or ln-likelihoods in detail, and terms this approach "the method of support" for making scientific inferences. In essence, this approach is to simply compare the ln-likelihoods of two models (say, a null and an alternative model) and classify the data (a single pedigree or an entire set of data) as "supporting" one model over the other to a certain degree, that is, the model with the larger ln-likelihood is better supported by the data.

However, one must remember the ln-likelihood function can almost always be increased by adding more parameters to the model, just as an R^2 can always be increased by adding higher-order polynomial terms to a multiple linear regression. This process is reflected in the observation that the maximum likelihood value of the "complete" model is greater (at least slightly) than that for any "reduced" model where constraints are placed on one or more parameters. Throughout science, there is always some penalty to be paid for adding unnecessary complexity, and the best model generally is taken as that which is most parsimonious (i.e., the one that best explains the data with the fewest parameters). Akaike (1974) proposed adding a penalty to each ln-likelihood to reflect the number of parameters estimated in a particular model. Specifically, Akaike's information criteria (AIC) is defined as

$$AIC = -2(\text{ln-likelihood}) + 2(\text{number of parameters}) \qquad (8\text{-}33)$$

and serves as a weighted measure of the fit of any given model. The best fitting model is that with the largest ln-likelihood (i.e., the smallest $-2 \ln L$ value), while the most parsimonious model is that with the smallest AIC value. While comparisons among nonhierarchical models remain without formal tests of statistical significance, the AIC does provide guidelines for identifying the most parsimonious model among a series of competing models.

8.4.4 Strategies for Inferring Genetic Control

The goal of segregation analysis is to identify genetic mechanisms that may be controlling the distribution of a disease or a quantitative trait in families. To successfully discern the presence of a genetic mechanism, some comparison against nongenetic alternatives must be made. This must be followed by discrimination among competing genetic explanations for observed familial aggregation.

While it is true that environmental factors lead to distinct phenotypes which cluster in families, there is no universal mechanism dictating how an environmental factor could lead to familial aggregation. Relevant environmental factors influencing a phenotypic trait might include the common immediate environment (e.g., diet); they also might represent the cumulative effects of a common exposure (e.g., where the length of time together is critical in determining similarity among relatives); they might also depend on a time-specific common exposure (e.g., one generation or one cohort only may have been exposed to a particular environmental factor); or any combination of these and other plausible nongenetic mechanisms can contribute to familial aggregation of a disease or trait. Such a broad array of plausible alternatives makes it difficult to specify decisively the most appropriate nongenetic model.

Commingling Analysis

A common strategy for dealing with quantitative traits is to look explicitly for evidence of distinct phenotypic groups in the family data, and test for equal proportions of such groups across generations. This search for evidence of commingling of underlying distributions can be done as a separate step or as part of the series of nongenetic and genetic models fit to the data, since fitting Mendelian models also depends on analyzing mixtures of distributions for a quantitative trait. It is also possible to estimate the coefficients of a power transformation that will remove any skewness in the underlying distributions (Morton, 1982). This has important advantages, since the occurrence of skewness in the underlying distribution can increase the rate of erroneously inferring single-locus mechanisms (MacLean et al., 1975). It should be understood, however, that the power of commingling analysis alone to detect mixtures of genetically determined distributions is quite low. Given some evidence that the overall phenotypic distribution is indeed a mixture of two or more underlying distributions, one can attempt to test whether the proportion of different groups is compatible with Hardy-Weinberg expectations in randomly mating population. However, the power to detect such deviations is again low. Studies have shown that formal segregation analysis can detect the presence of Mendelian loci even in the absence of any evidence of commingling in the overall distribution (Kwon et al, 1990).

A similar approach for testing hypotheses about possible commingled distributions is to estimate the proportion in each component distribution separately among founders and nonfounders, regardless of generation. This is accomplished by first fitting a model where the frequency of the essential "types" (or ousiotypes) is controlled by a common binomial process among both founders and nonfounders. Thus the "reduced" model requires specifying that the allele frequency in founders (p) be equal to the transmission parameters $(\tau_1 = \tau_2 = \tau_3)$ controlling the distribution among nonfounders. The "complete" model relaxes this constraint and estimates a separate allele frequency among founders and a separate (but single) transmission probability among nonfounders (i.e., $\tau = \tau_1 = \tau_2 = \tau_3$). If these obviously nongenetic models give a better fit to the data than do Mendelian models, then one is forced to conclude distinct phenotypic subgroups do exist in the data, but the trait itself is not under the control of a single major locus.

When analyzing qualitative traits, one can use a similar strategy of estimating the risk to founders and nonfounders in pedigree data. Evidence for "high-risk" and "low-risk" types of individuals may not represent genetic control if their frequency among founders and nonfounders is identical in a given data set. Even if the allele frequency were exactly .5 (i.e., $p = \tau_2$), the estimated transmission parameters cannot be equal for all essential "types" (ousiotypes) of founders under any Mendelian model; and it should be possible to discriminate between truly genetic and nongenetic models in this manner.

Single-Locus and Polygenic Components in "Mixed Models"

Beyond considering an admittedly modest selection of nongenetic models, the usual process of segregation analysis involves fitting both single-locus and polygenic models of inheritance, because these are the two most commonly considered genetic mechanisms. The relationship between single-locus models of inheritance and commingled distributions is clear: single-locus Mendelian models represent a particular class of commingled distributions where the transmission parameters are constrained to Mendelian values. The proportion of phenotypic subgroups among founders may fit with Hardy-Weinberg expectations, but that is not required. The transmission parameters that dictate the proportion of phenotypic subgroups among nonfounders must be compatible with Mendelian transmission, however, before inferring genetic control.

Polygenic inheritance does not require detectable commingling of underlying distributions, rather it dictates certain patterns of familial correlations. As discussed in Chapter 7, the expected covariance (or correlation) under a polygenic model is a simple function of kinship coefficients and the additive genetic variance. To the extent that familial correlations are present in a data set, the final maximum likelihood estimator for polygenic heritability (h^2) will reflect this correlation regardless of the true etiologic mechanism. Specifically, the usual additive polygenic model interprets any observed correlation between first-degree relatives as twice the narrow-sense heritability.

As discussed earlier, because the LRT can be invoked only to compare hierarchical models, a "complete" model incorporating both single-locus and polygenic control was developed and termed the "mixed model" (Morton and MacLean, 1974). When originally developed, this model was limited to nuclear families where the conditional likelihood of children given their parents could be computed. Later, a more general approach for computing the likelihood function of this mixed model was developed under the same sequential conditioning or "peeling" process described above (Hasstedt, 1982). Essentially, just as the likelihood function of single-locus models is accumulated by summation over all possible genotypes, the likelihood of the mixed model is computed by integrating over the range of possible polygenotypes for each single-locus genotype considered. While this approach is computationally intense, an approximation for this method was developed which is no more cumbersome than the calculations necessary for single-locus models themselves (Hasstedt, 1982). This mixed-model approach can also incorporate a limited array of components representing specified environmental factors that may contribute to the correlations over and above that due to the single locus (Hasstedt et al., 1985). Flexible estimation strategies for jointly considering effects of observed shared environments and genetic factors (both single-locus and polygenic) have been developed (Hasstedt, 1991).

Since a number of workers have been involved in the development and implementation of this "mixed model," different parameterizations are employed by various widely used computer programs. These different notations do not alter the underlying model, but they can generate confusion when comparing reports in the literature. Figure 8–2 diagrams the Mendelian "mixed model" and Table 8–8 shows the relationship between parameters developed for the conditional likelihood of children given their parents (used in the computer program POINTER) and those for the general likelihood approach (used in the program Pedigree Analysis Package (PAP), as well as the package Statistic Analysis for Genetic Epidemiology, S.A.G.E.). In either situation, the Mendelian "mixed model" (with both a single-locus component and a polygenic component) is fit as the penultimate model in a series. If this Mendelian "mixed" model gives a nonsignificant improvement in ln-likelihood compared to the simpler Mendelian model (where the polygenic heritability is fixed at zero), while comparing the straight polygenic model to the Mendelian "mixed model" leads to rejecting the null hypothesis that the single-locus component can be completely ignored, one can infer that a single

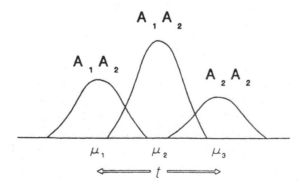

Figure 8–2. The Mendelian "mixed model," used in the computer programs POINTER and PAP. See Table 8-8 for details.

Table 8–8. Relationship between parameters in the Mendelian "mixed model": Figure 8–2 under the program PAP and POINTER

PAP*	POINTER†	Conversion
p frequency of A allele	q frequency of low allele	None if μ_1 is "low"
μ_1 mean of genotype A_1A_1	μ population mean	$\mu = p^2\mu_1 + 2pq\mu_2 + q^2\mu_3$
μ_2 mean of genotype A_1A_2	V population variance	$V = \sigma_W^2 + \sigma_{ML}^2$‡
μ_3 mean of genotype A_2A_2	t displacement between homozygotes	$t = \mu_3 - \mu_1$
σ_W^2 within genotype variance	d deviation due to dominance	$d = \mu_2 - \left(\dfrac{\mu_3 - \mu_1}{2}\right)$
H_p proportion of σ_W^2 attributed to additive polygenes $= (\sigma_A^2/\sigma_W^2)$	h^2 narrow-sense heritability $= \dfrac{\sigma_A^2}{V}$	$h^2 = H_p\left(\dfrac{\sigma_W^2}{\sigma_W^2 + \sigma_{ML}^2}\right)$

*Pedigree Analysis Package (Hasstedt and Cartwright, 1981).
†POINTER computer program (Lalouel et al., 1983).
‡Variance due to major locus, $\sigma_{ML}^2 = p^2(\mu_1 - \mu)^2 + 2pq(\mu_2 - \mu)^2 + q^2(\mu_3 - \mu)^2$.

Mendelian locus is influencing the phenotype in question. Conversely, if the null hypothesis that the single-locus component is zero cannot be rejected, while the simple polygenic model fits almost as well as the Mendelian "mixed model," then one could say that there was substantial familial correlation likely controlled by many loci, but there was no evidence of "major gene effects."

Frequently in the analysis of quantitative traits, however, both of the simpler "reduced" models are rejected in favor of this "complete" model containing both single-locus and polygenic components. In such situations, one is forced to conclude that at least a subset of the families appear to be segregating for a Mendelian locus exerting a major effect on the phenotype, but this "major gene" cannot account for all the observed correlations among relatives. While such additional unexplained correlations may indeed be a result of independently segregating "polygenes," it is also possible that nongenetic factors may underlie these correlations. Such ambivalent results showing some evidence of genetic control definitely warrant further investigation, but the additional unexplained familial correlations should warn the investigator that other forces, possibly environmental factors, must be operating at least in some families.

Estimating Transmission Parameters From Family Data

When there is evidence of single-locus control obtained from fitting both Mendelian single-locus and "mixed models," it is best to test directly for evidence of Mendelian transmission in the data. This is accomplished by estimating transmission parameters (τ_1, τ_2, and τ_3) along with the penetrance and frequency parameters. This is usually accomplished in two steps, first to test the null hypothesis that $\tau_2 = 0.5$ and, second, to fit the complete model where all three transmission parameters are simultaneously estimated. Frequently, this latter model is difficult to fit because the null hypothesis values of τ_1 and τ_3 represent boundary values, and obtaining valid estimators for the rarer "types" or ousiotypes can be problematic.

It must be recognized that most small to moderate-sized sets of families contain limited amounts of information for estimating these various parameters. Fitting ever more complicated models frequently leads to flat ln-likelihood surfaces, to problems with estimators on boundaries, or both. The particular structure of the data set always places limits on the amount of information it carries. Samples of many nuclear families with modest numbers of children may give good estimates of allele frequencies and possibly even transmission parameters (if the parents represent a balanced mixture of the different essential "types" or ousiotypes). Extremely large pedigrees with relatively few founders cannot be expected to give good estimates of population parameters, such as allele frequencies, but are likely to provide good estimates of transmission parameters. While the ideal analytic approach is to fit the full range of models of inheritance from the simplest to the most complex (see Table 8–9 for such a list), this is not always possible. Furthermore, the final model selected as "best" based either on ln-likelihoods or the AIC must also be judged by its biologic plausibility. When segregation analysis of a quantitative trait predicts mixtures of apparent genotypic distributions that are not compatible with the observed distribution, or when segregation analysis of a rare disease predicts a common allele is responsible for the "high-risk" genotype, the overall interpretation falls under suspicion.

8.4.5 Correcting for Ascertainment in Pedigree Analysis

Just as sampling sibships through a proband alters the expected distribution of affected and nonaffected offspring in the final sample, so too will sampling extended pedigrees through an affected proband (or a proband with an extreme value for a quantitative phenotype) induce a bias of ascertainment. Unfortunately, it is not feasible to write the expected likelihood function of a general model of inheritance in any simple fashion for a "general" pedigree because the likelihood function depends on both the model and the particular structure of the individual pedigree. As a consequence, it is not possible to write any simple form for the joint likelihood function for the proband (or the subset involved in the ascertainment) and the remainder of the pedigree, as it was for the analysis of sibship data.

Elston and Sobel (1979) have shown theoretically how to condition the usual likelihood of a model on a pedigree by multiplying this by the likelihood that the pedigree contains at least one proband (among all individuals eligible to be probands). In the simplest case of nuclear families where only offspring are eligible to be probands and assuming independent ascertainment of all probands, this approach will give the equivalent of the classic binomial likelihood function for sibships drawn from a single parental mating type discussed in section 8.3 (Elston, 1981). These results suggest the general likelihood approach for pedigree analysis may be able to adopt a relatively straightforward method to correct for ascertainment bias, one in which pedigrees of variable size need not be broken up into smaller units for analysis.

Bonney and Demenais (1991) have developed a theoretical framework for conditioning on ascertained subsets of extended pedigrees as part of a sequential sampling design, where a series of rules is established in which more

Table 8–9. Models commonly fit in segregation analysis of a quantitative trait on a set of pedigrees

Model	Parameters				Comments
	Means	*Variances*	*Correlations*	*Frequencies*	
1. Sporadic	μ	σ^2	(0)	(1.0)	Should be equal to sample mean and variance
2. Commingled distributed	μ_i	σ_i^2 (often = σ^2)	(0)	$p = \tau$	Equal mixtures among founders and nonfounders
3. Equal τ model	μ_i	σ_i^2	(0)	p	Different mixtures among founders and nonfounders
4. Polygenic	μ	σ^2	$\rho = h^2/2$	(1.0)	Forces all correlations to conform to genetic expectations
5. Familial correlations	μ	σ^2	$\rho_{SP}, \rho_{PO}, \rho_{SS}$	(1.0)	Must specify correlation structure for extended families (e.g., regressive models)
6. Mendelian single locus	μ_i	σ_i^2	(0)	p	Assume $\tau_1 = 1$, $\tau_2 = 0.5$, $\tau_3 = 0$
7. General single locus	μ	σ_i^2	(0)	Estimate τ_2, τ_3 p	Estimate τ_1
8. Mendelian "mixed" models	μ_i	σ^2	$\rho = h^2/2$	p	Assume $\tau_1 = 1$, $\tau_2 = 0.5$, $\tau_3 = 0$
9. General "mixed" models	μ_i	σ^2	$\rho = h^2/2$	p	Estimate τ_1, τ_2, τ_3
10. General familial correlation	μ_i	σ^2	$\rho_{SP}, \rho_{PO}, \rho_{SS}$	p	Estimate τ while specifying correlation structure (e.g., regressive model)

Symbols: μ_i: "type" or ousiotype specific means ($i = 1, 2, 3$); σ_i^2: "type" specific variance; ρ: correlations among all first-degree relatives, between parent-offspring (ρ_{PO}), among sibs (ρ_S) or between spouses (ρ_{SS}); p: allele frequency; τ_i: probability of ith "type" transmitting as A_1 allele. See text for further discussion of parameters.

distant relatives are sampled if, and only if, an affected individual is identified in the immediate family. In other words, a family study could be designed to identify probands from a defined source (preferably a registry or a survey of a target population) and sample all available first-degree relatives, while second-degree relatives would be sampled only for those families with one or more affected 1° relatives. Similarly, 3° relatives would be sampled only in those branches with an affected 2° relative, and so on. The final data set would, therefore, consist of pedigrees of varying sizes; but, in part, these differences would be due to deliberate choices made by the investigators. Cannings and Thompson (1977) show how such a sequential sampling design should not induce any further bias due to ascertainment (beyond that created by the ascertainment of the original proband), as long as all pedigrees regardless of their size are included in the final data to be analyzed.

The best approach for correcting for ascertainment bias when analyzing pedigrees is still a matter of debate. Shute and Ewens (1988b) propose identifying that subset of the pedigree which is relevant to ascertainment and then employing a two-stage maximum likelihood procedure for estimating parameters of the model (first in the subset and then in the remainder of the pedigree). Bonney and Demenais (1991) point out that this robust approach is equivalent to a partial likelihood approach. The more general approach of conditioning the full likelihood function on the likelihood of the proband (or ascertained subset) appears more tractable and has gained wider acceptance. As Elston (1981) points out, this full likelihood approach is equivalent to dividing the unconditional likelihood function by the probability of that a random individual is affected or otherwise eligible to be a proband, assuming all probands are indeed independently ascertained. This presupposes the individual is the unit of original ascertainment. Although no general consensus has yet been reached, the effect of improperly specifying a correction for ascertainment bias is likely to be greatest on estimators for population parameters (allele frequencies, heritability), and the bias might be expected to have a smaller effect on parameters such as penetrance and transmission.

8.4.6 Covariate Effects in Segregation Analysis

While the goal of segregation analysis is to identify evidence of genetic control over a phenotype using family data (either sibships or pedigrees), it is unrealistic to assume there are no external, observable factors influencing the phenotype in question. Frequently, when dealing with a quantitative trait, there are differences both between the sexes and across age groups, and these factors should be included as covariates in the analysis. Measurable environmental exposures are also candidates for covariates when dealing with quantitative phenotypes (e.g., smoking influences pulmonary function, contraceptives influence serum lipid levels), and these must be considered in segregation analysis. If such covariates truly exert simple, constant effects on the phenotypes of all individuals, one can use multiple linear regression models to remove fixed effects of covariates prior to fitting genetic models. Under this approach, residual values are computed for each individual prior to the segregation analysis; and the genetic analysis itself is the second step. Such residual values are computed as the difference between the observed phenotype and a predicted value based on the best-fitting regression model obtained from the entire sample (possibly excluding probands).

Interpretation of the results of such analysis ideally should include some reconversion to the original scale both in terms of means and variances, and this is usually straightforward. In terms of Mendelian models, this may mean simply adding a constant to the genotypic mean of one gender or the other. In terms of polygenic models, this may mean rescaling the components of variance. For example, a narrow-sense heritability of 80% seems much less impressive if covariates such as age, gender, and observable environmental exposures account for 85% of the observed phenotypic variation in the original trait. A large role for covariates in no way invalidates findings from genetic analysis; however, the relevance of genetic differences that account for 12% ($=0.8*(1 - 0.85)$) of variation in a quantitative trait seems minor compared to nongenetic factors. Clearly, if the covariates in such a situation were amenable to manipulation (age and gender are not), it would be wise to focus initial intervention strategies on them. On the other hand, it is important to realize that even a small genetic component represents a source of variation that is often resistent to intervention, but one which can be exploited to identify high-risk individuals. Further investigation to identify such groups is always warranted.

There is always some potential for bias when a two-stage strategy is adopted. For example, standard multiple regression models used for adjustment assume each individual is independent of all others; an assumption obviously inappropriate for family data. Furthermore, if unobserved genotypes do exist and have different means, the preliminary regression model will not correctly model the data as a mixture of distributions. Therefore, one can never be sure that the coefficients used to compute residual values are optimal estimators for these fixed effects of covariates. Bonney (1984) proposed a family of regressive models for quantitative traits that allowed simultaneous estimation of fixed effects for covariates and the parameters of Mendelian models. These models can be thought of as multiple regression models, which allow genotype specific intercepts, that is, the model can be written as

$$Y = \mu_i + \beta'X + e, \qquad (8\text{-}34)$$

where i indexes the means for the three essential "types" (or ousiotypes) of a generalized single-locus model. Note that the vector of covariates X is still assumed to have a fixed effect on the phenotype Y. The chief advantage that these regressive models provide is that a simple maximum likelihood procedure is used to estimate β and the parameters of the genetic model (i.e., the μ_i's, their variances, allele frequencies, and transmission parameters). It sometimes simplifies the interpretation of these regressive models if ($X - \overline{X}$) is used as a covariate, because then the genotype-specific means (i.e., the μ_i's) then represent phenotypic values at the mean covariate values rather than intercept values (i.e., when all $X = 0$). For example, if X included age and height, it may not be of interest to estimate genotype-specific means (μ_i) at age zero and height zero, but rather at the mean height and age for the sample. This approach is in keeping with the general rule that the estimated parameters of genetic models should be expressed in the original scale of measurement whenever possible.

It is important to note that originally these regressive models were not formulated to accommodate separate Mendelian and polygenic components as developed under the "mixed model." Rather, they were proposed as a general method for analyzing dependent data where each individual is sequentially conditioned on those preceding him or her in the nuclear family, that is, in the full regressive model the mother is conditioned on the father, the offspring are conditioned on the parents, younger sibs are conditioned on older sibs. The simplest regressive models condition sibs only on their parents, and correspond nicely with the Mendelian predictions that full sibs are independent given the parental mating type. More general regressive models condition each sib on both the parents and all preceding offspring; and these have been shown to be mathematically and numerically equivalent to the "mixed model" for quantitative traits for nuclear families (Demenais and Bonney, 1989). Regressive models, therefore, allow estimation and testing for both types of genetic components (i.e., Mendelian and polygenic), as well as simultaneous estimation of covariate effects.

The question of more complex effects of covariates often arises both from a biologic standpoint and from analysis of data on individuals with an identifiable genotype. It is quite plausible to envision a differential impact of a covariate in one genotype versus another, and the entire concept of genetic susceptibility requires such genotype-specific patterns of covariate effects. In an analysis of a large French Canadian pedigree segregating for familial hypercholesterolemia (FH), Moll and colleagues (1984a) illustrated how the effects of age on low-density lipoprotein (LDL) cholesterol levels were different between heterozygotes and normal homozygous individuals and heterozygous FH carriers (there were no homozygotes for the *FH* allele in this one large pedigree). Furthermore, if a simple, constant effect of age on LDL cholesterol were assumed to be operating, and fit in a two-stage procedure as described above, the final interpretation would have been quite different.

In general, therefore, statistical models used in segregation analysis should be made as flexible as possible to accommodate not only "type" (or ousiotype) specific means and variances, but also different covariate effects. This genotype specific covariate effect is, in effect, one form of genotype-by-environment interaction (where the covariate is an observed environment). Dealing with such interactions represents a major challenge in genetic epidemiology and can be critical in interpreting segregation analysis. For example, Perusse and coworkers (1991) showed how results of an analysis of systolic blood pressure in families ascertained through schoolchildren was ambiguous until genotype-dependent age and gender effects were included in the model. Once these covariates were considered, effects of a single Mendelian locus on blood pressure became obvious. Genotype-dependent covariate effects can also be incorporated into "mixed models" (Blangero et al., 1990). In an analysis of LDL cholesterol in baboons, Konigsberg and colleagues (1991) showed how a modest, but significant, fraction of variation could be attributed to a greater increase in LDL-cholesterol with age among mutant homozygotes. This form of genotype-by-covariate interaction may be important in a number of traits associated with chronic diseases.

While such flexibility in statistical models is desirable, it often leads to models with so many parameters that the information content of virtually any set of family data is quickly exhausted. Furthermore, the question of whether or when to transform data (before or during the analysis) becomes more complex when "type" (or ousiotype)-specific parameters are estimated. The goal of transformation is to assure normality of residual values (i.e., after covariate effects have been considered) as assumed by the underlying models. Large changes in the phenotypic scale, resulting from log- or power-transformations, may obscure or conceal the presence of underlying "type" (or ousiotype)-specific distributions, and may mask or obliterate the effects of covariates. Caution should always be exercised when using transformations on biologic measures, and final interpretation of the resulting models should make every attempt to convert estimated parameters back to a biologically meaningful scale.

8.5 LIMITATIONS OF SEGREGATION ANALYSIS

As described above, the usual procedure in segregation analysis is to fit a series of models ranging from the simplest nongenetic model to the most general single-locus model with arbitrary transmission of essential "types" (or ousiotypes) and possibly "type"-specific variances and regression coefficients (see Table 8–9). Statistical evidence from segregation analysis can only offer circumstantial evidence about a biologic mechanism, and two critical limitations must be considered: statistical power and etiologic heterogeneity.

8.5.1 Statistical Power

Relatively little is known about the statistical power of segregation analysis of pedigrees because there is no single nongenetic alternative model, but instead a range of competing models beginning with the simplest sporadic model (which assumes all individuals are independent of one another) to models of cultural inheritance with arbitrary transmission between parents and offspring along with possible sibship correlations. It is relatively straightforward to exclude a strictly nongenetic model even for modest samples of small families, if there are correlations among biologic relatives or an excess recurrence risk. However, it is much more difficult to estimate minimum sample sizes needed to reject a false genetic model when the alternative nongenetic model cannot be easily specified. In addition, one must consider the information content of families in the sample. Families, of course, vary in both size and structure, and this dictates their information content for any particular comparison between models. Even among nuclear families, the number of offspring per family dictates the information content of the sampling unit (with larger sibships being generally more informative).

An important contrast of interest is testing for Mendelian models against a polygenic or more general "mixed-model" alternative. As early as 1960, Edwards showed how difficult it could be to distinguish between these competing genetic models by using simple prevalence and recurrence risk data for a qualitative phenotype (Edwards, 1960).

However, quantitative traits carry far more information about the mode of inheritance and several workers have used simulation studies to estimate rates of type I and type II errors when comparing simple Mendelian and polygenic models for quantitative traits. If there is skewness in the underlying distribution, the "mixed model" tends to spuriously indicate a major gene is present even though all familial correlations are strictly due to an additive polygenic component (MacLean et al., 1975; Go et al., 1978). By incorporating explicit tests of the transmission parameters, however, the rate of such false conclusions can be substantially reduced when analyzing nuclear families (Demenais et al, 1986). Conceptually, such skewness is interpreted as evidence for a second distribution under Mendelian models, and explicit tests of the transmission parameters are required to avoid making a wrong inference. Ideally, Mendelian models should be tested against a generalized single-locus model where the complete τ vector is estimated. Estimating the null hypothesis that $\tau_2 = 0.5$ may not provide sufficient discrimination by itself (Demenais et al., 1986). It is also useful to include a test for commingling with constant transmission, that is, where mixtures of distributions are fit but equal transmission probabilities are assumed for all essential "types" (ousiotypes), for example, models 2 and 3 in Table 8-9. By requiring such a set of criteria be met before inferring the presence of a Mendelian mechanism, it may not be necessary to rely on power transformations to remove skewness in the data. This is important because fitting arbitrary power transformations to family data to insure normality in the underlying distribution reduces the ability to detect the effects of single-locus mechanisms controlling quantitative traits (MacLean et al., 1975; Demenais et al., 1986).

Many factors determine the rate of statistical errors in segregation analysis; these range from violations of key assumptions (e.g., skewness violates the assumption of normality) to the structure of the data itself. A key question in designing family studies is what size and kind of families should be recruited and examined. Nuclear families are easier to recruit, but may not be as informative as larger pedigrees. With little additional effort, a nuclear family can be expanded into a large pedigree (by examining grandparents, aunts and uncles, cousins, etc.), but when is this worthwhile? Burns and colleagues (1984) looked at the statistical power to detect segregation at a dominant Mendelian locus controlling a quantitative trait for pedigrees of variable sizes. In this simulation study, samples of extended pedigrees (45 members each) were generated, and then subsets of nuclear families (5 individuals each) and intermediate-sized pedigrees (9 to 15 individuals consisting of grandparents and aunts/uncles of the basic nuclear family) were examined separately. Samples of intermediate-sized pedigrees ascertained through a proband with an extreme quantitative phenotype (9 to 15 members over three generations) provided more power to identify a dominant Mendelian locus compared to either nuclear families or to the complete extended pedigrees. The benefit gained by drawing intermediate-sized pedigrees likely derives from two forces determining the information content of each pedigree. First, intermediate-sized pedigrees contain the maximum proportion of carriers for the rare dominant allele per unit without including uninformative branches of the full pedigree (i.e., branches where the mutant allele is not segregating). Second, the intermediate-sized pedigree spanning three generations offers much more information on transmission parameters compared to nuclear families that include only one mating.

Boehnke and associates (1988) extended this work and suggested a sequential rule for sampling nuclear families within an extended pedigree ascertained through a proband with an extreme quantitative phenotype. Again comparing a simple polygenic model to a mixed dominant Mendelian model, they showed that a sequential sampling strategy provided a greater probability of identifying a Mendelian dominant component with smaller final sample sizes than strategies where the entire pedigree was sampled. This sequential sampling strategy for quantitative traits involves first sampling all first-degree relatives and spouses of a proband with an extreme quantitative phenotype (say beyond the 90th or 95th percentile), and then sampling all additional first relatives and spouses of any previously sampled individual found to have a similarly extreme phenotypic value. At any point where none of the newly sampled relatives have extreme values, no further pedigree members are recruited. This sequential sampling design appears to maximize the statistical power for segregation analysis for dominant (and possibly codominant) Mendelian traits by increasing the ratio of the distinct phenotypic groups. For recessive traits, however, it is not clear that this design would be more efficient than simply ascertaining nuclear families through an affected offspring, because so few of the relatives (beyond the initial sibship) picked up as part of the sequential sampling would be homozygotes.

It must be understood, however, that the limitations of segregation analysis of pedigrees remains poorly defined with respect to rates of type I and type II errors. In part, this deficiency results from the fact that these statistical properties are dependent entirely on the particular models being compared and on the particular pedigree structures at hand. No simple rules can be devised to define a minimum sample size needed for a particular study without specifying the models to be considered. Also, pedigrees vary in their information content about any given contrast, both as a function of their size and structure. Pedigrees informative for tests between two particular models may not be informative for other contrasts. Availability of relatives in one or another branch of the family determines how much missing data are present in the final pedigree used in an analysis. Patterns of missing data sometimes vary by sex and age, and this alone may reduce a large and potentially informative pedigree to one that carries no information on the contrast between two particular models. While it is always desirable to spell out rules for both ascertainment and sampling used by a particular study, by in large, pedigrees available for segregation analysis are often collected on an "as available" basis.

8.5.2 Etiologic Heterogeneity

Many genetic diseases show etiologic heterogeneity in that more than one genetic form of the disease exists, and often nongenetic forms as well. Retinitis pigmentosa is a classic example of genetic heterogeneity with multiple well-documented autosomal dominant, autosomal recessive, and X-linked recessive forms, as well as an excess of simplex families suggestive of one or more nongenetic causes for this degenerative eye disease (Humphries et al., 1992). Such nongenetic cases are frequently termed phenocopies or sporadics. Since much of genetic epidemiology focuses on common, chronic diseases where both genetic and nongenetic factors contribute to the phenotype, etiologic heterogeneity must be accepted as the rule rather than the exception.

In some models for segregation analysis of sibships, penetrance parameters are set up to allow estimation of the proportion of phenocopies (affected individuals among those without the "high risk" genotype) (Morton, 1982), but even here the assumption is that this risk to the "normal" genotypes is constant over all families. Greenberg and Hodge (1985) reexpressed the likelihood function for a simple Mendelian recessive model with such a fixed proportion of affecteds among both normal homozygotes and heterozygotes to show that a maximum likelihood estimator for the degree of admixture between truly genetic and truly nongenetic forms of a disease could be obtained. Although their example was quite specialized, the concept of looking for etiologic heterogeneity within a sample of families or pedigrees is extremely important.

Whenever a set of pedigrees is fit to a single model of inheritance (be it a nongenetic, polygenic, Mendelian, or a "mixed" model) there is the implicit assumption of true etiologic homogeneity, however, it is still possible to test for etiologic heterogeneity. One approach is to stratify a set of pedigrees by some observable character and test for statistically significant heterogeneity using the likelihood ratio test. In this approach, a single model is fit to each of I subsets of pedigrees separately and to the combined set, and a chi-square test for heterogeneity is computed as

$$\chi^2 = 2[\ln L(\text{model}|\text{all data}) - \sum_{i=1}^{I} \ln L(\text{model}|\text{subset } i)], \quad (8\text{-}35)$$

which has degrees of freedom $k(I - 1)$ for a model with k parameters. Typically, subsets of families are defined by characteristics of the proband, but could also include sources of the data, ethnic groups, etc. Williams and Anderson (1984) used the cohort in which the proband was born to stratify pedigrees ascertained through a patient with breast cancer and showed no evidence of etiologic heterogeneity among families in a genetic study of breast cancer from a Danish population. Goldstein and coworkers (1988) used a similar model on pedigrees ascertained through a bilateral breast cancer case and showed evidence for heterogeneity among families ascertained through different types of cancer in the proband.

A second approach is more subjective and involves selecting the best model fit to the overall set of pedigrees and looking for evidence of heterogeneity based on the fit to this model. This approach can be very useful for identifying segregating families when the best-fitting model is a "mixed model" with both Mendelian and polygenic components. Pedigrees which show strong evidence for Mendelian segregation may be identified from phenotypic observations alone or by actually computing genotypic probabilities on their members. Moll and colleagues (1984b) used this latter approach to demonstrate that evidence for a Mendelian component controlling cholesterol levels in families ascertained through schoolchildren came from a small subset of families.

Whenever the comparison of interest is between two specific models, a "model choice" approach can also be used to create subgroups of pedigrees. In this approach, the ratio of ln-likelihoods for two particular models on each pedigree is used to group pedigrees into subsets that favor or support one model over another. Moll and colleagues (1989) found this ad hoc approach useful when both a nongenetic model and a Mendelian mixed model gave adequate descriptions for Apo A_1 levels in a group of 283 randomly selected pedigrees. By sorting these pedigrees on their degree of support for a genetic versus a nongenetic model, two distinct subgroups could be identified each of which gave internally consistent evidence for quite different patterns of familial aggregation in Apo A_1 levels. One group of pedigrees appeared to be segregating for a single Mendelian locus controlling Apo A_1, while the other showed evidence of distinctive phenotypic groups, but was not compatible with any genetic pattern of transmission. While appropriate caution must be exercised when grouping pedigrees on the basis of which model they best support, this "model choice" approach can be useful in identifying families segregating for Mendelian traits for further biochemical and genetic analysis.

8.6 CONCLUDING REMARKS

Segregation analysis can provide the statistical evidence for Mendelian control of a trait or disease, although this remains circumstantial evidence. In experimental situations, the predictions of segregation analysis can be confirmed by designed matings, but in observational studies, this is far more difficult and one must rely on "experiments of nature." As discussed in this chapter, segregation analysis frequently requires correction for biases due to ascertainment and ideally should include some explicit evaluation of etiologic heterogeneity.

Information from genetic markers can theoretically be incorporated into a formal segregation analysis and thereby jointly test for segregation at an underlying Mendelian locus and cosegregation with a specified marker. This joint approach requires more information from family data, but has great potential for yielding detailed answers about genetic mechanisms. Each approach, however, imposes its own requirements and has its own set of limitations. The principles of linkage analysis are presented in Chapter 9, where the limitations of combining linkage and segregation approaches are discussed in more detail.

9

Genetic Approaches to Familial Aggregation

III. Linkage Analysis

WITH DEBORAH A. MEYERS

9.1 INTRODUCTION

Linkage analysis has an important role in genetic epidemiology because it identifies a biologic mechanism for transmission of a trait or disease. Classically, the term "linkage" has been used to denote the situation where alleles from two loci segregate together in a family, that is, where they are passed as a single unit from parent to child, thus departing from Mendel's law of independent assortment. The most obvious biologic explanation for such an observation is that the two loci are physically located near one another on the same chromosome. Elston (1981) argues that demonstrating linkage is the highest level of statistical "proof" that a disease is due to a genetic mechanism. While final proof of genetic control must await identification of the gene product and a biologic explanation for pathogenesis, confirmation of reported linkage in multiple studies can quickly establish genetic transmission of a complex disease. Appropriate knowledge of the position of markers linked to a disease on the genetic or physical map of the human genome automatically uncovers further areas for research at the molecular level. The concept of "reverse genetics" or "positional cloning" requires linked markers to localize and identify genes controlling a disease. On the practical side, clear demonstration of genetic linkage also provides a basis for preventive steps through genetic counseling.

It is important to note that genes can be localized on the human gene map not only with the statistical methods of linkage analysis, but also with a variety of other physical methods. In fact, most of the autosomal loci compiled in McKusick's catalog have been mapped by experimental methods, and a small proportion have been mapped solely with linkage analysis. Physical techniques include in situ hybridization, somatic cell hybridization, and examination of specific chromosomal aberrations in affected individuals (see Table 9–1). Such methods are the tools used to localize or map genes, and complement

Table 9–1.   List of selected methods used to localize traits in the human genome

1. Linkage analysis involving statistical tests for cosegregation
2. Somatic cell hybridization testing for synteny
3. Chromosome sorting followed by hybridization
5. Fine scale restriction endonuclease mapping
6. Homology mapping
7. Deletion mapping
8. Chromosome aberration involving translocations and deletions
9. Techniques special to the X chromosome
   a. Lyonization studies
   b. X-autosome translocation
10. Other techniques
    a. Gene fusion based on "Lepore"-like gene products
    b. Radiation induced hybrids
    c. Cell-mediated gene transfer
    d. Exclusion mapping

Adapted from McKusick (1988).

the traditional linkage studies in families (for further detail see McKusick, 1990).

When there is linkage between two loci, it is important to remember that the specific alleles segregating together in one family may well differ from alleles at these same loci segregating together in another family. For example, if a disease were linked to the *ABO* locus, one family may have a disease allele segregating with the *A* allele at the *ABO* locus, while the next family may have this same disease allele cosegregating with the *B* allele. Unless certain combinations of alleles at different loci (i.e., certain haplotypes) predominate in the population (i.e., unless there is considerable *linkage disequilibrium*), there will always be such differences across families. Consequently, family studies are *always* necessary to measure genetic linkage. While population studies can be used to detect general "associations" between a given allele at a marker locus and a disease, they cannot test for genetic linkage or estimate the recombination fraction between different loci. When distinguishing between association and linkage, it is useful to remember that *association* is a property of alleles, while *linkage* is a property of loci and must involve all alleles at the marker locus.

Linkage analysis is now being widely used to map markers on each chromosome in the human genome, to map genetic diseases, and to identify genetic forms of common diseases. The basic methodology used to achieve these goals largely remains identical to that developed along with the very foundations of genetics. However, there are several critical questions that arise, in part, because of the large number of linkage studies now being undertaken and because these techniques are being extended to diseases of complex etiology where genetic transmission of the disease is not established. Issues of how to incorporate genetic marker information and linkage analysis into studies of complex diseases, where both genetic and nongenetic factors may jointly control pathogenesis, represent a major challenge in genetic epidemiology (Risch, 1990a). The objectives of this chapter are (1) to cover the basic principles of linkage analysis, both at the two-point and multipoint level; (2) to address various methodologic issues in linkage studies; (3) to present alternative sampling designs involving sets of relatives; and (4) to discuss ways in which linkage analysis studies can be incorporated into epidemiologic studies.

9.2   FUNDAMENTALS OF LINKAGE ANALYSIS

The type of family data needed to detect linkage is shown in Figure 9–1. It is assumed that the genetic mechanism is known and all segregation is Mendelian for both the disease locus and the marker locus. There must be one parent who is a double heterozygote for the two loci being studied (e.g., both the disease locus and the marker locus). Obviously, therefore, the probability of a marker being informative for linkage analysis is a function of the frequency of heterozygotes, which in turn is a function of the number of marker alleles and their frequencies. The polymorphic information content (PIC) is used to summarize the probability of a marker locus being informative (Botstein et al., 1980), and highest PIC scores are attained by markers with many, equally frequent, alleles.

In Figure 9–1, the father (II-1) has a rare Mendelian dominant disease (so he is most likely heterozygous for this locus). He is also heterozygous for the marker locus denoted as "+ −." Therefore, it is easy to determine whether all his offspring who inherit the disease allele have also inherited the same allele at the marker locus (i.e., whether these two alleles at different loci cosegregate), and whether all his unaffected offspring have consistently inherited the other allele at the marker locus. In this particular pedigree, the

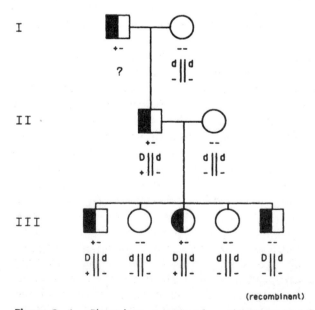

Figure 9–1.   Phase-known mating for a dominant Mendelian disorder

father has inherited the disease and the " + " allele at the marker locus from his own father. Therefore, this represents a *phase-known* mating, that is, if the loci are linked, the " + " allele and the disease allele must be on the same chromosome. Knowing the phase of this parent is important because it permits explicit classification of all offspring as recombinants or nonrecombinants. A *nonrecombinant* is an individual who inherited a haplotype identical to that the parent received from one grandparent; a *recombinant* is an individual who inherited a haplotype not identical to that inherited by his or her parent. The first four children shown in Figure 9–1 must all be nonrecombinants, having received one or the other paternal haplotypes intact. The two affected children have inherited the " + " allele from their affected father, while the two unaffected children have inherited the " − " allele. However, the last child inherited the " − " allele but is affected; therefore, genetic recombination has occurred during meiosis in the father. This fifth child is termed a recombinant, because he does not carry one of the paternal haplotypes. It should be noted that if two loci are being considered, only an odd number of crossovers can ever be detected. If there had been two crossing-over events between the disease and marker locus, the original parental phase would be restored, and this child would have been classified as a nonrecombinant.

Linkage analysis itself is straightforward when, as in this example, recombinant offspring can be counted directly. It is equally straightforward in experimental genetics where matings can be arranged. In these situations, questions of sample size and statistical power are addressed by relying on the familiar binomial distribution, and counts of recombinant versus nonrecombinant children can be tallied over all families of a single mating type. However, in human genetics, there are several reasons why this process is generally more complicated:

1. Not all matings are "phase-known" (for example, phase in the example in Figure 9–1 is established through examining the grandparents who may not always be available or informative).
2. Diseases with incomplete penetrance or age-dependent penetrance make it impossible to identify accurately all carriers of the disease allele.
3. If carrier detection is impossible, as with strictly recessive diseases, linkage analysis becomes uniformly more difficult because less information on genotypes of critical individuals is available.

9.2.1 Maximum Likelihood Methods for Linkage Analysis

Two-point or two-loci analysis described above still serves as the foundation for linkage analysis, although multipoint analysis (considering three or more loci) is becoming increasingly important as ever larger numbers of genetic markers become available. The maximum likelihood approach to linkage analysis dates back to Haldane and Smith (1947), but did not become widely used until Morton (1955) published tables of log-odds (or LOD) scores that could be used in the sequential analysis of family data. Several widely available computer software packages for two-point or multipoint analyses now exist

(Lathrop et al., 1985; Ott, 1985). Nonetheless, it is critical to understand the basis of this maximum likelihood approach to linkage analysis before results from such automated programs can be interpreted.

As seen in Table 9–2, the probability of a child inheriting the disease and the "+" allele at the marker is simply $\frac{1}{2} \times \frac{1}{2} = \frac{1}{4}$ if the disease locus and the marker locus are not linked, i.e., if there is independent assortment. There is a probability of $\frac{1}{4}$ for each of the four possible gametes formed in the double heterozygous parent. Therefore, if these loci are linked and the phase is as shown in Figure 9–1, the probability of inheriting the disease allele and the "+" allele, or inheriting the normal allele and the "−" allele should be greater than $\frac{1}{4}$ (children with these allelic combinations would be nonrecombinants given the phase-known mating shown in Figure 9–1). The actual probability of cosegregation is dependent on the genetic distance between these loci, typically measured by the recombination fraction Θ. Also, the probability of a child inheriting the disease allele and the "−" allele at the marker or inheriting the normal allele and the "+" allele should be less than $\frac{1}{4}$, again dependent on the actual recombination fraction between the loci. These probabilities effectively determine the likelihood function on a family where r is the number of recombinant children out of a total of n children and Θ is the recombination fraction, that is,

$$L(\Theta) = \left(\frac{\Theta}{2}\right)^{r} \left(\frac{1 - \Theta}{2}\right)^{n-r}. \tag{9-1}$$

Terms representing the probability of the mating type itself, the birth order of children, and so on, have been omitted here, so this likelihood is merely proportional to the actual probability of observing any one family. Note the null hypothesis of independent assortment (i.e., no linkage) corresponds to a recombination value of $\Theta = .5$. The log-odds or LOD score serves as a useful summary of all information on linkage, that is,

$$\text{LOD} = \log \frac{L(\Theta)}{L(\Theta = 0.5)} = \log \left(\frac{(\Theta/2)^{r}[(1 - \Theta)/2]^{n-r}}{(0.25)^{n}}\right)$$
$$= \log 2^{n}\Theta^{r}(1 - \Theta)^{n-r}. \tag{9-2}$$

Table 9–2. Probability of receiving alleles at two loci*

	Independent Assortment Disease		Linkage Disease	
Marker	D	d	D	d
+	1/4	1/4	$\dfrac{1 - \Theta}{2}$	$\dfrac{\Theta}{2}$
−	1/4	1/4	$\dfrac{\Theta}{2}$	$\dfrac{1 - \Theta}{2}$

*(A dominant disease locus with alleles D and d, a marker locus with alleles + and −, under independent assortment and linkage.

This quantity is the conventional measure of the strength of evidence for linkage at a specified value of Θ. Since the denominator is constant, varying Θ to maximize the LOD score is equivalent to obtaining the maximum likelihood estimator (MLE) for Θ (Ott, 1974).

In Figure 9–2, the parents of the affected father were not studied; therefore the "phase" of the disease allele and the marker alleles in this father cannot be known. Linkage information can still be obtained even from a *phase-unknown* mating such as this, however. In this type of family, the children are classified as possible recombinants or not in relationship to one another. For example, in Figure 9–2 the first three children are all nonrecombinants *if* the father inherited the disease and the " – " allele from his affected parent. In this situation, only the last child would be a recombinant. *If*, however, the father carried these alleles in the opposite phase, the first three children would be recombinants and the fourth child would be a nonrecombinant. When dealing with phase unknown matings, it is critical to consider both possibilities, otherwise tests for linkage will be biased. The log-likelihood for this family is therefore written as

$$L(\Theta) = \frac{1}{2}\left(\frac{\Theta}{2}\right)^{r}\left(\frac{1-\Theta}{2}\right)^{n-r} + \frac{1}{2}\left(\frac{\Theta}{2}\right)^{n-r}\left(\frac{1-\Theta}{2}\right)^{r} \qquad (9\text{-}3)$$

for any value of Θ, where r is the number of apparent recombinant offspring under one phase. Note that under this formulation both phases are equally likely, and the children classified as "recombinants" under one phase are classified as "nonrecombinants" under the other phase. Writing this as an LOD score gives

$$\begin{aligned}
\text{LOD} &= \log \frac{L(\Theta)}{L(\Theta = 0.5)} \\[2mm]
&= \log \frac{\frac{1}{2}\left[\left(\frac{\Theta}{2}\right)^{r}\left(\frac{1-\Theta}{2}\right)^{n-r} + \left(\frac{\Theta}{2}\right)^{n-r}\left(\frac{1-\Theta}{2}\right)^{r}\right]}{(0.25)^{n}} \qquad (9\text{-}4) \\[2mm]
&= \log\{2^{n-1}[\Theta^{r}(1-\Theta)^{n-r} + \Theta^{n-r}(1-\Theta)^{r}]\}.
\end{aligned}$$

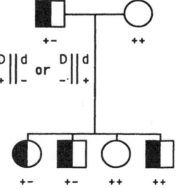

Figure 9–2. Phase-unknown mating for a dominant mendelian disorder.

Since the likelihoods of independent families are multiplied to accumulate a total likelihood for any one sample, these log-likelihoods or LOD scores are simply summed over all independent matings. Table 9–3 gives the LOD scores over a number of possible Θ values from six example families shown in Figure 9–3. The summed LOD scores over all families can be used to obtain the MLE of the recombination fraction (here $\Theta = .12$, at a LOD = 4.78). The total LOD curve for these six families is displayed in Figure 9–4, showing the MLE of Θ and their approximate 95% confidence limits. Such approximate 95% confidence limits or *support limits* can be derived from plots such as this by subtracting 1.0 from the maximum LOD value and calculating the corresponding recombination fractions, either explicitly or by interpolation (Conneally, 1985).

A LOD of 3.0 or more has been traditionally considered strong evidence *for* linkage, while a LOD score of -2.0 or less has been taken as evidence *against* linkage. These critical values correspond to 1000:1 odds for linkage and 100:1 odds against linkage, respectively, at some specified value of Θ. The actual rate of type I error (i.e., rejecting the true hypothesis that $\Theta = \frac{1}{2}$) using these values is very close to the conventional 5% level of significance, once the prior probability of two loci being linked is considered. The prior probability of two loci being linked has been estimated at approximately 5% based on the relative length of all autosomes (Renwick, 1971). If this prior probability of autosomal linkage were ignored, selecting a critical value for LOD scores with a nominal type I error rate of 5% (i.e., setting the critical value to reflect odds of 20:1) would produce an unacceptably high rejection rate for the null hypothesis that $\Theta = \frac{1}{2}$ (Smith, 1953). The approach used in linkage analysis has evolved as a compromise between statistical principles and recognized biologic constraints. Morton (1955) originally developed these critical values in the context of sequential testing for linkage, where families were sampled until conclusive evidence either for or against linkage was accumulated. Even though the framework of sequential testing has not been strictly followed, and often estimation of Θ is a primary goal, most tests of significance in linkage analysis still rely on this critical value of 3.0 (Ott, 1985). The probability of a type I error (i.e., falsely identifying two loci as linked)

Table 9–3. Log-odd (LOD) scores for six example families over a range of recombination fractions

Family	Recombination fractions									
	.01	*.05*	*.10*	*.15*	*.20*	*.25*	*.30*	*.35*	*.40*	*.45*
1	0.38	0.95	1.09	1.09	1.03	0.93	0.80	0.64	0.46	0.24
2	0.89	0.81	0.72	0.62	0.52	0.41	0.30	0.19	0.09	0.03
3	0.37	0.93	1.04	1.02	0.93	0.81	0.65	0.46	0.26	0.08
4	0.38	0.95	1.09	1.09	1.03	0.93	0.80	0.64	0.46	0.24
5	−0.89	0.81	0.72	0.62	0.52	0.41	0.30	0.19	0.09	0.03
6	−1.62	0.35	0.09	0.27	0.33	0.33	0.28	0.21	0.11	0.03
Total	1.28	4.11	4.75	4.71	4.36	3.82	3.13	2.33	1.48	0.65

$\Theta = 0.12$, LOD = 4.78.

Family 1

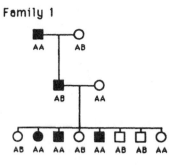

Family 2

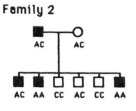

Family 3

Family 4

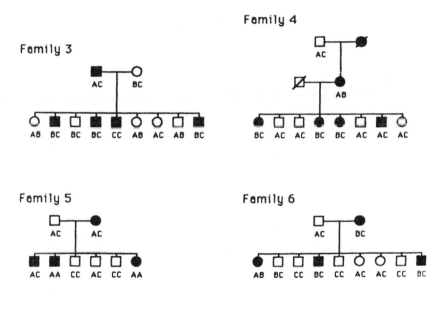

Family 5

Family 6

Figure 9–3. Six example pedigrees.

must always consider the low prior probability of linkage, and from theoretical grounds this probability of nonlinkage at an LOD score of 3.0 seems to be 3 to 4% (Smith 1986; Conneally and Rivas, 1980). Empirical evidence suggests that less than 2% of linkages giving LOD $\geq$ 3.0 are spurious (Rao et al., 1978). As multiple loci are considered in linkage analysis, however, strict reliance on this critical LOD value of 3 may be less appropriate. Strategies for valid tests in multipoint analysis are still evolving (Lander, 1988; Weeks et al., 1990).

In a linkage analysis, the distinction between hypothesis testing and estimation of the recombination fraction is often lost. When two loci have been physically mapped close to each other, the purpose of the linkage study is strictly to estimate Θ, the recombination fraction. For example, if two loci are known to be X linked, they must automatically be *syntenic* (i.e., on the same chromosome) and the primary focus becomes estimation of the recom-

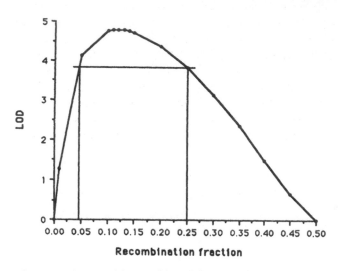

Figure 9-4. Total long odds (LOD) curve for six example families.

bination fraction (synteny does not automatically imply linkage as several linkage groups may be on the same chromosome). On the other hand, when there is little or no prior information about linkage, then the primary purpose becomes establishing linkage through tests of significance, using the LOD score or the likelihoods themselves, although an estimate of recombination may also be desirable. Maximum likelihood approaches to linkage analysis have very little power to detect loose linkage ($.25 < \Theta < .45$), and the critical values discussed above were deliberately chosen to maximize the probability of detecting tight linkage. Therefore, building a comprehensive genetic map requires sequentially identifying tightly linked markers and building up linkage groups.

9.2.2 Recombination in Males Versus Females

Sex differences in recombination have been observed in many species. Typically there is increased recombination in the homogametic sex compared to the heterogametic sex, often corresponding to up to a threefold increase in recombination in females compared to males in humans. Therefore, recombination in males (Θ_M) and recombination in females (Θ_F) should be estimated separately. Details for standard methods of reporting linkage results in humans are given by Conneally (1985). A simple test for heterogeneity in recombination fractions between males and females is computed as

$$X^2 = 4.6[\text{LOD}(\hat{\Theta}_M, \hat{\Theta}_F) - \text{LOD}(\hat{\Theta})], \qquad (9\text{-}5)$$

which compares a model with sex-specific recombination rates (i.e., Θ_M is the male recombination fraction and Θ_F is the female recombination fraction) to one with a single recombination fraction common to both sexes (i.e., the null hypothesis states $\Theta = \Theta_M = \Theta_F$). This difference is simply a likelihood ratio test, where $4.6 (= 2 \times 2.30)$ is twice the constant for converting from common to natural logs. As the sample size increases, the approximation to a true chi-square distribution improves. One of the first documented differences in recombination between the sexes was seen in the linkage analysis of the ABO locus and nail-patella syndrome (NPS1) (Schleutermann et al, 1969). The MLE for recombination in males (Θ_M) was 0.10 and the corresponding MLE in females (Θ_F) was .15, with LOD = 43.804. If male and female recombination fractions were forced to be equal, the MLE for the common recombination rate was .10, with LOD = 43.015. Therefore the chi-square test statistic would be 4.6 (43.804 − 43.015) = 3.633, and p = .06. As discussed by Ott (1985), the power to detect differences in recombination fraction using this approach is relatively low. Therefore, it is not surprising that an apparent 50% difference in recombination between the sexes resulted in a marginally significant p value.

9.2.3 Multipoint Mapping

The term *multipoint mapping* refers to linkage analysis of more than two loci at a time. Considering multiple loci simultaneously gives substantial increases in information for both estimating the recombination fraction and establishing the order of linked loci. Not only are there more opportunities for identifying crossing-over events when considering multiple loci, but there is greater opportunity for encountering informative matings. In general, markers flanking a disease locus provide the most useful information for establishing risk in genetic counseling; therefore, it is important to establish the correct order of loci (i.e., is the order A-D-B or A-B-D for markers A and B relative to disease locus D?). There are several different approaches commonly used:

1. Constructing maps covering multiple loci by looking at two pairs of loci at a time
2. Analysis of multiple loci simultaneously based on joint likelihoods incorporating the corresponding recombination fractions between all loci
3. Testing whether a new locus (marker or disease) can be mapped onto an existing map of several marker loci

In the first two approaches, the amount of recombination between the different loci is varied simultaneously, while in the third approach a new locus is tested only in relation to a fixed map for all other loci.

Before any multipoint analysis is performed, two-point LODs for all possible pairs should be calculated. From these pairwise values, a first attempt at a multipoint map can be made. For example, consider six loci with the pairwise LOD scores displayed in Table 9–4. The MLE of the pairwise recombination fractions are shown in the upper right triangular portion of the table, with their corresponding LODs in the lower left triangular portion. An intuitive map of these loci can be constructed as shown in Figure 9–5, by starting with loci showing tight linkage and continuously checking for consistency of pairwise relationships.

There are several issues to be considered from this map:

Table 9–4. Results of two-point linkage analysis which can be used to construct a tentative map of six loci.

LODS	Recombination fractions (MLE)					
	A	B	C	D	E	F
A	—	0.10	0.26	NI	0.41	0.50
B	1.5	—	0.20	NI	0.22	0.25
C	2.0	2.7	—	0.01	0.05	0.11
D	NI	NI	10.5	—	0.05	0.09
E	0.4	1.7	8.2	8.6	—	0.07
F	0.0	1.6	6.0	5.5	7.7	—

Estimated recombination fractions are given in the upper triangular portion, while the corresponding LOD scores are given in the lower triangular portion.
LODs, log odds score; MLE, maximum likelihood estimator; NI, not informative.

i. The order of loci C and D in relationship to the other loci will be hard to determine because of their own very close linkage.
ii. The order of loci (C:D), E, F is more obvious. The LODs are higher (smaller confidence limits) and all pairwise estimates point to this order.
iii. The order of loci A and B in relationship to locus C is not clear. Because of the relatively low LODs (likely due to a relatively small number of informative families), the order B-A-C is still quite possible.
iv. In general, the pairwise estimate of recombination for nonsequential loci is smaller than the sum of the sequential pairwise estimates. This nonlinear relationship between recombination fractions reflects the limitation on detecting odd numbers of crossover events and the impact of *interference* among crossing-over events (where the occurrence of a crossing-over event in one region alters the probability of crossing-over in another regions).

Given such a preliminary order, these data could then be analyzed by several different methods.

The *first* method has been widely used to construct linkage maps of chromosomes based on summary LOD score data collected from multiple laboratories (Rao et al., 1979). In this case, the joint likelihood of all loci is determined, and maximum likelihood estimates of recombination between each pair of loci under a given order is obtained. The analysis is then repeated for different possible orders of the loci, and the likelihoods for each order determined to give odds in favor of one order versus another.

In the *second* and more general approach, the family data on all the loci would be analyzed to give a joint likelihood and estimates of the recombi-

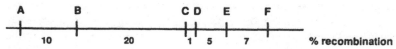
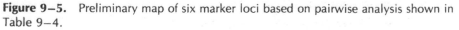

Figure 9–5. Preliminary map of six marker loci based on pairwise analysis shown in Table 9–4.

nation fractions under a given order (Lathrop et al., 1984, 1985, 1986). The difference between these two approaches is that data on parents informative for more than two loci can be included in this latter analysis. Frequently, this can be critical. For example, the family seen in Figure 9–6 provides clear indication that one order is better than another. As seen in this figure, the second child (III-2) must be a double recombinant if the order is D-C-E, while a single crossing-over event can explain these data if the order is C-D-E.

The third common approach in multipoint analysis is designed to assign a new marker or disease locus to a known map. Here the order and recombination fractions for a background group of markers is held constant, and the recombination fraction between a new locus and each member of this background set is varied to find the most likely genetic map. For example, if a large group of data from several sources has established the map for five markers to be A-B-C-E-F with reasonable certainty, it is of interest to establish where a new locus (D) falls in this map. By varying each recombination fraction involving D and one of these markers (but not those involving the five background loci, i.e., Θ_{AB}, Θ_{BC}, etc.), a new multipoint map can be

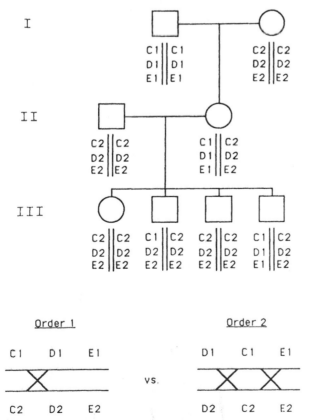

Figure 9–6. Mating informative for three markers. Note that under order 1, III-2 is a recombinant with a single crossover event between C and D. Under order 2, this individual must represent two crossing-over events. Therefore, order 1 is more likely.

constructed. An example of this type of analysis is shown in Figure 9–7. This shows the placement of a marker locus (D4S95) in relationship to the locus for Huntington disease (HD) and two loci previously linked to HD (Wasmuth et al., 1988). As seen in the graph, the new marker D4S95 is closely linked to HD and could be on either side of it. However, it is much less likely that the new marker D4S95 is further from the HD locus than the two established markers D4S10 and D4S62.

Although genetic maps of the human chromosomes are constantly being updated, it is worth examining one published map to compare different approaches. For example, the map of chromosome 2 by O'Connell and colleagues (1989) summarizes results from two-point and multipoint analysis of 20 loci. Different rates of recombination in males versus females were seen, as depicted in Figure 9–8. Also shown here is a combined map of chromosome 2 showing appropriate confidence intervals for each locus location.

It is important to note that recombination fractions are *not* equal to map distances (measured in centimorgans [cM]) because (1) the presence of multiple crossover events (involving any even number of crossovers) will restore the original parental haplotype, and (2) there is *interference* of crossing over. As noted previously, only an odd number of crossovers between any two loci can ever be detected. For example, two crossovers occurring in the region between any two loci restores the original parental haplotype. This tends to bias estimates of recombination between distant loci downward. However, when one crossover event has occurred in a region, it is less likely that another crossover will occur in that same region (i.e., there is *positive interference* between nearby crossover events). Although interference has been seen in

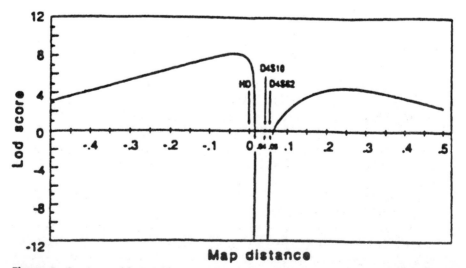

Figure 9–7. Log odds (LOD) scores for map location of a new marker (D4S95) and the fixed map of Huntington's disease (HD), D4S10, and D4S62. The HD locus was arbitrarily set at location 0 with the telomere to the left and centromere to the right. [Adapted from Wasmuth et al, (1988).]

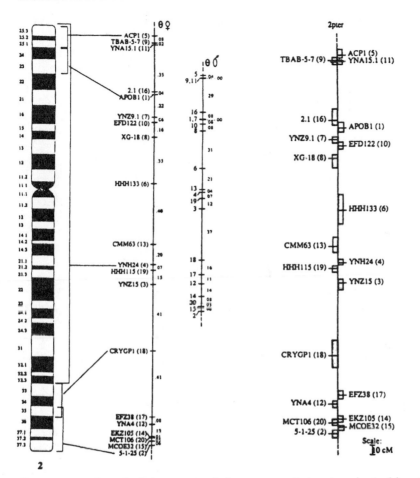

Figure 9–8. Genetic linkage map of chromosome 2 showing physical location, sex-specific genetic distances (based on Haldane's mapping function, and confidence limits for location of 20 marker loci). [Adapted from O'Connell et al. (1989).]

other species, it has not yet been well documented in humans. As more data on multiple-linked loci and better genetic maps become available, this will be a fruitful area of investigation.

Recombination fractions can be converted to map distances by the use of a mapping function. The oldest mapping function often used for human data is that of Haldane (1919), which takes multiple crossing over into account but does not consider interference. Kosambi (1944) and Carter and Falconer (1951) both derived mapping functions for the mouse that incorporate positive interference. Rao and coworkers (1977) have proposed a mapping function for human data that is essentially a weighted combination of these three functions and have applied this in a map of chromosome 1 (Rao et al, 1979). As a rule of thumb, for close linkage, map distances and recombination fractions can be assumed to be equal, although truly comprehensive genetic maps must be based on some mapping function.

9.3 METHODOLOGIC ISSUES IN LINKAGE ANALYSIS

As mentioned earlier, linkage analysis seeks to estimate the recombination fraction between different loci in identifiable meiotic events. The focus is strictly on the proportion of crossover events, and Mendelian inheritance of both the marker and disease is typically assumed. Linkage analysis alone is relatively insensitive to sampling biases because it does not attempt to estimate population parameters (e.g., allele frequencies), only the recombination fraction. Whenever linkage is carried out simultaneously with segregation analysis, however, the problem of ascertainment biases must be addressed.

Linkage studies impose their own requirements on family data. First of all, doubly heterozygous parents are obviously necessary, preferably in a backcross mating (i.e., a double heterozygote mated to a double homozygote). Matings between two double heterozygotes can be informative, especially if the parents are heterozygous for different alleles at the marker locus (e.g., an AB × CD mating for marker genotypes). Second, multiplex families are generally more informative than families with only one affected individual. Certain family structures are intrinsically uninformative (e.g., phase-unknown matings with a single offspring), while others depend on the genotypes of parents. A general strategy involves identifying potentially informative families, based on the pedigree structure obtained from interviewing one or more family members, and concentrating on these. A potentially informative pedigree structure may still turn out uninformative for recombination involving any one pair of loci, but this cannot be determined until the individuals are genotyped (the affected parent must be heterozygous at any marker locus to be informative). A sequential strategy may be adopted where parents are genotyped first and then children. By constantly checking the genotypic structure of the family, some laboratory effort can be saved (i.e., little will be gained by genotyping the children of two homozygotes). For practical reasons and as a quality control check, however, it may be easier to genotype all members of a family as a single unit.

9.3.1 Statistical Power in Linkage Studies

As in all other aspects of genetic epidemiology, it is important to determine whether there is a reasonable chance of identifying genetic linkage for the disease in question, given the available sample of families. Calculations of statistical power are difficult to perform in human genetics because there is no single "standard" family unit, and different families contribute different amounts of information. In the simplest possible situation for linkage analysis (i.e., where all families represented phase-known matings), it is relatively easy to compute the number of children necessary to give an 80% probability of finding LOD = 3.0, the most commonly used critical value for establishing linkage. This situation reduces to a binomial distribution for the number of recombinants among all children. However, this ideal situation is rarely attained as there is usually a mixture of phase-known and phase-unknown families from any one study.

It is important to understand that the unit of interest in testing for linkage is the number of identifiable meiotic events in an informative mating, not the number of offspring or the number of matings. Indeed within a single pedigree, there may be both phase-known and phase-unknown matings, and not all offspring will necessarily be informative. If an investigator does not have access to family information before undertaking the linkage study, then sample size determinations must be based on a prespecified family structure. For example, the expected amount of information can be determined for offspring of phase-known matings, and the minimum number of such offspring sufficient to demonstrate linkage can be estimated for a specified recombination fraction (Ott, 1989).

Often, however, there is some information available on the actual families before their marker genotypes are determined. In this situation, power calculations can be performed based on the structure of the particular families at hand, including who are affected with the disease in question and which family members are available for typing. Boehnke (1986) proposed a bootstrap approach, which has shown to be an efficient method for answering the question: "Will my families be sufficient to demonstrate linkage if it exists?" Under this approach, 1000 replicates of a given family structure can be simulated for a marker, given the number of alleles, their frequencies, and the recombination fraction with the disease locus. These simulated families can then be analyzed, and the mean LOD scores computed over all simulated replicates. From these simulated data, the probability of LOD > 3.0 for a prespecified value of Θ can be easily determined. If the investigator is interested in determining whether a candidate gene (or one of a set of candidate genes) is linked to the disease, then simulations are performed with very tight linkage, that is, a recombination fraction at or near zero (Ploughman and Boehnke, 1989). If the goal of the study is to map the disease using a spanning set of markers, then these simulations would be performed based on the overall genetic map to be used. For example, if a set of markers known to be no more than 20 cM apart are chosen, the disease locus can be at the most 10 cM from one of the markers.

9.3.2 Etiologic Heterogeneity

The same test statistic used to test for homogeneity in the recombination fraction between males and females can be used to test for heterogeneity of linkage within a single data set (Ott, 1989). If it is possible to divide families into groups based on clinical features of the disease or trait in probands (or possibly all relatives), this same test for heterogeneity can be done to see whether only one clinical form of the disease is linked to the marker in question. Absence of detectable linkage or evidence against linkage in a subset of families indicates heterogeneity in the disease. The subset of families providing evidence for linkage may represent the only genetic form of the disease.

Even when dividing families based on clinical features of the disease is not feasible, it is still possible to test for heterogeneity through linkage analysis. Morton (1956) proposed a general test for heterogeneity among all families based on the deviation of the separate maximum LODs from the maximum obtained from the overall sample. This test statistic is computed as

$$2 \ln (10) \left[\sum_{i=1}^{I} Z_i(\hat{\theta}_i) - Z(\hat{\theta}) \right], \qquad (9\text{-}6)$$

where $\hat{\theta}_i$ is the MLE for the recombination fraction obtained in the ith family and $Z_i(\hat{\theta}_i)$ is its corresponding LOD score, while $Z(\hat{\theta})$ is the maximum LOD score obtained from the total sample of I families. This statistic should approximate a chi-square distribution with $I - 1$ degrees of freedom. Risch (1988) points out that this statistic is sensitive to small sample sizes, however, and can be too liberal in rejecting the null hypothesis at small values of Θ.

An alternative test for a mixture of families with linkage and families without linkage was first proposed by Smith (1963). Here the proportion (α) of families demonstrating linkage is estimated along with the recombination fraction, while the remaining proportion ($1 - \alpha$) is assumed to be completely unlinked (Ott, 1977; Risch and Baron, 1982). This is a one-sided test, that is, the null hypothesis is $\alpha = 1$ versus the alternative $\alpha < 1.0$, and the likelihood ratio test approximates a chi-square distribution with 1 degree of freedom. Recently, Risch (1988) proposed another likelihood ratio test for heterogeneity that incorporates a β distribution to describe the prior probability of heterogeneity among families. Comparisons of the observed critical values over a variety conditions of sample size and true recombination fraction revealed that these two approaches for detecting heterogeneity do not differ much in their statistical power, although both are conservative at small values of Θ (i.e., the empirical critical values are less than that of the usual chi-square distribution) (Risch, 1988).

9.3.3 Incomplete Penetrance

So far, only linkage analysis between a simple dominant disease with complete penetrance or a codominant disease and a codominant marker has been discussed. Linkage studies of dominant disorders with incomplete penetrance are also feasible, but the probability of each genotype in at-risk subjects must be estimated or assigned. This approach invariably results in a loss of information relative to the situation with a fully penetrant disease, because an unaffected at-risk family member cannot be definitively classified as a recombinant or nonrecombinant, since his or her genotype for the disease locus is no longer known with certainty. Therefore, it is necessary to collect data from more families to establish linkage than would be needed for a dominant disease with complete penetrance. Even for phase-known double backcross matings, Ott (1989) showed the reduction in statistical efficiency depends on both the recombination fraction and the penetrance itself. Their combined effects can be dramatic. For example, if a disorder closely linked to a marker (i.e., $\Theta = .01$) showed 90% penetrance, the relative efficiency drops 50%; if the penetrance was 50%, this relative efficiency becomes only 25% compared to a fully penetrant disease. Note that these lower efficiencies require a doubling and quadrupling of the sample size, respectively (Ott, 1989).

Frequently penetrance of the disease is age-dependent, with at-risk offspring below a certain age contributing very little information to the linkage analysis because they have not yet entered the age of risk. Conversely, in these situations the probability of actually being an unaffected carrier declines with age, so it may be possible to classify older unaffected individuals as true noncarriers (and, therefore, establish their status recombinants or nonrecombinants). In such situations, it is extremely helpful, and almost imperative, to have some externally supplied age-of-onset function. These are usually obtained from studies of clinic populations, and thus, it becomes important to ask whether the disease is homogeneous. Diseases which are etiologically heterogeneous must be treated with caution, as the family used in the linkage analysis may or may not be representative of the larger population of all affected patients. Also, sources of bias in age-of-onset curves derived from clinic populations must also be addressed, especially if a substantial fraction of gene carriers never become affected.

9.3.4 Traits With Recessive Inheritance

Recessive traits present a unique set of difficulties for linkage analysis. In studies of rare recessive disorders, both unaffected parents are potentially informative for linkage because both are obligate heterozygotes for the disease allele. Therefore, if markers with multiple alleles are tested, there is a high probability that segregation at both the disease and marker loci can be detected in gametes from both parents. However, there is also a loss of information, since phase-known matings are rarely available for recessive diseases. Typing grandparents of an affected child will not help, because their genotypes at the marker locus does not automatically establish phase in the parents (the carrier status of the two pairs of grandparents remains uncertain for truly recessive diseases).

To optimize the chances for successfully mapping a recessive disease, families with multiple affected children are needed. Although some information can be gained from the unaffected sibs of a proband with a recessive disease, they are not fully informative, since their genotype at the disease locus is also not known (although, on average, two-thirds of these unaffected sibs should be heterozygous at the disease locus). However, multiple unaffected children in a sibship can still provide some useful information. As an example, consider a family with nine unaffected children and no living affected children other than the proband. For a three-allele marker locus where the parents are ab and ac, the affected proband is aa, and $none$ of the eight unaffected children are aa, a LOD as high as 1.12 can be obtained at $\Theta = 0$. Conversely, if the unaffected children of such a mating show all possible marker genotypes (including aa), this $alone$ is evidence for recombination, and there is little need to search further for tight linkage.

In addition, two other approaches can be utilized either separately or in conjunction with the standard method of linkage analysis. The first alternative is "homozygosity mapping," which is based on the use of inbred families to map rare recessive lethal diseases (Lander and Botstein, 1987). The main problem in dealing with a truly lethal genetic disease is that families with multiple affected children may never be available if affected children die early. However, even if a single affected child is available from an inbred family, information on linkage can still be obtained. Lander and Botstein (1987) showed that under certain, rather strict, assumptions the LOD score is directly related to the coefficient of inbreeding for an inbred child. For example, with a first-cousin marriage, the coefficient of inbreeding is 1/16, and the odds in favor of tight linkage are also approximately 16:1 (LOD = 1.20 at Θ = 0) if the affected child is homozygous for a rare allele at a marker locus. However, this is calculated assuming an extremely polymorphic marker system where the probability would be high that the affected child is homozygous by descent for both the disease and the marker loci. Unfortunately, if the marriage is between second or third cousins (or more distantly related individuals), relatively little information is obtained under this approach. Similarly, if the allele frequencies at the marker locus are such that automatically assuming the affected child carries alleles that are identical by descent (*ibd*) is unjustified, the ability to detect linkage declines dramatically.

The second alternative is to look at rare recessive diseases in a closed population where there are multiple affected children from different nuclear families but all such families can be traced back to a single founder couple (Meyers et al., 1989). This approach allows information on phase to be obtained, but, more importantly, linkage analysis is possible even though separate multiplex nuclear families may never be available. In this situation, information on linkage is available from single affected children even though the degree of inbreeding is much less than second or third cousins. Of course, combinations of these approaches can also be utilized, since LOD scores are calculated directly. A critical limitation is imposed by the frequencies of the alleles at the marker loci, however, and most information is obtained when markers are highly polymorphic. An additional assumption to these approaches for linkage analysis of recessive diseases is that the disease is completely homogeneous. While this may occur in closed populations, several recessive diseases have been shown to be genetically heterogeneous in outbred populations.

9.4 ALTERNATIVE METHODS FOR DETECTING LINKAGE

The maximum likelihood approach to linkage analysis described above is strictly dependent on the specified model of inheritance. When the model is not known, either in some detail or at a broader level (i.e., it may not even be clear whether the disease is genetic or not), estimation of the recombination fraction and tests for linkage become suspect. There are, however, alternative methods for testing for genetic linkage and these have great potential for use with many of the common diseases thought to be at least partially genetic. Most commonly used methods arose from early work by Penrose (1935), who reasoned that if linkage existed it would be reflected in the nonrandom association of two traits (for a disease and a marker, or for two markers) in independent pairs of sibs. Table 9–5 shows the layout for Penrose's original sib-pair method for two codominant markers. It is important to note that the test statistic for this analysis is more specific than the usual chi-square tests for independence. In particular, Penrose's original test looked for excess concordance in the four corner cells representing concordance for marker loci (Li, 1961). One spin-off of this approach was to examine only pairs of affected sibs, who could either be alike or different at the marker locus. The chief advantage of both the sib-pair and the affected sib-pair methods is that they can be used *without* knowing the exact genetic mechanism, and both hold the potential for identifying previously unrecognized genetic forms of common diseases.

9.4.1 Sib-Pair Methods

The original sib-pair design exploits the fact that full sibs are expected to share alleles or haplotypes in defined patterns. Specifically, assume the marker loci being considered are sufficiently polymorphic to establish four distinct parental haplotypes (i.e., the mating can be denoted $AB \times CD$ as in Figure 9–9, and the proband has genotype AC). Siblings may share no haplotypes by descent with the index case (e.g., genotype BD), or one haplotype (e.g., AD or BC), or two (e.g., AC). In the absence of linkage between the unknown susceptibility locus and the marker locus, the expected distribution of these haplotypes shared by descent among siblings is 25%, 50%, and 25%, respectively. Tests for deviations from these Mendelian expectations can be easily incorporated into epidemiologic studies of sibships in either a case-control or cohort design (see section 9.5).

Penrose (1935) considered only discrete phenotypes and independent pairs of sibs in his original approach, but later extended this to quantitative traits

Table 9–5. Layout of sib-pair data for Penrose's test for linkage between two markers

		Marker phenotype 2 in sib pair		
		$+\,+$	$+\,-$	$-\,-$
Marker phenotype 1	$+\,+$	n_{11}	n_{12}	n_{13}	$n_{1.}$
in sib pair	$+\,-$	n_{21}	n_{22}	n_{23}	$n_{2.}$
	$-\,-$	n_{31}	n_{32}	n_{33}	$n_{3.}$
		$n_{.1}$	$n_{.2}$	$n_{.3}$	N

If the null hypothesis of no linkage is true, the expected cell size is simply a product of the marginal probabilities, i.e., $e_{ij} = n_{i.} \, n_{.j}$. While a standard chi-square test for independence can be used to test for association between two markers, it ignores the specific predictions of genetic linkage for full sibs. In particular, if there were genetic linkage, one should see higher than expected values in the four corner cells and in the center cell, and correspondingly smaller than expected values in the remaining cells (where there is discordance for either marker alleles between the sibs).

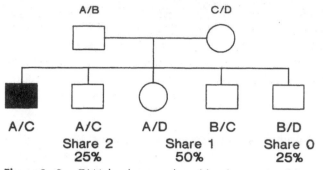

Figure 9–9. DNA haplotypes shared by descent in siblings of affected individuals.

(Penrose, 1938). Later, Haseman and Elston (1972) showed how regressing the squared within-pair difference for a quantitative phenotype on the number of marker alleles shared *ibd* by two sibs (which provides an estimator for the number of *ibd* alleles at the trait locus) can serve to identify linkage between the marker and a major locus controlling a quantitative phenotype. Other types of biologic relatives can be considered in this approach by merely specifying the probability of their sharing 0, 1, or 2 alleles *ibd* at the marker locus (see Table 9–6), but full sibs are the most readily available relationship with nonzero probabilities for all three combinations of shared alleles (Elston, 1990).

This regression of the squared within-pair difference on the number of alleles shared *ibd* can serve as a useful screening tool to quickly identify markers likely to be linked to a locus exerting a major effect on a quantitative trait (Elston, 1988). Amos and associates (1990) extended this approach to include multiple quantitative traits. The null hypothesis is that the slope of these squared within-pair differences is zero (compared to the alternative hypothesis under linkage that this slope is negative, that is, the difference within pairs declines as the number of *ibd* marker alleles increases). Black-welder and Elston (1982) have shown this approach to have acceptable power for situations of tight linkage and high heritability at the locus controlling the quantitative trait. Although the statistical power of later sib-pair statistics is

Table 9–6. Probabilities that a pair of relatives share 0, 1, or 2 alleles identical by descent (*ibd*) at an autosomal locus

Type of relative pair	Probability of sharing *ibd* alleles		
	0	*1*	*2*
Monozygotic twins	0	0	1
Full sibs	1/4	1/2	1/4
Parent-offspring	0	1	0
First cousins	3/4	1/4	0
Double first cousins	13/16	1/8	1/16
Grandparent-Grandchild*	1/2	1/2	0

* Also half-sibs and avuncular pairs (aunt/uncle–niece/nephew pairs).

much better than Penrose's original one, large sample sizes are nonetheless required to detect even tight linkage (see Table 9–7). Furthermore, statistical power drops precipitously in the presence of recombination.

9.4.2 Methods Based on Pairs of Affected Relatives

A variation on the sib-pair method is to consider only pairs of affected sibs in a test for linkage between a marker locus and a disease locus (Penrose, 1953). There are several advantages to limiting the sampling design to affected relatives. First, if an extensive search of a large array of markers is to be done, it may be extremely important to minimize the number of individuals to be typed to hold down costs. Second, limiting sampling to individuals already known to be affected minimizes errors of misclassification (i.e., it eliminates false negatives). This is particularly critical in diseases with an age-dependent onset or reduced penetrance because there may be a substantial number of sibs who carry the disease gene but have not yet expressed it. Third, by focusing on multiplex families (i.e., where more than one relative is affected), the chances of including nongenetic cases of the disease (phenocopies) are reduced. These advantages may overcome some of the statistical disadvantages of this approach, especially considering these methods *do not* require prior specification of the model of inheritance for the disease. Thus, methods of linkage analysis based on pairs of affected relatives can be used to define the role of genetic factors in disease. This opportunity has led to increased interest in using DNA polymorphisms to identify genetic forms of common diseases.

The affected sib-pair method can be applied most successfully in situations where the marker locus is extremely polymorphic, where it is possible to count directly the number of alleles shared *ibd* in pairs of affected sibs (this still requires typing the parents or other sibs, although the analysis itself is done only on affected sibs). If the marker locus is completely independent of the disease locus, sampling only pairs of affected sibs will not alter the probabilities for sharing *ibd* marker alleles (i.e., they remain .25, .50, .25 for

Table 9–7. Approximate number of sib pairs required for 80% power at the 5% significance level to detect linkage between a codominant genetic marker (with two equally frequent alleles) and a single locus controlling a quantitative trait (allele frequency $P = .5$) with varying levels of heritability

Major locus heritability (σ^2_{MG}/σ^2)	Strictly codominant locus $(\mu_{AB} = (\mu_{AA} + \mu_{BB})/2)$	Complete dominance $(\mu_{AA} = \mu_{AB} > \mu_{BB})$
.2	5343	5561
.4	1066	1191
.6	371	464
.8	161	238
.9	112	184

Adapted from Blackwelder and Elston (1982).

sharing 0, 1, and 2 alleles *ibd*). If, on the other hand, the marker locus is linked to the disease locus, there should be an excess of sibs sharing two marker alleles *ibd* in any sample of affected sibs, and a corresponding deficiency of sibs sharing no alleles *ibd* at the marker locus. A number of statistics have been developed to test for such deviations from expected values (Suarez and Van Eerdewegh, 1984; Blackwelder and Elston, 1985; Thomson, 1986). Statistical power depends partially on the model of inheritance and the prevalence of the disease, but in situations of tight linkage and high relative risk among those carrying the disease genotype(s), the affected sib-pair approach offers an attractive sampling design. It should be remembered that some useful information can be obtained from unaffected sibs in the same family, however, and it is often worthwhile to sample parents and all full sibs (affected or not). Risch (1990c) pointed out that incorporating information on other family members increases the power of affected-pair methods greatly.

Recently, the "affected pairs" design has been expanded to consider all possible types of biologic relatives. Weeks and Lange (1988) relied on identity by state (*ibs*) relationships, where two individuals carry the same allele (but they may not be copies of a common ancestral allele), to test for association between marker alleles and disease status. Several factors influence the statistical power of these methods, including the type of relative pairs used, the polymorphism of the marker, the probability of *ibd* at the trait locus for a particular type of relative, and the recombination between the marker locus and the disease locus (Bishop and Williamson, 1990). Unfortunately, these factors interact in a manner that precludes establishing simple guidelines for designing family studies. For example, if a recessive disease shows incomplete penetrance, affected sib pairs are the most informative sampling design. Also, for dominant diseases with incomplete penetrance, full sibs are the relationship of choice whenever the disease gene frequency is low. On the other hand, for a simple dominant disease with complete penetrance, other types of relative pairs (e.g., grandparent-grandchild) may actually carry more information than do full sibs. Among all second-degree relatives, grandparent-grandchild pairs are frequently far more informative than half-sibs or avuncular pairs (i.e., uncle/aunt and niece/nephew pairs). Occasionally, pairs of distant relatives may be more informative than first- or second-degree relatives, but this occurs only when the allele frequency is very low and there is tight linkage. In general, the power of these affected-pair methods drops precipitously even with modest rates of recombination (Bishop and Williamson, 1990), although the grandparent-grandchild pairs are less affected by recombination than other types of relatives (Risch, 1990c).

9.5 INCORPORATING THE LINKAGE APPROACH INTO EPIDEMIOLOGIC STUDIES

An increasing number of genetic markers has become available in recent years and more will be forthcoming as techniques of molecular biology continue to improve. The amount of polymorphism in the human genome appears greater than previously detectable by examining gene products alone. The increasing number of "anonymous" DNA markers scattered throughout the genome should soon permit development of a complete linkage map of the human genome. This information will, in turn, permit mapping susceptibility loci without prior knowledge of either the function of these susceptibility genes or their products. A "fishing expedition" of this type is similar in principle to the one used by epidemiologists in many case-control studies. Here a large array of genetic markers is examined with the hope that one or more will be tightly linked to a disease susceptibility locus.

9.5.1 Study Designs

Genetic markers can be incorporated into epidemiologic studies of disease etiology, although one must recognize the limitations on using such information. Typically, family study designs are based on evaluation of disease recurrence in relatives of affected individuals (index cases or probands). Ideally, such family studies should be based on complete ascertainment of incident disease cases in population-based registries (Dorman et al., 1988). At a minimum the standards for case definition, the method for ascertainment, and criteria for determining if cases are representative should be specified. Although the study of single large pedigrees with multiple affected members provides the most information for linkage analysis, such families may not be representative of the universe of cases and, therefore, permit only limited inferences about disease in the general population. While simplex families may be far more common, the need for multiplex families necessitates conducting almost all linkage studies on selected subgroups of families.

As discussed in Chapter 5, an epidemiologic study of recurrence among siblings of probands may be viewed either as a cohort study or a case-control study (Table 9–8). Under either design, the null hypothesis of no linkage predicts equal risks when sibs are stratified by the number of haplotypes shared *ibd* with the proband. This approach requires testing all siblings of

Table 9–8. Testing for susceptibility locus using full sibs of affected proband

| Haplotypes shared *ibd* | Case-control design* (affected sib-pair method) | | | Cohort design | |
	*Proportion of affected sibs**	*Expected proportion under H_0*	*Odds ratio*	*Recurrence risk*	*Relative risk*
0	P_0	.25	1	I_0	1
1	P_1	.50	$P_1/2P_0$	I_1	I_1/I_0
2	P_2	.25	P_2/P_0	II_2	I_2/I_0

ibd, identical by descent.

The number of haplotypes shared by descent can be used to stratify sibs for analysis as a cohort or case-control design. If the observed proportion of affected sibs is compared to its expected proportion, the case-control design becomes the affected sib-pair method.

* If no controls are used, and the test is based on expected proportion, the case-control design becomes the affected sib-pair test.

affected cases. Under this case-control strategy, affected sibs of the proband may be viewed as *cases*, while a sample of unaffected siblings could serve as *controls*. The number of haplotypes shared *ibd* with the proband serves as the exposure variable for comparing "case" and "control" sibs. However, the control group is technically unnecessary, since the theoretical distribution is known explicitly (unless there is differential survival of individuals with different haplotypes). Without the sib control group, this design becomes the classic affected sib-pair method. In either situation, the odds ratios obtained by comparing the odds of sharing one and two versus no haplotypes among cases with their theoretical expectation can measure relative risk.

As also shown in Table 9–8, a cohort approach can be used to evaluate whether the risks of disease in sibs sharing one or two haplotypes *ibd* with the proband is increased compared with the risk of disease in siblings sharing no haplotypes *ibd* with the proband. Relative risks for the "share1" and "share2" groups can be statistically evaluated for departure from unity. This approach was used by Cavender and colleagues (1984) to show the increased risk to IDDM among sibs of cases sharing HLA haplotypes.

9.5.2 Genotype-Environment Interaction and Linked Genetic Markers

When the presence of disease requires some interaction between genetic and environmental factors, relative risk values associated with the susceptibility genotype tend to be diluted toward unity by the proportion of susceptible individuals who are *not* exposed to the environmental factor. Therefore, it is important to provide information about environmental factors relevant to a disease in studies, including genetic markers. Under the cohort approach, sibling recurrence risks stratified by the number of haplotypes shared with the index case can also be stratified by other risk factors of interest. Evidence of interaction between the exposure and the number of haplotypes shared can then be examined.

Similarly, in the affected sib-pair method, environmental exposures thought to play a role in disease etiology should be measured whenever possible. In the presence of interaction between the susceptibility genotype and an environmental factor, haplotype analysis of affected sib pairs, where both members are exposed to the putative environmental factor, may be more revealing than the analysis of all pairs combined. This is illustrated in the hypothetical example given in Table 9–9. The distribution of the numbers of haplotypes shared *ibd* is compared between all affected sib pairs and those sib pairs concordant for exposure. Here, the underlying assumption is that the excess disease risk is seen only in the presence of *both* the susceptible genotype and exposure (Khoury et al, 1990). In this simple example, a fixed exposure frequency of 5% is assumed for the population, and no familial clustering of the exposure is considered. It can be seen that more noticeable departures from the theoretical distribution are obtained by limiting the analysis to affected sib pairs concordant for exposure.

Table 9–9. Distribution among affected sib pairs of number of haplotypes shared *ibd* for a genetic marker tightly linked with the susceptibility trait where an environmental factor is also required

Allele frequency	No. of haplotypes shared by descent	Autosomal dominant		Autosomal recessive	
		All affected sib pairs (exposure 5%)	*Affected sib pairs with exposure*	*All affected sib pairs (exposure 5%)*	*Affected sib pairs with exposure*
.01	0	.21	.02	.25	.20
	1	.50	.50	.50	.41
	2	.29	.48	.25	.39
.05	0	.17	.05	.25	.05
	1	.50	.49	.50	.16
	2	.33	.45	.25	.79
.10	0	.17	.09	.23	.03
	1	.50	.49	.48	.20
	2	.34	.42	.29	.77
.25	0	.20	.16	.19	.05
	1	.49	.49	.45	.33
	2	.31	.35	.36	.62
.40	0	.22	.20	.18	.09
	1	.49	.49	.46	.41
	2	.29	.31	.36	.50

Assumptions: Relative risk associated with susceptibility genotype = 100; no familial clustering of exposure and disease frequency = .001

Adapted from Khoury et al. (1990).

9.5.3 Illustration of the Linkage Approach for Known Genetic Trait-Disease Associations

The use of linked genetic markers is illustrated with three examples of marker-disease associations discussed in Khoury and colleagues (1990) (Table 9–10). In these examples it is assumed that the associations are truly causal in nature. For a marker locus tightly linked with the susceptibility locus (i.e., no recombination), values of sibling recurrence risks were computed over the three strata (i.e., 0, 1, or 2 haplotypes shared *ibd* with the proband), as well as computing the haplotype distribution expected between pairs of affected sibs. A further assumption was made here that genetic susceptibility is the sole reason for all familial aggregation in these diseases. Note that this last assumption may not be realistic.

For ankylosing spondylitis and the *HLA-B27* allele, very high relative risks (about 100) and attributable fraction (close to 90%) are seen. In this example, a 10-fold gradient in recurrence risk is observed over the strata of shared haplotypes (0 to 2), and there is a marked departure from the .25, .50, .25 haplotype distribution among affected sib pairs. In the case of chronic obstructive pulmonary disease, in spite of the relatively strong association with the homozygous *PiZ* genotype (relative risk of 20), this particular genetic trait accounts for very little of the disease in the population (attributable fraction less than 1%). Therefore, the addition of a linked marker can hardly

Table 9–10. Illustration of the use of hypothetical tightly linked genetic markers in the case of reported genetic trait disease associations

	Disease		
	Ankylosing spondylitis	*Chronic obstructive pulmonary disease*	*Bladder cancer*
Disease risk	0.002	0.05	0.019
Marker allele	HLA-B27	α_1-Antitrypsin deficiency	Slow acetylator phenotype
Type of trait	Autosomal Dominant	Autosomal Recessive	Autosomal Recessive
Allele frequency	.036	.02	.75
Genotype relative risk	100	20	1.6
Attributable fraction (%)	87.5	0.8	25.2
	Sibling recurrence risks		
No. of haplotypes shared *ibd*			
0	0.002	0.0501	0.0190
1	0.012	0.0501	0.0194
2	0.022	0.0571	0.0199
	Expected distribution among affected sib pairs		
0	.04	.24	.24
1	.50	.48	.50
2	.46	.28	.26

Adapted from Khoury et al. (1990).

be expected to identify differences in recurrence risks or in the distribution of shared haplotypes among affected sib pairs. The same can be said about bladder cancer and the slow acetylator phenotype. Here, the relative risk is small (1.6), and examining the haplotype distribution in affected sib pairs is unlikely to be rewarding. The analysis might be more revealing, however, if affected sib pairs were stratified into those concordant and discordant for the suspected environmental exposure (e.g., occupational exposures).

9.6 CONCLUDING REMARKS

In summary, technical advances are providing more opportunities to incorporate genetic markers into etiologic studies. Linkage analysis holds potential for identifying the genetic contributions to common diseases, but the intrinsic limitations of traditional linkage studies must be recognized. Both association and linkage approaches can be used to search for disease-susceptibility genes in the broader context of epidemiologic studies. These approaches are clearly complementary, and each has its own strengths and limitations. When considering genetic markers, epidemiologists can evaluate the role of specific candidate genes (measured through either a gene product or a DNA marker) in disease etiology in terms of both relative and attributable risks. This approach will not detect all possible mutations involving such susceptibility genes, although its utility is expected to increase as marker resolution improves. While in principle, genetic markers can be treated as conventional risk factors, there are definite limitations on the interpretation of any observed associations between a genetic marker and disease, imposed by problems of confounding, a high rate of type 1 errors, linkage disequilibrium, and etiologic heterogeneity. Linkage analysis can be used to search for markers tightly linked to disease susceptibility genes in population-based epidemiologic studies of familial recurrence. These can, in turn, lead to better identification of genetic mechanisms, and offer the opportunity for intervention through genetic counseling. Finally, when dealing with diseases of complex etiology where both environmental and genetic factors contribute to pathogenesis, it is important to recognize that inclusion of specific environmental exposures can enhance the ability to detect disease-susceptibility genes.

10

Applications of Genetic Epidemiology in Medicine and Public Health

10.1 INTRODUCTION

Throughout this book the approaches of genetic epidemiology have been discussed in terms of the contributions of the individual disciplines of genetics and epidemiology. Both population and family studies seek to identify the role of genetic factors in disease etiology and pathogenesis, and to quantify the impact of genetic factors along with environmental factors on disease distribution in human populations. This chapter is concerned with the applications of genetic epidemiology in medicine and public health, including the evaluation of diagnostic tests, disease heterogeneity, disease natural history, therapeutic efficacy, and safety, as well as disease prevention in families and populations, and in public health surveillance. With continuing advances in DNA technology, ethical considerations will assume an increasingly significant role in applications of genetic epidemiology in human populations. Because of the current burgeoning of knowledge in this area, only an introduction to these complex topics can be presented here. The reader is encouraged to consult other sources (e.g., Emery and Rimoin, 1983; Holland et al., 1984; Lappe, 1986; Last, 1986; Murray, 1986; Porter, 1986; Vogel and Motulsky, 1986; Weiss, 1986; Gordis, 1988c; Holtzman, 1989; Suzuki and Knudston, 1989).

10.2 APPLICATIONS OF GENETIC EPIDEMIOLOGY IN CLINICAL MEDICINE

Although individually rare, classical Mendelian disorders contribute significantly to pediatric morbidity and mortality. A number of studies have found that a significant proportion (4% to 7%) of pediatric hospital admissions are due to recognized Mendelian diseases, and another 0.4% to 0.7% due to chromosomal abnormalities. Patients with genetic diseases tend to have a larger number of hospital admissions compared to either the total pediatric population or to patients with nongenetic diseases. Furthermore, the families of pediatric patients with genetic disorders have to shoulder more of the actual cost of health care than does the average family (Hall et al., 1978).

One study reviewed the scientific literature on a sample of 351 randomly selected Mendelian diseases to provide an estimate of the "average" effects of a genetic disease (Costa et al., 1985). From this survey, a general picture of the overall impact of genetic disease clearly shows that Mendelian diseases are life-threatening and result in significant handicaps. Genetic diseases represent a significant burden on the health-care system largely because they are relatively intractable and largely not amenable to simple cures or treatment.

Hayes and colleagues (1985) took these same Mendelian diseases and developed a pre- and posttreatment score for the affected phenotype, considering seven different areas of "health" (life span, reproductive capacity, somatic growth, intellectual development, learning ability, work ability, and cosmetic impairment). A total score was computed by summing these seven individual measures for the untreated phenotype and for the treated phenotype based on *reported* successes in the literature. These observations on response to treatment are historical in nature, highly selected, and tend to overstate the impact of the treatment. Even focusing on a set of metabolic genetic diseases where the gene product was known and where the treatment should be most effective, 70% of these genetic diseases showed no change in life span or reproductive capability in response to treatment, 80% showed no change in intellectual development, and 65% to 76% showed no change in measure of social adaptation in response to treatment. Of the selected 65 metabolic diseases, 8 could be completely cured (however, some of these diseases had a relatively mild "affected" phenotype), treatment had some effect in 26 diseases, and treatment had no demonstrable effect in 31 diseases. In general, success was more likely when the treatment consisted of delivery of a normal gene product (e.g., factor VIII in hemophilia A) or by environmental manipulation to restore physiologic homeostasis (e.g., restriction of phenylalanine restores a normal physiologic state to homozygotes affected with PKU). In general, treatment was ineffective when the deviant gene product was intracellular in location, was expressed prenatally, or conferred a complex cascade of metabolic and cellular effects. The outcome of treatment is likely to be poor for genetic mutations affecting metabolic systems, such as glycolysis or energy metabolism, and for genetic diseases affecting development. For the majority of genetic diseases, there is still no effective treatment.

The new genetic techniques are finding increasing applications not only in the classical single-gene disorders, but for a variety of common diseases such as cancer and coronary heart disease. With most diseases involving genetic components, it is becoming feasible to describe patients not only in terms of "classical" or typical "cases" (Childs et al., 1988), but to improve diagnostic specificity by using DNA techniques. For example, with the recent identification of the cystic fibrosis (CF) gene, it became possible to identify the distinct mutations responsible for this disease. It turns out, however, that the most common mutation accounts for about 75% of CF chromosomes, while numerous other "private" mutations may be involved (Riordan et al., 1989; Rommens et al., 1989; Lemma et al., 1990). Thus, even with this relatively homogeneous Mendelian disorder, it is a major challenge to identify the molecular alterations leading to the disorder, to correlate molecular variation with phenotypic variability, and to implement effective population screening and prevention programs. The challenge is even greater for common disorders that undoubtedly manifest etiologic heterogeneity, involve several genetic loci, and/or incomplete penetrance for any particular gene (Childs et al., 1988; Holtzman, 1989).

Methods of genetic epidemiology provide medical researchers with the tools to evaluate (1) screening and diagnostic tests, (2) disease heterogeneity, (3) disease natural history, and (4) therapeutic efficacy and safety.

10.2.1. Screening and Diagnostic Tests

The quantitative evaluation of laboratory tests for measuring genetic traits was considered in Chapter 4. The validity of tests (sensitivity and specificity) was discussed with respect to correct classification of the underlying genotypes and the impact of misclassification errors on epidemiologic studies of genetic traits. These approaches are useful in assessing the role of specific genetic factors in disease outcomes. In particular, one is interested in the clinical and screening usefulness of data on genetic traits and other risk factors with respect to accurate prediction of specific diseases in individuals (Khoury et al., 1985b; Baron, 1989). One might question the usefulness of family history in making a diagnosis of a specific genetic form of the disease (e.g., family history of coronary heart disease in relation to familial hypercholesterolemia). Information considered for differential diagnosis, clinical judgement, or screening programs (see below) usually includes clinical data, such as age at onset, severity of the disease, and clinical manifestations, as well as laboratory data. It is important to distinguish between the use of genetic testing for diagnostic purposes (where the individual is already clinically affected) versus predictive purposes (where the individual has no clinical manifestation at the time of testing but is at some risk of developing disease related to family history or other risk factors. For example, linked DNA markers can be used to predict the presence of Huntington's disease in offspring of affected individuals long before the development of clinical signs and symptoms (Gusella et al., 1983; Hayden et al., 1988; Brandt et al., 1989; Bloch and Hayden, 1990). Also, DNA testing can be used in the differential diagnosis of a disease once some clinical manifestations became apparent.

Whether genetic testing is carried out for prediction, diagnostic, or screening purposes, quantitative evaluation of such testing can be done in terms of sensitivity, specificity, and predictive values defined with respect to the occurrence of disease (rather than the underlying genotype as in Chapter 4).

Here, sensitivity refers to the proportion of individuals with the trait among those who will develop the disease; specificity refers to the proportion of individuals without the trait among those who will not develop the disease; positive predictive value (PPV) refers to the proportion of individuals who develop the disease among those who have the trait. These parameters depend on the frequency of the genetic trait in the population (g), the lifetime risk of disease (p), as well as the epidemiologic relationship between the genetic trait and the disease (presented in terms of relative risk R). The relationships of sensitivity, specificity, and PPV with p, g, and R can be derived (Khoury et al., 1985b) as shown in Table 10–1.

It has been indicated that many risk factors identified in epidemiologic studies are of limited usefulness for clinical prediction, even with high relative risks (Baron, 1989; Khoury et al., 1985b). To illustrate, refer to Table 10–2, where Newill and colleagues (1986) use the example of three genetic markers (PiZ homozygosity, ABH nonsecretor status, and blood group A antigen) in the clinical prediction of chronic obstructive pulmonary disease. These three markers have been shown to be risk factors for COPD, and the assumption made here is that their association with COPD is causal and not due to confounding, chance, or population stratification. As can be seen with mark-

Table 10–1. Relationship of sensitivity, specificity, and positive predictive value of a genetic trait to the frequencies of disease and the trait, and relative risk

Genetic trait	Will develop disease	Will not develop disease	Total
Present	bp	$(1 - a)(1 - p)$	g
Absent	$(1 - b)p$	$a(1 - p)$	$1 - g$
Total	p	$(1 - p)$	1

Sensitivity: $b = \dfrac{Rg}{1 + g(R - 1)}$

Specificity: $a = 1 - g\,\dfrac{1 - (Rp)/[1 + g(R - 1)]}{1 - p}$

Positive predictive value: $PPV = \dfrac{Rp}{1 + g(R - 1)}$

where g = the frequency of the genetic trait
  p = the frequency of the disease
  R = relative risk relating genetic trait to disease

Adapted from Khoury et al. (1985b).

Table 10–2. Sensitivity, specificity, and positive predictive value (PPV) of three genetic traits for chronic obstructive pulmonary disease (COPD)*

Genetic marker	Marker frequency	Relative risk	Sensitivity (%)	Specificity (%)	PPV (%)
PiZ homozysity	.0005	20	1.0	99.99	99.1
ABH nonsecretors	.25	1.5	33.3	75.4	6.7
Blood group A antigen	.45 (whites)	1.3	51.5	55.3	5.7

* The expected lifetime risk of COPD is assumed to be 5%.

Adapted from Newill et al. (1986).

ers such as PiZ homozygosity that are rarer than the disease, sensitivity is very low, even though relative risks and PPV may be high. This reflects etiologic heterogeneity of COPD and the relatively small contribution of PiZ to the total disease prevalence. On the other hand, for markers that are more frequent than the disease (such as blood group A antigen), while sensitivity of the test may be higher, PPV will always be low. This is true even in the presence of high relative risks (Khoury et al., 1985b).

10.2.2. Disease Heterogeneity

Heterogeneity of disease is a fundamental concept in genetics as well as in epidemiology. As indicated by Childs and Motulsky (1988): "We sometimes forget that diseases have no intrinsic being; that their names represent only convenient rubrics, classes that have logistic uses but no precise conceptual content, particularly as to cause." Even in single-gene diseases with well-defined mutations, such as phenylketonuria, heterogeneity at the molecular level has been documented. The presence of several genetic mutations either within the same locus or involving different loci and/or environmental factors producing phenotypically similar clinical presentations has been termed etiologic heterogeneity. With the more common disorders, such as psychiatric disease and coronary heart disease, heterogeneity of disease can be seen at the clinical, pathophysiologic, and molecular levels. To approach disease heterogeneity, cases of disease can be classified into subgroups that appear homogeneous in regard to clinical, pathologic, biochemical, or molecular characteristics, with the eventual goal of identifying sufficient causes underlying each subgroup. Clinically, several disease characteristics can be used to distinguish subgroups of cases, including age at onset, signs and symptoms, progression of disease, natural history of complications, response to therapy, radiologic findings, and other laboratory tests. Once subgroups of a particular disease or condition have been identified, investigators can attempt to determine whether these groups differ with respect to their descriptive epidemiologic characteristics (in time, place, and persons), associations with exposures, and familial patterns of recurrence, and eventually characterize susceptibility genes along with environmental determinants.

Consider the example of neural tube defects (NTD). Clinically, about 20% of affected infants appear to have one or more serious defects unrelated to the presence of the neural tube defect. Some of these cases have been associated with Mendelian syndromes and chromosomal abnormalities (Holmes et al., 1976; Khoury et al., 1982a), but most have no underlying known etiology. Because of the clinical suspicion that the disease process in infants with isolated NTDs might be different from that of NTDs with other defects, epidemiologic and genetic analyses were performed to compare these subgroups. In fact, as shown in Table 10–3, the two groups do have different patterns of occurrence by race, gender, ethnicity, geographic variation, secular trends, and familial recurrence risks. This strongly indicates underlying etiologic heterogeneity among these subgroups. Although the basic defects have not been identified for either group, it is highly likely that further

Table 10–3. Heterogeneity of neural tube defects according to the presence or absence of other defects

Characteristic	Type of neural tube defect	
	Isolated	*Associated with other defects*
Race/ethnicity	Rates higher in whites than blacks	Rates similar for whites and blacks
Gender	Rates higher in females than males	Rates similar for males and females
Geographic variation	Rates in the U.S. higher in the east than the west	Rates similar in east and west
Secular trends	Rates declining over time	Rates relatively stable over time
Sibling recurrence risks	1%–2%	0%

Adapted from Khoury et al. (1982a, 1982b) and Holmes (1976).

heterogeneity can be expected within these subgroups. In the isolated group, heterogeneity may be related to the type of the NTD (anencephaly, spina bifida), level of lesion (cervical, thoracic, and lumbosacral), type of lesion (open/closed), and so on. On the other hand, NTDs with associated defects may also be a mixed group that can be further characterized, based on the types of associated defects.

10.2.3. Disease Natural History

Natural history has been broadly defined as the consequences of a disorder, an account of the sequence of events, onset of the manifestation and the complications. Hall (1988a) has suggested that the evaluation of natural history is important in five areas in medical genetics. Although these areas are primarily viewed in the context of Mendelian disorders and congenital anomaly syndromes, they can be applied to all diseases in general. They include the following:

1. *Diagnosis*: For many conditions, clinical manifestations change with age. Natural history can be important to make an accurate diagnosis of a disease.
2. *Heterogeneity and expression of disease*: Differences in natural history and rate of complications can provide important clues to underlying differences in basic defects.
3. *Definition of the basic defect*: The evaluation of the course of disease often provides clues to underlying mechanisms of pathophysiology and can help in directing the search for the basic defect.
4. *Management*: The study of natural history of disease permits better recognition, prediction, and clues to intervention strategies, as well as the prevention of complications that may occur during the course of the illness.

5. *Genetic counseling*: Knowledge of risks regarding the course of a disease allows more accurate genetic counseling for both patients and their families.

The evaluation of natural history can be approached by using classical epidemiologic study designs (Weiss, 1986). Both cohort and case-control studies can be performed (Table 10–4). Here, the disease itself becomes the risk factor of interest. The outcome can be any complication or event occurring during the course of illness ranging from mild sequelae to death. In a cohort study, the clinical outcome of interest is measured among persons with the disease and compared with controls. Incidence and cumulative incidence measures can be used, as well as measures of association (relative risks, risk differences, and odds ratios) between the disease and the outcome. On the other hand, case-control studies start with "cases" being persons with the outcome of interest and "controls" being persons without the outcome. The frequency of antecedent disease is then compared between cases and controls and measures of association calculated (odds ratios and attributable fraction). As in any observational study, possibilities of bias have to be considered in the design, analysis, and interpretation of these studies (Weiss, 1986).

For example, the relationship between trisomy 21 and childhood leukemia has been well documented (Miller, 1968, 1969). Children with trisomy 21 are at a greatly increased risk of developing leukemia during childhood. To quantitate this relationship in a cohort study, one would have to follow up a group of trisomy 21 newborns throughout childhood (up to a certain age) and a comparable group of healthy infants and compare the incidence of leukemia between the two groups. Like any cohort study, such studies are costly and involve follow-up of large samples. One alternative to this type of study is to link data from existing population-based birth defects and cancer registries in relatively stable populations. For example, Mili and colleagues (1992) recently identified records of 532 infants with trisomy 21 from the Metropolitan Atlanta Congenital Defects Program and linked these records with the SEER cancer registry in the same population (Table 10–5). Of the Down syndrome cases, three were found to have developed leukemia by age 15. The cumulative incidence of leukemia in Down syndrome by age 15 years was found to be .95% which is about 26 times the background cumulative incidence of leukemia for children born in this same population. The assumption here, of course, is that follow-up was available on all infants with Down syndrome (which is almost certainly incomplete, leading to an underestimate of the magnitudes of absolute and relative risks). Measures of ab-

Table 10–4. Epidemiologic study designs for assessing natural history

Group	N	Cohort study outcome frequency	Case-control study	
			Persons with outcome	*Persons without outcome*
With disease	N_1	f_1	a	b
Without disease	N_2	f_2	c	d

Table 10–5. A cohort study of Down syndrome and childhood leukemia by age 15 yrs

Group	N	Cohort study		
		Number with leukemia	Cumulative incidence	Relative risk
Down syndrome	532	3	.95%	26.2
Livebirths	544,304	116	.04%	1.0

Adapted from Mili et al. (1992).

solute risk from this type of study can be used in counseling families regarding the risk of leukemia in a Down syndrome child.

On the other hand, a case-control study of childhood leukemia can be conducted by using population-based cancer registries. The exposure of interest, the presence of Down syndrome in a child diagnosed with leukemia can be compared with the frequency of Down syndrome in a population of children without leukemia. The measure of odds ratio obtained here closely approximates that of relative risk in a cohort study. Also, this type of study can measure the proportion of childhood leukemia that are attributable to trisomy 21.

Both cohort and case-control designs can incorporate the impact of measured cofactors (genetic or environmental) on the natural history of disease. The general outline for such an analysis is shown in Table 10–6. Essentially, the analysis shown in Table 10–4 is now stratified by the presence or absence of a single cofactor (e.g., a genetic marker or an exposure to an environmental factor). Measures of dose and other covariates, as well as assessment of interaction between the disease and the cofactor can also be incorporated in the analyses (Chapters 4 and 5). In the example of Down syndrome and leukemia stated earlier, cofactors that may interact with the trisomy 21 genotype in leading to leukemia may include radiation exposures, viral infections, blood group antigens, and racial/ethnic groups. Finally, outcomes need not be categorical in nature (condition absent/present) but may be polychotomous or continuous.

Like all observational studies, epidemiologic studies of natural history are subject to potential biases and limitations including recall bias, confounding,

Table 10–6. Epidemiologic study designs for assessing natural history in relation to the impact of a cofactor

Group	Cofactor	N	Cohort study frequency of outcome	Case-control study	
				Persons with outcome	Persons without outcome
With disease	Present	N_{11}	f_{11}	a_1	b_1
	Absent	N_{12}	f_{12}	a_2	b_2
Without disease	Present	N_{21}	f_{21}	c_1	d_1
	Absent	N_{22}	f_{22}	c_2	d_2

misclassification and selection. The association between a disease and an outcome may well be due to hidden confounding effects especially if groups are not comparable with respect to other risk factors of interest. For the leukemia-Down syndrome association, if one assumes, for the sake of the argument, that advanced maternal age per se is a risk factor for childhood leukemia, then the relationship between Down syndrome and leukemia could be confounded by the maternal age-leukemia association, since advanced maternal age may be also associated with the risk of Down syndrome. Thus, stratification and adjustment for maternal age may be important in these analyses.

Selection bias is another potential limitation in studies that assess clinical outcomes in relation to the presence or absence of a given condition. This is particularly relevant in hospital-based studies (the so-called Berksonian bias, Lilienfeld and Lilienfeld, 1980). Consider again the example of the Down syndrome-leukemia association in a hypothetical situation (Table 10–7). In a population-based study where all children with Down syndrome and leukemia are ascertained in a hypothetical population of 100,000 children followed from birth, it is assumed that the risk of Down syndrome is 1/1000, the risk of leukemia is 1/1000, and the risk of leukemia in Down syndrome is 2%. This leads to an odds ratio of 20.8 relating leukemia with Down syndrome (Table 10–7). On the other hand, if one conducts a hospital-based case-control study where the sample includes all hospitalized children, it is assumed that

1. all children with Down syndrome and/or childhood leukemia are hospitalized, and
2. only 4.8% of children without Down syndrome or leukemia are hospitalized.

Table 10–7. Hypothetical example of selection bias in the study of Down syndrome-leukemia association using hospital-based case-control studies

Down syndrome	Childhood leukemia		
	Yes	*No*	*Total*
Population			
Yes	2	98	100
No	98	99,802	99,900
Total	100	99,900	100,000
Hospital study			
Yes	2	98	100
No	98	4,802	4,900
Total	100	4,900	5,000

Odds ratio in a population-based case-control study is $[2 \times 99{,}802]/[98 \times 98] = 20.8$.

Under the severe assumptions that the hospitalization proportion of children with Down syndrome and/or childhood leukemia is 100%, while the hospitalization proportion of children without leukemia or Down syndrome is 4802/99,802 or 4.8%, the resulting odds ratio relating Down syndrome and leukemia is $[2 \times 4802]/[98 \times 98] = 1.0$.

In this situation, the resulting odds ratio relating leukemia and Down's syndrome is 1.0. This extreme example of Berksonian bias occurs because of different sampling fractions of individuals in the study design. The study of natural history is also a powerful tool to evaluate the heterogeneity of disease. If subgroups of a disease based on the presence or absence of clinical, genetic, epidemiologic, or laboratory characteristics have different natural histories (e.g., presence or absence of certain complications), this may point to underlying biologic mechanisms. Again, epidemiologic methods can be useful. Table 10–8 illustrates the extension of study designs of natural history for a hypothetical disease where two subgroups can be identified. In this situation, two subgroups of the disease are compared with each other as well as with a suitable control group with respect to the outcomes of interest. In the example of Down syndrome-leukemia association, it may be important to separate cases of trisomy 21 by the parental origin and the meiotic stage of the nondisjunction event. If the risk of leukemia is found to be increased in one subgroup of cases but not another, it may point to underlying molecular mechanisms leading to carcinogenesis in trisomies (e.g., imprinting).

10.2.4. Therapeutic Efficacy and Safety

Therapeutic interventions include drugs, medical devices, surgical operations, radiologic procedures, and behavior modification. Assessing their effects on individual patients requires the incorporation of knowledge of genetic variation in response into observational studies and clinical trials (Meinert, 1986; Weiss, 1986). While differential genetic susceptibility to both efficacy and safety of drugs has been long recognized (pharmacogenetics), this has received little, if any, attention in standard clinical trials. Several examples of recognized pharmacogenetic traits in relation to drug response or toxicity are shown in Table 10–9. More recently, epidemiologic methods are being applied in the evaluation of pharmacologic agents. The discipline of pharmacoepidemiology, which has grown at the interface of epidemiology and clinical pharmacology (Strom, 1989), should consider genetic differences among individuals.

The role of genetic factors in differential response to drugs and other interventions is at the heart of human biochemical individuality (Childs et

Table 10–8. Epidemiologic study designs for assessing natural history in the context of disease heterogeneity

Group	N	Cohort study outcome frequency	Case-control study Persons with outcome	Case-control study Persons without outcome
With disease				
Group 1	N_{11}	f_{11}	a_1	b_1
Group 2	N_{12}	f_{12}	a_2	b_2
Without disease	N_0	f_0	c	d

Table 10–9. Examples of pharmacogenetic traits in drug response

Genetic trait	Drug	Clinical effect
Acetylator phenotype	Isoniazid	
Slow		Prone to develop peripheral neuropathy
Rapid		Less favorable results for treatment of tuberculosis
Pseudocholinesterase deficiency	Succinylcholine	Prolonged postoperative apnea
G6PD deficiency	Primaquine	Hemolytic crises when receiving this and other related drugs

G6PD, glucose-6-phosphate dehydrogenase
Adapted from Price-Evans (1983).

al., 1988; Scriver and Childs, 1989). As with the individuality of disease, genetic epidemiology attempts to answer questions such as

1. Why do certain patients have an adverse reaction to a particular drug while others do not?
2. Why do certain patients require larger or smaller doses of a specific medication than the "average" dose to achieve adequate therapeutic response?
3. Why does a certain drug prevent a disease or cure a clinical disease in some individuals, but not in others?

As with other aspects of genetic epidemiology, both genetic and epidemiologic methods are applied in intervention studies to assess the role of measured and nonspecific genetic factors and their interaction with other factors in drug response. These studies must consider a variety of clinical and laboratory parameters, such as drug absorption, excretion, blood levels, occurrence of clinical endpoints, such as a disease, or a subclinical disease state, as well as the presence of clinical complications, and laboratory markers of injury to various organ systems.

Intervention studies are usually done on individuals with certain illnesses. Prevention efforts have also been extended to individuals without illness to test whether certain therapeutic agents reduce the risk of occurrence of certain diseases. Some examples here include vitamin A in cancer risk reduction, aspirin to reduce the risk of coronary heart disease, and periconceptional multivitamin/folic acid supplementation in protecting against neural tube defects in offspring (Smithells et al., 1983; Wald and Polani, 1984; Mulinare et al., 1988; Bower and Stanley, 1989; Mills et al., 1989; Milunsky et al., 1989). In all these studies, genetic variation in response should be specifically evaluated.

The search for genetic susceptibility to the effects of drugs and other therapeutic interventions can be conducted within the framework of an epidemiologic study design (cohort or case-control). As shown in Table 10–10, a cohort study can be conducted on individuals who are using a therapeutic

Table 10–10. Epidemiologic study designs for assessing genetic factors in therapeutic efficacy and safety

		Cohort study frequency of outcome	Case-control study	
Group	N^*		Persons with outcome	Persons without outcome
With a genetic factor	N_1	f_1	a	b
Without a genetic factor	N_0	f_0	c	d

*All individuals are treated with a specific drug or intervention.

agent, where the frequencies of particular therapeutic or toxicity endpoints are compared among individuals with different genetic traits that are suspected to interact biologically with the agent of interest. Alternatively, a case-control study can be conducted where cases are all individuals who are on a specific therapeutic regimen and who have a certain clinical endpoint, while controls are individuals on the same regimen but without the endpoint of interest. Other confounding factors have to be considered in the design and analysis of these studies. For example, Strickler and colleagues (1985) searched for genetic susceptibility to the teratogenic effects of diphenylhydantoins. They classified 24 children exposed to phenytoins throughout pregnancy into two groups according to a lymphocyte assay that measured the arene oxide detoxification of phenytoin metabolites; 14 infants had a "positive" assay (i.e., a significant increase in cell death associated with phenytoins, presumably due to a genetic defect in arene oxide detoxification), and 10 infants had a "negative" assay. Using blinded examinations of these children, 10 of the 14 children with "positive" assays had major or serious birth defects, while only 2 of the 10 children with "negative" assays had major birth defects. This preliminary investigation suggested a role of genetic factors in the susceptibility to teratogenic effects of hydantoins. These findings were confirmed by a more recent study (Buehler et al., 1990) and may have important implications in the clinical management of pregnant women on phenytoins.

10.3 APPLICATIONS OF GENETIC EPIDEMIOLOGY IN DISEASE PREVENTION

Genetic epidemiology addresses the fundamental goals of preventive medicine and public health at the various levels of disease prevention. The practice of public health involves applications of methods of techniques of epidemiology, biostatistics, health policy, and other biomedical sciences toward promoting health and preventing disease in the population. While the goals of preventive medicine and public health are identical, namely, health promotion and disease prevention, a delicate balance is often struck between concern for individuals versus communities, with preventive medicine oriented toward preventing physical, mental, and emotional disease and injury in well individuals and their families (Last, 1986), and public health is directed to the maintenance and improvement of health of the population at large (Last, 1986). The prevention of disease at the community level depends on the complex interaction of prevailing social, political, legal, and ethical values regarding health and disease that occasionally may clash with approaches toward maintaining health at the individual level. This conflict is also apparent in human genetics, where misuse of genetics for social or political reasons and disregard of individual rights are strong reminders that extreme caution is necessary when considering widespread genetic testing in human populations (Holtzman, 1989).

10.3.1. Scope and Strategies of Disease Prevention

Applications of genetic epidemiology in disease prevention can be viewed in terms of the three levels of disease prevention (Table 10–11; Last, 1986; Chronic Disease Planning Group, 1986). Primary prevention refers to the prevention of the occurrence of the disease in the population. While the most straightforward example of primary prevention is immunization against infectious diseases, most chronic diseases do not have single identifiable etiologies. For such conditions primary prevention may be oriented toward elimination of potential risk factors for the disease in question (e.g., smoking cessation programs to reduce risk from coronary heart disease, lung cancer, and pulmonary disease). A genetic example of primary prevention would be screening programs to detect carriers for Tay-Sachs disease in high-risk populations (Kaback, 1981). Secondary prevention refers to the prevention of clinical manifestations by early detection of preclinical disease and intervention. Classical examples of secondary prevention in medical genetics are newborn screening for congenital hypothyroidism and phenylketonuria, with resulting early intervention. Finally, tertiary prevention is concerned with minimizing the effects of disease by preventing complications and deterioration. An example of tertiary prevention for a genetic disease is that of antibiotic prophylaxis and immunization for individuals with sickle cell anemia to prevent life-threatening bacterial infections. Another example of tertiary

Table 10–11. Levels of disease prevention: Some examples

Level	Description	Examples
Primary	Preventing the occurrence of disease	Carrier detection for Tay-Sachs disease in high-risk populations
Secondary	Prevention of sequelae of disease by early detection of persons with disease	Neonatal detection of congenital hypothyroidism and phenylketonuria
Tertiary	Prevention of complications and deterioration	Antibiotic prophylaxis or vaccination in preventing bacterial infections among patients with sickle cell anemia

prevention is the development of therapeutic procedures that have improved survival of patients with cystic fibrosis from early childhood to young adulthood.

The above classification of levels of prevention becomes more complex when viewed in the context of the pathogenesis and natural history of disease, especially in relation to genetic susceptibility. For classical Mendelian conditions with no effective treatment available (e.g., Tay-Sachs disease), primary prevention can be thought of in terms of preventing the conception and/or birth of affected individuals by using carrier detection, genetic counseling and prenatal diagnosis. For numerous chronic diseases that do not follow simple Mendelian inheritance, but nevertheless have a strong genetic component, susceptibility genotypes can also be thought of as risk factors that interact with environmental factors in the eventual development of clinical disease. For example, in the case of ankylosing spondylitis (AS) most cases are associated with the presence of the *HLA-B27* allele. Only a small proportion of persons with the *B27* allele, however, are expected to develop the disease, presumably because of other genetic and environmental cofactors. In this situation, primary prevention for AS can be thought of as the identification and interruption of cofactors that lead to clinical disease among persons with the *B27* allele. This ambiguity in defining primary prevention results from the quantitative distinction of risk between disease genotypes (with disease risk of 100%) and disease susceptibility genotypes (with disease risk less than 100%) discussed in Chapter 5.

Once determinants of a disorder are identified in a specific population in terms of genetic and environmental risk factors, three overlapping strategies for prevention are available (Table 10-12; Breslow, 1983; Detels and Breslow, 1984; Chronic Disease Planning Group, 1986).

Education and Behavior Modification

The first strategy involves education and behavior modification. This strategy is based on the assumption that basic knowledge of facts regarding risks is essential to influence behavior. Unfortunately, communication of the concept of risk to the general public is a difficult task, especially in the face of weak or conflicting scientific evidence (Nelkin, 1989). Behavior modification may therefore not always be attainable. Despite impressive evidence regarding the deleterious effects of smoking on health, smoking cessation and reduction have been slow in the United States and throughout the world (McGinnis and Shopland, 1987). As noted by Mattson and coworkers (1987): "Segments of the public may have a false sense of security from the observation that 'not all smokers get cancer'." HIV infection provides an additional example where behavior modification is sought by educating the public regarding methods of transmission. As education and behavior modification can sometimes be most effective in population groups at highest risk for the disease in question, intervention programs for the control of HIV infection have been efficient in decreasing the rate of seroconversion in homosexual men (Berkelman and Curran, 1989). In genetic epidemiology, the basic premise is that education and behavior modification programs can be targeted toward indi-

Table 10–12. Strategies for disease prevention: Some examples

Strategy	Description	Examples
Education	Influencing the behavior of individuals for the purpose of risk reduction	Drug and dietary counseling in G6PD deficiency; cholesterol screening in families with familial hypercholesterolemia
Social/ environmental measures	Reducing the risk of disease by providing environmental control measures and changes in societal attitudes	Curtailing the promotion of cigarettes, reducing occupational exposures to carcinogens, mutagens
Health care service delivery	Delivery of quality medical care with emphasis on preventive medicine	Prenatal care in reducing pregnancy complications; prenatal diagnosis and genetic counseling in the prevention of Down syndrome in women ≥35 years of age and in inborn errors of metabolism

G6PD, glucose-6-phosphate dehydrogenase.

viduals, families, and population subgroups with differential genetic susceptibilities to specific environmental factors in order to reduce risks of disease (see sections 10.3.2 and 10.3.3).

Social and Environmental Measures

The second strategy (Table 10–12) involves social and environmental control measures to reduce disease risks in specific populations. As more and more environmental pollutants and occupational exposures are implicated in risks of genetic damage, some prevention strategies are increasingly oriented toward reducing global exposures to carcinogens and mutagens in the workplace and in the home, as well as reducing disease risks by food supplementation with certain essential nutrients. Because many risk factors for chronic disease are associated with cultural habits and societal mores (such as smoking, drinking), intervention should be focused on changing society's attitudes and actions toward unhealthy behaviors (Chronic Disease Planning Group, 1986), such as the promotion of cigarettes (Breslow, 1983). It should be noted that environmental strategies for intervention are geared toward the population as a whole and do not inherently address genetic differences among individuals. Sometimes, global programs such as food supplementation, while beneficial to most people, may be deleterious to a relatively small fraction of genetically susceptible individuals who may be sensitive to adverse effects from this intervention. In a discussion of reducing risks from environmental hazards and the differential genetic susceptibility to environmental exposures, Omenn points out that "the recognition of individuals or groups of persons at increased risk for adverse effects from chemical exposures should lead us to redouble our efforts to reduce or eliminate those exposures" (Omenn, 1988).

Preventive Health Care Service Delivery

The third strategy (Table 10–12) involves health care delivery with emphasis on preventive medicine. For most chronic diseases, the delivery of high quality preventive care is essential. This includes preventive examinations, screening, laboratory testing, and medical procedures (Chronic Disease Planning Group, 1986). Nevertheless, barriers still exist in the access and the delivery of quality health care in different countries and in subgroups of the population within a single country (Meade, 1986; Mahler, 1988).

In medical genetics, the availability of genetics centers, genetic counseling, and prenatal diagnosis are essential in the diagnosis, management, and family counseling for many genetic diseases. An example of the increasing attention to genetics in health-care delivery in genetics is the widespread use of prenatal testing for trisomy 21 among older pregnant women. Because of the increasing birth prevalence of Down syndrome with advancing maternal age, it has become common medical practice to offer prenatal diagnosis and genetic counseling to all older pregnant women. Nevertheless, widespread utilization of prenatal diagnosis of trisomy 21 in older women has been slow (Adams et al., 1981), and the effect of prenatal diagnosis on the birth prevalence of trisomy 21 has been modest (Kallen and Knudsen, 1989).

How can the methods of genetic epidemiology be applied toward disease prevention? Prevention requires the ability to educate individuals regarding risks for diseases in themselves, their progeny, and their relatives, based on the unique combination of their genetic background and their lifetime experience. While genes and genotypes of individuals remain largely unmodifiable, environments can be modified either at level of individuals or populations; and prevention can be targeted toward elimination, reduction, or change of the environmental experience of individuals. As indicated by Childs and Motulsky (1988):

> a great deal of epidemiologic work is necessary before it will be apparent what genetic risk factors, singly or in combination, mean to individuals. Odds ratios based on case-control studies, even when well done, can never stand as precise risks for individuals . . . and then it is not apparent what an individual is to do with them, particularly, when the provocation that makes risk a reality is unknown.

Thus, an important goal of genetic epidemiology is to refine risk estimates of disease to individuals beyond average relative risks and population risks.

10.3.2. Family-Based Prevention

Family-centered approaches can be employed to predict risk of disease in relatives of individuals affected with disease. These approaches include (1) use of empirical family history information without specification of underlying models, (2) use of family data in the context of well-defined genetic models, and (3) use of linked genetic markers in the context of family data.

Use of Empiric Family History Information

Even without the knowledge of specific biologic mechanisms, empirical recurrence risks can help direct preventive efforts. For example, recurrence risks for many isolated birth defects, such as neural tube defects, oral clefts, and pyloric stenosis are on the order of 2% to 5% (Carter, 1976). These estimates, although compatible with any number of genetic and environmental models, are often used in genetic counseling to inform parents who already have an affected infant regarding the risk of recurrence in subsequent pregnancies and the availability of prenatal diagnosis. However, crude recurrence risks are averages that are pooled over the population, and may be markedly influenced by etiologic heterogeneity. If a subset of cases involves an autosomal dominant trait with complete penetrance, the recurrence risk will be on the order of 50% rather than the population average. For another subset, where the defect was associated with a unique pregnancy exposure, the recurrence risk could be negligible. Yet, for another subset of cases, where a single gene effect along with an environmental trigger is needed to induce the defect, the recurrence risk depends both on the presence of the exposure and on Mendelian segregation. It is, therefore, recommended medical genetic practice to have a full clinical, laboratory, and family evaluation of each patient to identify subgroups of disease that could have different recurrence risks.

Similarly, epidemiologic studies of chronic adult-onset diseases that use family history information can yield estimates of disease risks to individuals, which can in turn be used to direct prevention strategies. As an example, Table 10–13 shows data from the case-control study of breast cancer of Sattin and colleagues (1985). This population-based investigation examined the relationship between family history of breast cancer in first-degree relatives (mothers and sisters) and the risk of breast cancer. Odds ratios for breast cancer were 2.1, if either a mother or a sister were reported to be affected, but increases to 13.6 if both are reportedly affected. Again, these odds ratios

Table 10–13. Estimation of lifetime risks of breast cancer by family history of breast cancer in mothers and sisters from a case-control study

Family history of breast cancer	No. of cases	No. of controls	Odds ratios	Lifetime* risk (%)
None	1804	2139	1.0	7.0
Mother	364	196	2.1	14.7
Sister	136	74	2.1	14.7
Both affected	35	3	13.6	95.2

*Overall lifetime risk in the population is assumed to be 8%. This corresponds to the sum of stratum-specific risks by family history weighted by the proportion of controls in each stratum. This leads to computation of stratum-specific risks.

Adapted from Sattin et al. (1985).

are population averages that could conceal underlying disease heterogeneity. Also, the interpretation of an odds ratio is difficult for individuals with different ages, menopausal status, and lifetime reproductive and hormonal experiences. However, with an estimated lifetime risk of 8% for breast cancer in U.S. women (Sattin et al., 1985), one can translate odds ratios into estimates of lifetime risks of breast cancer for individuals with one first-degree relative affected as 14%, and for those with both mother and a sister affected as more than 90%. Certainly these estimates should be viewed with caution because they are subject to assumptions behind estimates of lifetime risk, and limitations of the original study design, sample size, possible recall bias, and the use of odds ratios instead of relative risks for a relatively common disease. Also, risk estimates are best refined by type of familial cancer, estrogen receptor status, laterality, age of the woman, and other cofactors that are important for disease prediction.

Use of Family Data in the Context of Genetic Models

When an underlying genetic model for the condition is known, family data can be used to inform individuals regarding their risks of carrying disease alleles, even in the absence of genetic markers or biochemical tests. For classical Mendelian conditions with complete penetrance, risk predictions have long been provided by geneticists within the context of genetic counseling. Estimation of risk has a firm theoretical basis in Mendelian principles and relies on Bayesian methods (Murphy and Chase, 1974). For example, in the case of Huntington disease, the prior risk of inheriting the disease allele in offspring of affected individuals is 50% based on Mendelian expectations (without use of any DNA linkage information). Because the disease has a variable age at onset, the probability of a currently unaffected offspring being a gene carrier varies with age. As children of patients with Huntington disease grow older and remain asymptomatic, their probability of being a carrier declines. A 40-year-old individual who is so far unaffected has a probability close to 0.43, while a 60-year-old unaffected individual has a probability of about 0.15 (Vogel and Motulsky, 1986).

Quantitative estimates of risk can be developed for susceptibility genes with incomplete penetrance. In this situation, the risk function can be modeled, incorporating any number of covariates such as age, sex, and other exposures that may be associated with disease risk (Chase et al., 1986). For complex diseases, results of segregation analysis of pedigree data can be used to provide estimates of risk. To illustrate, results of a study involving complex segregation analysis of breast cancer in 200 Danish families (Williams and Anderson, 1984) are presented in Table 10–14. The investigators found statistical evidence for an autosomal dominant susceptibility allele. These data can be used to estimate lifetime cumulative risks for women with and without the susceptibility allele in this population. According to these analyses, by age 80, women carrying the putative allele have a 52% risk of developing breast cancer, compared with a cumulative risk of 5% in women who do not carry this allele.

Table 10−14. Estimation of cumulative risk of breast cancer by age, and presence of putative autosomal susceptibility allele: results of complex segregation analysis of Danish families

	Cumulative risk		
Age	With susceptible allele	Without susceptible allele	Total population
30	0.01	0.00	0.0001
40	0.07	0.00	0.0016
50	0.20	0.00	0.0081
60	0.33	0.02	0.0195
70	0.43	0.03	0.0342
80	0.52	0.05	0.0544
80+	0.57	0.06	0.0662

Adapted from Williams and Anderson (1984).

Use of Linked Genetic Markers in Family Data

Advances in molecular technology have made it possible to refine risk estimates for many Mendelian diseases and increasingly for complex adult-onset disorders. Linkage methods using DNA markers such as restriction fragment length polymorphisms (RFLPs) are applied to map disease loci as well as genes that confer susceptibility to diseases (Chapter 9). These methods have found growing applications in prenatal diagnosis, genetic counseling and heterozygote detection (Ostrer and Hejtmancik, 1988; Antonarakis, 1989). For example, the DNA marker D4S10 that is genetically linked to the Huntington disease locus can be used to predict the occurrence of the disease in individuals at risk before they develop symptoms (Jenkins and Conneally, 1989). Family studies are needed to evaluate the patterns of cosegregation between the marker and disease loci within families. Using linkage analysis in pedigrees, the risk of the disease in offspring of affected individuals can be refined from the prior probability of 50% mentioned earlier to a much higher or much lower figure. Some level of uncertainty remains because of the small amount of recombination (4%) that occurs between the marker locus and the disease locus. Although such predictive testing for Huntington disease is being increasingly applied in clinical medicine (Meissen et al., 1988; Brandt et al., 1989), numerous ethical, psychological, and societal concerns are raised by these applications, as the disease remains essentially incurable (Jenkins and Conneally, 1989).

It should be noted that a number of problems still exist in the application of DNA technology in predicting familial risks, even for simple Mendelian disorders (Holtzman, 1989). These include the availability of the extended family for testing, misinformation regarding pedigree structure and reported paternity, the availability of informative probes and informative family members, recombination, and the possibility of etiologic heterogeneity in the disease.

When dealing with diseases that do not have a simple Mendelian basis, applications of DNA technology in family-based prevention becomes more tenuous. Here, research methods of linkage analysis, coupled with epidemiologic designs (Chapters 5 and 9), should permit investigators to use a reductionist approach to identify disease susceptibility genes that increase risk of disease, by interacting with other genes as well as with environmental exposures. An example is the relatively recent linkage of early-onset familial breast cancer to genetic markers on chromosome 17 (Hall et al., 1990). Family-centered risk prediction for relatives of affected individuals will thus depend on the genetic relationship to the affected person, the number of linked DNA haplotypes shared with the affected individual and other covariates (both genetic and environmental) that are important in determining risk.

To illustrate, consider a hypothetical example of a disease that shows evidence of linkage with a DNA marker locus in the absence of knowledge of its gene product. Assume a certain environmental exposure is assumed to be a risk factor for the disease. As indicated in Table 10–15, the recurrence risk for particular relatives of probands can be estimated empirically, using information on the number of haplotypes identical by descent at the marker locus (see Chapters 5 and 9) as well as by the presence or absence of the environmental exposure. This approach can be extended to any number of single-gene systems and environmental exposures (including dose information). Again, to use the example of isolated birth defects (such as cleft lip and palate) with empirical sibling recurrence risks of 2% to 5% (i.e., $P(D)$ in Table 10–15), assume that the transforming growth factor α ($TGFA$) gene locus plays a role in the pathogenesis of the condition as suggested by the study of Ardinger and colleagues (1989) (see Chapter 5), and that maternal cigarette smoking is a risk factor (Khoury et al., 1989b). With these assumptions, the use of linked DNA markers at the $TGFA$ locus, and knowledge of smoking status of the mother, will allow refinement of the crude recurrence risk into at least six risk estimates, according to number of haplotypes shared by descent with the proband and maternal smoking information. Depending on the pattern of interaction between smoking and the $TGFA$ locus, if any, recurrence risks may differ across subgroups. Prevention strategies can then be targeted directed at the subgroups with highest recurrence risks. Further data are needed to confirm the role of the $TGFA$ locus, as well as to evaluate

Table 10–15. Refinements of familial recurrence risks using closely linked DNA markers and the presence of an exposure

Number of haplotypes identical by descent with proband	Exposure		Total
	No	*Yes*	
0	$P_0(D\|E-)$	$P_0(D\|E+)$	$P_0(D)$
1	$P_1(D\|E-)$	$P_1(D\|E+)$	$P_1(D)$
2	$P_2(D\|E-)$	$P_2(D\|E+)$	$P_2(D)$
Total	$P(D\|E-)$	$P(D\|E+)$	$P(D)$

D, disease; E, exposure.

whether there is a biologic interaction between its gene product(s) with cigarette smoking or other drugs and environmental exposures.

10.3.3 Population-Based Prevention

With ongoing efforts in gene mapping and sequencing and with the long-term promises of the human genome project, it may not be unreasonable to expect in the foreseeable future that most, if not all, human genes will be mapped and sequenced. The next step will be to understand the function of these genes as reflected in the structure and function of their products and their relationship to other genes and the environment at large, with respect to disease processes. Although this is a goal for the future, the technology is moving at a rapid pace, at least for selected genes that are directly associated with disease (such as cystic fibrosis and Huntington disease) or with susceptibility to disease (e.g., growth factor genes, cytochrome P-450 genes, HLA system). The identification of mutations that are associated with disease or disease susceptibility will permit the application of preventive efforts on a population scale in addition to family-based prevention.

One major difference between population-based strategies and family-based strategies for prevention is that the former requires direct identification of the allele(s) responsible for disease or susceptibility, either at the level of gene products or at the molecular level (Chapter 5), while the latter relies on indirect approaches such as linkage and segregation analyses. Compared with family-based prevention strategies, population-based prevention has a more significant potential impact on the reduction of disease risks. For example, as periconceptional multivitamin/folic acid supplementation has been found to reduce the occurrence of neural tube defects, implementation of this prevention in the population will reduce the overall occurrence of NTDs much more than implementation only among families with a previously affected infant. The latter group accounts for only a small fraction (less than 5%) of all cases.

Genetic Screening

The application of population-based prevention strategies requires genetic screening, the systematic search for persons with certain genotypes that (1) are associated with disease or predispose to disease, (2) are associated with disease in progeny (National Academy of Sciences, 1975; Erbe and Boss, 1983). Genetic screening has found increasing applications in medical practice, including (1) newborn screening for certain inborn errors of metabolism such as PKU and galactosemia, (2) heterozygote detection in high-risk subpopulations (e.g., Tay-Sachs disease among Ashkenazi Jews), and (3) prenatal screening for the presence of certain birth defects and chromosomal abnormalities (e.g., maternal serum α-fetoprotein for the detection of open neural tube defects, and advanced maternal age and other biochemical indices for the detection of Down syndrome [Wald et al., 1988]). The prerequisites, usefulness, and limitations and pitfalls of genetic screening have been discussed (Holtzman, 1978, 1989; Kazazian, 1978; Thomas, 1978; Kaback, 1983;

Carter and Willey, 1986; Vogel and Motulsky, 1986). Important issues to be considered include the incidence of the disorder, the sensitivity and specificity of the screening test, the cost of the screening test, and the availability of intervention strategies to reduce morbidity and mortality. Although strides are being made in the development of gene therapy (Friedman, 1989), advances in molecular technology continue to outpace advances in therapeutic intervention (Holtzman, 1989); as yet, the early detection of many Mendelian disorders, such as Huntington disease and cystic fibrosis does not provide hope for cure or improved survival for affected individuals. For the most part, the only available modes of intervention involve reproductive planning, carrier detection, and prenatal diagnosis, sometimes leading to ethical and personal dilemmas.

The situation is even more complex for diseases with no simple Mendelian involvement. For such diseases, the reductionist approach to the identification of single genes in disease occurrence will lead to identifying genes that are "risk factors" singly or in combination for the disease of interest. As discussed in Chapter 5, however, many genetic marker-disease associations that are found in population studies are noncausal and secondary to population stratification (confounding), linkage disequilibrium, or chance (type I errors). The challenge to genetic epidemiology will be to identify those associations that are biologically meaningful in disease pathogenesis (e.g., PiZ polymorphism in chronic lung disease). For such associations, once the necessary environmental determinants that interact with genetic susceptibility are identified, disease risks in the population can be stratified according to the number of susceptibility alleles carried by the individual, and the presence of relevant environmental exposure (Table 10–16). This can be extended to any number of genetic systems and environmental exposures (accounting for dose information). Depending on the pattern of interaction between the exposure and the susceptible genotype (see Chapter 5), disease prevention may or may not be more effectively targeted to the high-risk group by eliminating or reducing exposures. Examples of the high-risk approach in disease prevention include the reduction of phenylalanine in the diet of individuals with PKU. In this situation, phenylalanine produces deleterious effects causing mental retardation only in individuals with the enzyme deficiency. Intervention can easily be targeted to the genetically susceptible individuals. However, for many

Table 10–16. Refinements of disease risks in the population according to the presence of disease susceptibility alleles and the presence of an exposure

Genotype at susceptibility locus	Exposure		Total
	No	*Yes*	
NN	$P_0(D|E-)$	$P_0(D|E+)$	$P_0(D)$
NS	$P_1(D|E-)$	$P_1(D|E+)$	$P_1(D)$
SS	$P_2(D|E-)$	$P_2(D|E+)$	$P_2(D)$
Total	$P(D|E-)$	$P(D|E+)$	$P(D)$

N, normal allele; *S*, susceptible allele.

common diseases with etiologic heterogeneity, the situation is far more complex and different patterns of interaction may be observed. A notable example is cigarette smoking, where the deleterious effects are observed in a large proportion of smokers (Mattson et al., 1987). It is likely that multiple genetic systems (as well as other environmental exposures) interact with the numerous biochemical toxicants in cigarette smoke, leading to various diseases. Moreover, because the overall deleterious effects of smoking (both in smokers as well as among nonsmokers passively exposed to smoking) are so great, regardless of genetic susceptibility ($P(D|E+)$ compared with $P(D|E-)$ in Table 10–16), the best prevention strategy is the abolition or reduction of cigarette smoking in the whole population. It is to be emphasized, however, that extreme caution needs to be exercised in applying epidemiologic data on risks from exposures to different subgroups of the population that can be distinguished on the basis of genetic susceptibility. As discussed in section 10.5, applications of genetic testing to identify "hypersusceptible" individuals have ethical, social, and political ramifications.

Thus, an emerging application of genetic screening lies in the identification of healthy individuals in the population with genotypes that make them more susceptible to the development of certain diseases. Interest in such applications has been mounting in industry (Holtzman, 1989). Reasons for such an interest include concerns regarding the individual's safety, job performance, compensation, and liability. Again, the utility of these programs can be evaluated quantitatively in terms of sensitivity, specificity, and predictive values of genetic tests with respect to the development of the disease. On the other hand, several authors have expressed concern about the utilization of genetic testing in the occupational setting (Lappe, 1986; Murray, 1986; Omenn, 1988; Holtzman, 1989). The potential exists for stigmatization and discrimination as well as for increased tendency to remove the "susceptibles" from the workplace rather than eliminating hazardous exposures. These issues should be considered before instituting widespread genetic testing for disease susceptibility in the workplace and other population settings.

Environmental Health Risk Assessment

Finally, methods of genetic epidemiology are increasingly applied in the area of health risk assessment from environmental hazards (Omenn, 1988). With growing concern among scientists, politicians, and the public, regarding environmental risks from pollutants and other chemical and physical agents, epidemiologic methods are used to estimate levels of disease risks from occupational and environmental exposures (Gordis, 1988a). Risk assessment is one of four sequential steps involved in the response to environmental hazards: (1) hazard identification, (2) quantitative risk assessment, (3) exposure assessment, and (4) risk management (Stallones, 1988). These steps require multidisciplinary cooperation from many fields of the biomedical sciences such as toxicology, biochemistry, and genetics, in addition to reliance on epidemiologic methods. The ultimate response to the control of an environmental hazard requires implementation of public policy, and therefore quantitative methods of risk assessment are inevitably associated with public health policy (Stallones, 1988).

Two applications of genetic epidemiology in environmental risk assessment have been considered (Omenn, 1988). The first is in the genetic variation in susceptibility to exogenous agents (ecogenetics). As discussed earlier, the quantification of risks associated with exposures can be further refined, according to the presence or absence of specific genetic traits that interact biologically with the exposure. Several polymorphic genetic traits have been shown to affect the metabolism of, or tissue sensitivity to, certain chemicals and could potentially alter risk estimates from such exposures. These include, for example, the cytochrome P-450 system (such as the debrisoquine hydroxylation phenotype), the acetylator phenotype, plasma paraoxonase activity (related to parathion inactivation), glucose-6-phosphate dehydrogenase (G6PD) deficiency and α_1-antitrypsin deficiency (Omenn, 1988).

The second application in environmental risk assessment lies in the evaluation of genetic damage (both in somatic and germinal cells) induced by environmental exposures (genetic toxicology; Omenn, 1988). The evaluation of endpoints, reflecting genetic damage endpoints, such as sister chromatid exchange and chromosomal aberrations, mutagenicity assays, protein and DNA adducts (Wilcosky and Rynard, 1990; Schwartz, 1990; Goldring and Lucier, 1990) involves quantification of the effects of the exposures on the frequency of these endpoints, as well as the relationship between these biologic markers and the occurrence of specific disorders, notably cancer.

10.4 APPLICATIONS OF GENETIC EPIDEMIOLOGY IN PUBLIC HEALTH SURVEILLANCE

Finally, genetic epidemiology closely interfaces with the surveillance activities that are a vital link in the control and prevention of disease in communities. Although concepts of surveillance have traditionally started with infectious diseases, increasing attention is being focused on chronic diseases, cancer, birth defects, injuries, and environmental hazards (Thacker and Berkelman, 1988). The Centers for Disease Control (1986) defines surveillance as the "ongoing systematic collection, analysis, and interpretation of health data, essential to the planning, implementation, and evaluation of public health practice, closely integrated with the timely dissemination of these data to those who need to know." Surveillance programs are continuing systems of data collection, analysis, and dissemination, and not simply one-time epidemiologic or genetic studies (Thacker and Berkelman, 1988). In the United States, many surveillance programs have been essentially carried out at either the federal level (public health service) or at the local level (state and county health departments). An essential function of these programs is to provide data for the evaluation of intervention and prevention programs in communities.

Three interrelated surveillance activities involve the human genome: teratogenesis, mutagenesis, and carcinogenesis. The interaction of the genome with the environment at large may lead to both somatic mutations (potentially associated with long-term risk of cancer), and germinal cell mutations (many of which are associated with structural birth defects and malformation syndromes). The objectives of surveillance programs in these areas are as follows:

1. To provide baseline information on the incidence of cancers, birth defects and mutations in different communities
2. To evaluate variation in frequencies of these events (such as space-time clusters and long-term secular changes) that can be attributed to environmental agents
3. To provide a repository of epidemiologic data that can be used in follow-up studies to test hypotheses regarding etiologic factors and to conduct genetic investigations
4. To assess the impact of public health programs on the frequency of various endpoints

For example, population-based surveillance systems for birth defects (including structural defects, chromosomal abnormalities) have continued to proliferate and expand both in the United States and throughout the world (Kallen et al., 1984; Holtzman and Khoury, 1986; Flynt et al., 1987). Collaborative epidemiologic studies are being done as part of the International Clearinghouse for Birth Defects Monitoring Systems (1985, 1987), the research of Bjerkedal and colleagues (1982), and the EUROCAT project (1988), including the work of DeWals and colleagues (1985). This intensive activity in birth defects surveillance was propelled by the thalidomide tragedy that underlined the need to develop early warning signals for the introduction of new teratogens into the environment. The accomplishment and limitations of birth defects surveillance systems have been reviewed (Klinberg et al., 1983; Kallen et al., 1984; Holtzman and Khoury, 1986; Khoury and Holtzman, 1987; Kallen, 1988).

Birth defects surveillance systems are becoming invaluable resources as population-based registries for the evaluation of health services and for the conduct of descriptive epidemiologic studies, family studies, and case-control studies, either to generate hypotheses about risk factors for specific defects or to test already suggested ones regarding suspected new and old teratogens. One example is the large-scale case-control study conducted by the Centers for Disease Control between 1982 and 1984 to test whether the offspring of male Vietnam veterans were at greater risk of having serious birth defects than the offspring of men who did not serve in Vietnam (Erickson et al., 1984). The study was conducted relatively more efficiently because cases were ascertained as part of the existing Metropolitan Atlanta Congenital Defects Program, which has been in operation since 1968 (Edmonds et al., 1981).

In the future, the scope and applications of genetic epidemiology in public health surveillance may expand beyond the areas previously discussed to include, for example, (1) changes in the human genome (somatic and germinal) that are not necessarily associated with the immediate onset of disease, but could lead to cancers and other pathologies in the future, and (2) systematic population searches for inherited polymorphic genetic traits that are associated with disease susceptibilities. The latter expansion clearly overlaps with genetic screening and raises several issues regarding the objectives of surveillance, how information concerning genomic information on individuals will be used, and problems of confidentiality.

10.5 CONCLUDING REMARKS: ETHICAL ISSUES IN GENETIC EPIDEMIOLOGY

The avalanche of genomic information expected to be accrued over the next decades has already led to concerns regarding the use and misuse of such information in society (Suzuki and Knudston, 1989; Holtzman, 1989). Un-doubtedly, information regarding genetic variation at the DNA level will be employed in genetic epidemiology to refine risks of diseases in individuals and their relatives according to their genetic background and environmental experiences. Who should be informed about genetic risks to individuals? How will various sectors of society react to such knowledge? What are the risks of discrimination by employers, medical care providers, insurance companies, and policymakers against individuals because of their genetic background? These and many other questions remain largely unaddressed at the present time, although many authors have expressed concern regarding ethical issues resulting from the unrelenting advances in genetic technology (Vogel and Motulsky, 1986; Lappe, 1986; Murray, 1986; Holtzman, 1989; Suzuki and Knudston, 1989).

In his discussion of the perils of the new genetic technology, Holtzman (1989) argues that there is a great need to "proceed with caution" in applying genetic testing in human populations because

1. Misuse of genetics in the recent past (or more appropriately eugenics) by society has led to human rights abuses in the form of sterilization laws, immigration restrictions, and even mass genocide.
2. There is an accelerated trend toward commercialization of the DNA technology. Motivation for profit could lead to differential development of testing for some diseases but not others, and an indiscriminate application of genetic tests without understanding the limitations in interpreting their results.
3. Finally, discrepancies exist between the ability to detect disease-susceptibility genes and the ability to provide effective intervention after detection.

On the one hand, the triumph of medical genetics in the secondary prevention of mental retardation as a result of newborn screening for inborn errors of metabolism (such as PKU, galactosemia, and congenital hypothyroidism) illustrates the potential benefits of prevention. It is imperative, however, to keep in mind the ethical issues involved in preclinical detection of Huntington disease that has a progressive and devastating course with no current effective therapeutic intervention. Persons at risk of inheriting the Huntington disease gene can be tested by using linked DNA probes to assess the risk of carrying the *HD* allele. The value of predictive testing in the absence of effective intervention is open to question, however. Who should be tested and for what purpose? What is the psychological impact on the tested persons? Who should know the result of such testing? Will knowledge of test results lead to discrimination problems in the workplace or by providers of medical and life insurance? (Bloch and Hayden, 1990). Some persons in the early stages of the disease or even in the preclinical state seek predictive testing using DNA markers (Meissen et al., 1988). Programs offering such testing have largely followed ethical principles of autonomy founded on the respect for individuals' right to decide what is best for themselves.

The application of predictive testing on children and fetuses becomes even more controversial. Many feel that such testing should be avoided, since minors are unable to indicate their willingness or unwillingness to obtain such information (Bloch and Hayden, 1990). According to these authors,

> if we accede to the wishes of the parents for their children to be tested, we will have broken the primary principles of confidentiality, privacy, and individual justice that are owed to those children. This could be the thin edge of a wedge which could result in adoption agencies, educational institutions, insurance companies, and other third parties demanding genetic testing for another individual.

The ethical issues surrounding genetic testing in the workplace have also been discussed (e.g., Office of Technology and Assessment, 1983; Lappe, 1986; Murray, 1986; Holtzman, 1989; Suzuki and Knudston, 1989). Because of the increasing number of polymorphic genetic traits shown to increase susceptibility to the effects of certain chemicals and environmental agents, some employers have started, or have considered, implementing genetic testing programs designed to detect "hypersusceptible" individuals (Omenn, 1982; Murray, 1986; Holtzman, 1989). Several criteria have been discussed to justify programs to detect genetic susceptibility to environmental factors in the workplace: (1) a reasonable frequency of the susceptibility trait in the worker population exposed to the agent, (2) a considerable excess risk of disease among persons with the susceptible genotype compared with persons without the genotype at the same level of exposure, and (3) a sensitive and specific (predictive) test available to classify susceptible individuals (Omenn, 1982; Office of Technology and Assessment, 1983; King, 1984). As discussed by several authors (Office of Technology and Assessment, 1983, Khoury et al., 1985b; Holtzman, 1989), it appears that current genetic tests for hypersusceptibility have relatively poor predictive ability to identify susceptible persons who are likely to develop diseases with certain levels of exposure.

Given the growing interest in genetic testing in industry, ethical implications of such testing should be carefully evaluated. Could genetic testing lead not only to increased protection of individuals from harmful exposures, but also to discrimination against such individuals by denying them jobs or medical benefits, and so on? For example, for many years, genetic testing for sickle cell trait was carried out on applicants to the United States Air Force. Carriers for the sickle cell trait were denied entry because of the suggested theoretical risks of sickling crises at high altitude. While such practices have been abandoned (Uzych, 1986), a study by Kark and colleagues (1987) has shown an increased risk of sudden death during severely strenuous basic military physical training. It is unclear whether the results of this study and other similar studies could be used as a basis for policy changes in certain occupations, and it is also unclear what the impact of such changes might involve for individuals and society.

Another danger of genetic testing in the workplace is the potential for shifting the emphasis from making the work environment cleaner and healthier to blaming the workers for their susceptible genetic makeup. Even when genetic tests are found to predict reliably who is at risk from certain exposures, the fundamental issue remains as to whether genetic testing should be used to exclude susceptible individuals from the polluted work environment or to require elimination or reduction of toxic chemicals from the workplace (Suzuki and Knudston, 1989).

Clearly, in the coming decades, society will have to deal with ethical issues related to predicting disease risks according to genetic background. As suggested by several authors (Holtzman, 1989; Suzuki and Knudston, 1989), safeguards in the proper use of genetic testing should include: (1) protection of individual autonomy and the right to decide based on a proper informed consent process, (2) preservation of confidentiality of results of genetic testing, (3) limiting genetic testing in the workplace and by insurance companies, (4) careful scientific evaluation of the ability of genetic tests to measure the underlying susceptible genotype and of the biologic evidence for increased disease risks from certain exposures, and finally, (5) proper education of the medical profession and the general public regarding the importance of genetics in the practice of clinical and preventive medicine.

REFERENCES

Adams F (1939). *The Genuine Works of Hippocrates*. [Translated from the Greek]. Baltimore, Williams & Wilkins.

Adams MJ, Khoury MJ, James LM (1989). "The use of attributable fraction in the design and interpretation of epidemiologic studies." *Journal of Clinical Epidemiology* 42:659–662.

Adams MM, Finley S, Hansen H, et al. (1981). "Utilization of prenatal genetic diagnosis in women 35 years of age and older in the United States, 1977 to 1978." *American Journal of Obstetrics Gynecology* 139:673–677.

Ahearn JM, Hochberg MC (1988). "Epidemiology and genetics of ankylosing spondylitis." *Journal of Rheumatology, Supplement 16* 15:22–28.

Akaike H. (1974). "A new look at the statistical model identification." *IEEE Transactions on Automatic Control* AC-19:716–723.

Alfi OS, Chang R, Azen SP (1980). "Evidence for genetic control of nondisjunction in man." *American Journal of Human Genetics* 32:477–483.

Allen G (1965). "Twin research: Problems and prospects." *Progresss in Medical Genetics* 4:242–269.

Amos CI, Elston RC, Bonney GE, Keats BJS, Berenson GS (1990). "A multivariate method for detecting genetic linkage with application to a pedigree with an adverse lipoprotein phenotype." *American Journal of Human Genetics* 47:247–254.

Amos CI, Elston RC, Wilson AF, Bailey-Wilson JE (1989). "A more powerful robust sib-pair test of linkage for quantitative traits." *Genetic Epidemiology* 6:435–449.

Andreasen NC, Rice J, Endicott J, Reich T, Coryell W (1986). "The family history approach to diagnosis: How useful is it?" *Archives of General Psychiatry* 43:421–429.

Annest JL, Sing CF, Biron P, Mongeau JG (1979a). "Familial aggregation of blood pressure and weight in adoptive families. I. Comparisons of blood pressure and weight statistics among families with adopted, natural and both natural and adopted children." *American Journal of Epidemiology* 110:479–491.

Annest JL, Sing CF, Biron P, Mongeau JG (1979b). "Familial aggregation of blood pressure and weight in adoptive families. II. Estimation of the relative contributions of genetic and common environmental factors to blood pressure correlations between family members." *American Journal of Epidemiology* 110:492–503.

Antonorakis SE (1989). "Diagnosis of genetic disorders at the DNA level." *New England Journal of Medicine* 320:153–163.

Antonorakis SE (1990). "The mapping and sequencing of the human genome." *Southern Medical Journal* 83:876–878.

Antonorakis SE, Kazazian HH, Orkin SH (1985). "DNA polymorphism and molecular pathology of the human globin gene clusters." *Human Genetics* 69:1–14.

Antonorakis SE, Lewis JG, Adelsberger PA, et al (1990). "Parental origin of the extra chromosome in trisomy 21 revisited: DNA polymorphism analysis suggests that in 95% of cases the origin is maternal." *American Journal of Human Genetics, Supplement* 47:A207.

Ardinger HH, Buetow KH, Bell GI, Bardach T, Van Demark DR, Murray JC (1989). "Association of genetic variation of the transforming growth factor alpha gene with cleft lip and palate." *American Journal of Human Genetics* 45:348–353.

Armenian HK, Khoury MJ (1981). "Age at onset of genetic diseases: An application of Sartwell's model for the distribution of the incubation period." *American Journal of Epidemiology* 113:596–605.

Armenian HK, Lilienfeld AM (1983). "Incubation period of disease." Epidemiologic Reviews 5:1–15.

Astemborski JA, Beaty TH, Cohen BH. (1985). "Variance components analysis of forced expiration in families." *American Journal of Medical Genetics* 21:741–753.

Ayesh R, Idle JR, Ritchie JC, Crothers MJ, Etzel MR (1984). "Metabolic oxidation phenotypes as markers for susceptibility to lung cancer." *Nature* 312:169–170.

Azevedo ES, da Costa TP, Silva MC, Ribeiro LR (1983). "The use of surnames for interpreting gene frequency and past racial admixture." *Human Biology* 55:235–242.

Bailey NTJ (1975). *The Mathematical Theory of Infectious Diseases and its Applica tions*. London, Griffin.

Baldwin JA, Acheson ED, Graham WJ (eds) (1987). *Textbook of Medical Record Linkage*. Oxford, Oxford University Press.

Bale SJ, Chakravarti A, Strong LC (1984). "Aggregation of colon cancer in family data." *Genetic Epidemiology* 1:53–61.

Bao MZ, Wang JX, Dorman JS, Trucco M (1989). "*HLA-DQb* non-asp-57 allele and incidence of diabetes in China and the USA." *Lancet* 2:497–498.

Barbeau A, Cloutier T, Roy M, et al (1985). "Ecogenetics of Parkinson's disease: 4-Hydroxylation of debrisoquine." *Lancet* 2:1213–1216.

Barbujani G (1987). "Autocorrelation of gene frequencies under isolation by distance." *Genetics* 117:777–782.

Barbujani G (1988). "Diversity of some gene frequencies in European and Asian populations. IV. Genetic population structure assessed by the variogram." *Annals of Human Genetics* 52:215–225.

Barbujani G, Russo A, Farabegoli A, Calzolari E (1989). "Inferences on the inheritance of congenital anomalies from temporal and spatial patterns of occurrence." *Genetic Epidemiology* 6:537–552.

Baron JA (1989). "The clinical utility of risk factor data." *Journal of Clinical Epidemiology* 42:1013–1020.

Barrai I, Rosito A, Cappellozza G, et al (1984). "Beta-thalassemia in the Po-Delta: Selection, geography, and population structure." *American Journal of Human Genetics* 36:1121–1134.

Beadle GW (1945). "Biochemical genetics." *Chemical Reviews* 37:15.

Bean LL (1990). "The Utah population database: Demographic and genetic convergence and divergence." In Adams J. Hermalin AI, Lam DA, Smouse PE (eds), *Convergent Issues in Genetics and Demography*. New York, Oxford University Press, pp 231–244.

Beaty TH, Cohen BH, Newill CA, Menkes HA, Diamond EL, Chen CJ (1982). "Impaired pulmonary function as a risk factor for mortality." *American Journal of Epidemiology* 116:102–113.

Beaty TH, Liang KY (1987). "Robust inference for variance components models in families ascertained through probands. I. Conditioning on proband's phenotype." *Genetic Epidemiology* 4:203–210.

Beaty TH, Liang KY, Seerey S, Cohen BH (1987). "Robust inference for variance components models in families ascertained through probands. II. Analysis of spirometric measures." *Genetic Epidemiology* 4:211–221.

Beaty TH, Maestri NE, Meyers DA, Murphy EA (1988a). "Predicting recurrence risks under epistatic models." *American Journal of Medical Genetics* 28:631–645.

Beaty TH, Self SG, Liang KY, Connolly MA, Chase GA, Kwiterovich PO (1985). "Use of robust variance components models to analyze triglyceride data in families." *Annals of Human Genetics* 49:315–328.

Beaty TH, Yang P, Munoz A, Khoury MJ (1988b). "Effect of maternal and infant covariates on sibling correlation in birth weight." *Genetics Epidemiology* 5:241–253.

Beaudet AL, Scriver CR, Sly WS, et al (1989). "Genetics and biochemistry of variant human phenotypes." Scriver CR, Beaudet AL, Sly WS, Valle D (eds), *The Metabolic Basis of Inherited Disease*, 6th Ed. New York, pp 3–53.

Bennett JH, Rhodes FA, Robson HN (1959). "A possible genetic basis for kuru." *American Journal of Human Genetics* 11:169–187.

Bennett PH, Burch TA, Miller M (1971). "Diabetes mellitus in American (Pima) Indians." *Lancet* 2:125–128.

Berkelman RL, Curran JW (1989). "Epidemiology of HIV infection and AIDS." *Epidemiologic Reviews* 11:222–228.

Berkson J (1946). "Limitations of the application of the fourfold table analysis to hospital data." *Biometrics* 2:47–53.

Bernstein F (1931). *Comitato Italiano per lo Studio dei Problemi della Populazione.* Rome, Istituto Poligratcio dello Stato.

Bishop DT, Skolnick MH (1984). "Genetic epidemiology of cancer in Utah genealogies: A prelude to the molecular genetics of common cancers." *Journal of Cellular Physiology, Supplement* 3:63–77.

Bishop DT, Williamson JA (1990). "The power of identity-by-state methods for linkage analysis." *American Journal of Human Genetics* 46:254–265.

Bjerkedal T, Czeizel A, Goujard J, et al (1982). "Valproic acid and spina bifida" [Letter]. *Lancet* 2:1096.

Blackwelder WC, Elston RC (1982). "Power and robustness of sib-pair linkage tests and extension to larger sibships." *Common Stat Theor Method* 11:449–484.

Blackwelder WC, Elston RC (1985). "A comparison of sib-pair linkage tests for disease susceptibility loci." *Genetic Epidemiology* 2:85–98.

Blangero J, MacCluer JW, Kammerer CM, Mott GE, Dyer TD, McGill HC (1990). "Genetic analysis of apolipoprotein AI in two dietary environments." *American Journal of Human Genetics* 47:414–428.

Bloch M, Hayden MR (1990). "Predictive testing for Huntington disease in childhood: Challenges and implications." [Opinion]. *American Journal of Human Genetics* 46:1–4.

Blumberg BS, Melartin L, Gunito RS, Werner B (1966). "Family studies of a human serum isoantigen system (Australia antigen)." *American Journal of Human Genetics* 18:594–608.

Boehnke M (1986). "Estimating the power of a proposed linkage study: A practical computer simulation approach." *American Journal of Human Genetics* 39:513–527.

Boehnke M, Lange K (1984). "Ascertainment and goodness of fit of variance components models for pedigree data." In Rao DC, Elston RC, Kuller LH, Feinleib M, Carter C, Havlik R (eds), *Genetic Epidemiology of Coronary Heart Disease: Past, Present and Future*. New York, Alan R Liss, pp 173–192.

Boehnke M, Moll PP, Lange K, Weidman WH, Kottke BA (1986). "Univariate and bivariate analyses of cholesterol and triglyceride levels in pedigrees." *American Journal of Medical Genetics* 23:775–792.

Boehnke M, Young MR, Moll PP (1988). "Comparison of sequential and fixed structure sampling of pedigrees in complex segregation analysis of a quantitative trait." *American Journal of Medical Genetics* 43:336–343.

Boers GHJ, Smals AGH, Trijbels FJM, et al (1985). "Heterozygosity for homocystinuria in premature peripheral and cerebral occlusive arterial disease." *New England Journal of Medicine* 313:709–715.

Boerwinkle E, Chakraborty R, Sing CF (1986). "The use of measured genotype information in the analysis of quantitative phenotypes in man. I. Models and methods." *Annals of Human Genetics* 50:181–194.

Boerwinkle E, Sing CR (1987). "The use of measured genotype information in the analysis of quantitative phenotypes in man. III. Simultaneous estimation of frequencies and effects of the apolipoprotein E polymorphism on residual polygenic effects on cholesterol metabolism." *Annals of Human Genetics* 51:211–226.

Bonney GE (1984). "On the statistical determination of major gene mechanisms in continuous human traits: Regressive models." *American Journal of Medical Genetics* 18:73–749.

Bonney GE (1986). "Regressive logistic models for familial and other binary traits." *Biometrics* 42:611–625.

Bonney GE, Demenais FM (1991). Ascertainment and sampling units in the analysis of family data. In manuscript.

Bonney GE, Lathrop GM, Lalouel JM (1988). "Combined linkage and segregation analysis using regressive models." *American Journal of Human Genetics* 43:29–37.

Botstein D, White RL, Skolnick M, Davis RW (1980). "Construction of a genetic linkage map in man using restriction length polymorphisms." *American Journal of Human Genetics* 32:314–331.

Boughman JA, Conneally PM, Nance WE (1980). "Population genetic studies of retinitis pigmentosa." *American Journal of Human Genetics* 32:223–235.

Bourguet CC, Grufferman S, Delzell E, DeLong, Cohen HJ (1985). "Multiple myeloma and family history of cancer." *Cancer* 56:2133–2139.

Bower C, Stanley FJ (1989). "Dietary folate as a risk factor for neural tube defects: Evidence from a case-control study in western Australia." *Medical Journal of Australia* 150:613–619.

Box GED, Cox DR (1964). "An analysis of transformations." *Journal of the Royal Statistical Society, Series B* 26:211–252.

Bracken MB (1984). "Methodologic issues in the epidemiologic investigations of drug-induced malformations." In Bracken MB (ed), *Perinatal Epidemiology*. New York, Oxford University Press, pp 434–440.

Brandt J, Quaid KA, Folstein SE, et al (1989). "Presymptomatic diagnosis of delayed-onset disease with linked DNA markers: The experience in Huntington's disease." *Journal of the American Medical Association* 261:3108–3114.

Breslow L (1983). "The potential for health promotion." In Mechanic D (ed), *Handbook of Health, Health Care, and the Health Professsion*. New York, Free Press, p 50.

Breslow NE, Day NE (1980). *Statistical Methods in Cancer Research, Vol. 1: The Analysis of Case-Control Studies*. Lyon, France, IARC Scientific Publications.

Breslow NE, Enstrom JE (1974). "Geographic correlations between cancer mortality rates and alcohol-tobacco consumption in the United States." *Journal of the National Cancer Institute* 53:631–639.

Brewer GJ (1971). "Human ecology: An expanding role for the human geneticist." [Annotation]. *American Journal of Human Genetics* 23:92–94.

Browner WS, Newman TB (1989). "Sample size and power based on the population attributable fraction." *American Journal of Public Health* 79:1289–1294.

Brugge J, Curran T, Harlow E, McCormick F (eds) (1991). "The origins of human cancers: A comprehensive review." Cold Spring Harbor, NY, Cold Spring Harbor Laboratory Press.

Bryant HE, Visser N, Love EJ (1989). "Records, recall loss, and recall bias in pregnancy: A comparison of interview and medical records data of pregnant and postnatal women." *American Journal of Public Health* 79:78–80.

Buehler BA, Delimont D, van Waer M, Finnel RH (1990). "Prenatal prediction of risk of fetal hydration syndrome." *New England Journal of Medicine* 322:1567–1572.

Bulmer MG (1985). *The Mathematical Theory of Quantitative Genetics*. Oxford, Clarendon Press.

Burns TL, Moll PP, Schork MA (1984). "Comparison of different sampling designs for the determination of genetic transmission mechanisms in quantitative traits." *American Journal of Human Genetics* 36:1060–1074.

Calabrese EJ (1984). *Ecogenetics: Genetic Variation in Susceptibility to Environmental Agents*. New York, Wiley.

Cannings C, Skolnick MH, DeNevers K, Sridharan R (1976). "Calculation of risk factors and likelihoods for familial diseases." *Computers and Biomedical Research* 9:393–404.

Cannings C, Thompson EA (1977). "Ascertainment in the sequential sampling of pedigrees." *Clinical Genetics* 12:208–211.

Cannings C, Thompson EA, Skolnick MH (1978). "Probability functions on complex pedigrees." *Advances in Applied Probability* 10:26–91.

Caporaso N, Hayes RB, Dosemeci M, et al (1989a). "Lung cancer risk, occupational exposure and the debrisoquine metabolic phenotype." *Cancer Research* 49:3675–3679.

Caporaso N, Landi MT, Vineis P (1991). "Relevance of metabolic polymorphisms to human carcinogenesis: Evaluation of epidemiologic evidence." *Pharmacogenetics* 1:4–19.

Caporaso N, Pickle LW, Bale S, et al (1989b). "The distribution of debrisoquine metabolic phenotypes and implications for the suggested association with lung cancer risk." *Genetic Epidemiology* 6:517–524.

Carter CO (1976). "Genetics of common isolated malformations." *British Medical Bulletin* 32:21–26.

Carter TC, Falconer DS (1951). "Stocks for detecting linkage in the mouse and theory of their design." *Journal of Genetics* 50:307–323.

Carter TP, Willey AM (eds) (1986). *Genetic Disease: Screening and Management*. New York, Alan R Liss.

Cartwright RA, Glashan RW, Rogers HJ, et al (1982). "Role of *N*-acetyltransferase phenotypes in bladder carcinogenesis: A pharmacogenetic epidemiological approach to bladder cancer." *Lancet* 2:842–846.

Cassidy SB, Gainey AJ, Butler MG (1989). "Occupational hydrocarbon exposure among fathers of Parder-Willi syndrome patients with and without deletions of 15q." *American Journal of Human Genetics* 44:806–810.

Castilla EE, Adams JA (1990). "Migration and genetic structure in an isolated population in Argentina: Aicuña." In Adams J, Hermalin AI, Lam DA, Smouse PE (eds), *Convergent Issues in Genetics and Demography*. New York, Oxford University Press, pp 45–62.

Cavalli-Sforza LL, Bodmer WF (1971). *The Genetics of Human Populations*. San Francisco, CA, WH Freeman.

Cavender DE, Wagener DK, Orchard TJ, Laporte RE, Becker DJ, Kuller LE (1984). "Multivariate analyses of the risk of insulin-dependent diabetes mellitus for siblings of insulin-dependent diabetic patients." *American Journal of Epidemiology* 120:315–327.

Centers for Disease Control (1986). *Comprehensive Plan for Epidemiologic Surveillance* Atlanta, GA, Centers for Disease Control.

Chakraborty R (1984). "Relationship between heterozygosity and genetic distance in the three major races of man." *American Journal of Physical Anthropology* 65:249–258.

Chakraborty R (1985). "Some analytical explorations for detecting familial aggregation of disease traits." In Chakraborty R, Szathmary EJE (eds), *Diseases of Complex Etiology in Small Populations: Ethnic Differences and Research Approaches.* New York, Alan R Liss, pp 21–37.

Chakraborty R (1986). "The inheritance of pyloric stenosis explained by a multifactorial threshold model with sex dimorphism for liability." *Genetic Epidemiology* 3:1–15.

Chakraborty R, Chakravarti A (1977). "On consanguineous marriages and the genetic load." *Human Heredity* 36:47–54.

Chakraborty R, Ferrell RE, Stern MP, Haffner SM, Hazuda HP, Rosenthal M. (1986). "Relationship of prevalence of non-insulin-dependent diabetes mellitus to Amerindian admixture in the Mexican-Americans of San Antonio, Texas." *Genetic Epidemiology* 3:435–454.

Chakraborty R, Szathmary EJE (eds) (1985). *Diseases of Complex Etiology in Small Populations.* New York, Alan R. Liss, Inc, pp 3–8.

Chakraborty R, Weiss KM (1986). "Frequencies of complex diseases in hybrid populations." *American Journal of Physical Anthropology* 70:489–503.

Chakraborty R, Weiss KM, Majumber PP, Strong LC, Hershon J (1984). "A method to test excess risk of disease in structural data: Cancer in relatives of retinoblastoma patients." *Genetic Epidemiology* 3:229–244.

Chakravarti A, Chakraborty R (1978). "Elevated frequency of Tay-Sachs disease among Ashkenazi Jews unlikely by genetic drift alone." *American Journal of Medical Genetics* 30:256–261.

Chandley A (1991). "On the parental origin of de novo mutation in man." *Journal of Medical Genetics* 28:217–223.

Chapman M (1990). "Predictive testing for adult-onset genetic disease: Ethical and legal implications of the use of linkage analysis for Huntington disease." [Invited Editorial]. *American Journal of Human Genetics* 42:1–2.

Chase GA, Folstein MF, Breitner JC, Beaty TH, Self SG (1983). "The use of life tables and survival analysis in testing genetic hypotheses, with an application to Alzheimer's disease." *American Journal of Epidemiology* 117:590–597.

Chase GA, Markson LE, Brookmeyer R, Folstein SC (1986). "Covariate-dependent genetic counselling: Huntington's disease." *Journal of Neurogenetics* 3:215–223.

Childs B, Holtzman NA, Kazazian HH, Valle DL (eds) (1988). *Molecular Genetics in Medicine.* New York, Elsevier.

Childs B, Motulsky AG (1988). "Recombinant DNA analysis of multifactorial disease." In Childs B, Holtzman NA, Kazazian HH, Valle DL (eds), *Molecular Genetics in Medicine.* New York, Elsevier, pp 180–194.

Childs B, Scriver CR (1986). "Age at onset and causes of disease." *Perspectives in Biology and Medicine* 29:437–460.

Ching GHS, Chung CS (1974). "A genetic study of cleft lip and palate in Hawaii. I. Interracial crosses." *American Journal of Human Genetics* 26:162–176.

Christian JC, Kang KW, Norton JA. (1974). "Choice of an estimate of genetic variance from twin data." *American Journal of Human Genetics* 26:154–161.

Chronic Disease Planning Group, Centers for Disease Control (1986). *Positioning for Prevention: An Analytic Framework and Background Document for Chronic Disease Activities*. Atlanta, GA, U.S. Department of Health and Human Services.

Chung CS, Mi MP, Beechert AM (1987). "Genetic epidemiology of cleft lip with or without cleft palate in the population of Hawaii." *Genetic Epidemiology* 4:415–423.

Clarke CA (1961). "Blood groups and disease." In Steinberg AG (ed), Progress in Medical Genetics. Volume 1. New York, Grune-Stratton.

Claus EB, Risch NJ, Thompson WD (1990). "Age at onset as an indicator of familial risk of breast cancer." *American Journal of Epidemiology* 131;961–971.

Clifford CA, Hopper JL, Fulker DW, Murray RM (1984). "A genetic and environmental analysis of a twin family study of alcohol use, anxiety, and depression." *Genetic Epidemiology* 1:63–79.

Cohen BH (1980). "Chronic obstructive pulmonary disease: A challenge in genetic epidemiology." *American Journal of Epidemiology* 112:274–288.

Cohen BH, Ball WC, Bias WH, et al (1975). "A genetic epidemiologic study of chronic obstructive pulmonary disease. I. Study design and preliminary observations." *Johns Hopkins Medical Journal* 137:95–104.

Cohen BH, Diamond EL, Graves CH, et al (1977a). "A common familial component in lung cancer and chronic obstructive pulmonary disease." *Lancet* 2:523–526.

Cohen BH, Lilienfeld AM (1970). "The epidemiological study of mongolism in Baltimore." *Annals of the New York Academy of Sciences* 171:320–327.

Cohen BH, Lilienfeld AM, Kramer S, Hyman LC (1977b). "Parental factors in Down's syndrome: Results of the second Baltimore case-control study." In Hook EB (ed), *Population Cytogenetics*. New York, Academic Press, pp 301–352.

Cohen BH, Lilienfeld AM, Sigler AT (1963). "Some epidemiologic aspects of mongolism: A review." *American Journal of Public Health* 53:223–236.

Cole P (1979). "The evolving case-control study." *Journal of Chronic Diseases* 32:15–27.

Committee on Biological Markers of the National Research Council (1987). "Biological markers in environmental health research." *Environmental Health Perspectives* 74:3–10.

Conneally PM (1985). "Report of the committee on methods of linkage analysis." Eighth International Workshop on Human Gene Mapping.

Conneally PM, Rivas ML (1980). "Linkage analysis in man." *Advances in Human Genetics* 10:209–266.

Connolly M, Liang KY (1988). "Conditional logistic regression models for correlated binary data." *Biometrika* 75:501–506.

Cooper DN, Clayton JF (1988). "DNA polymorphisms and the study of disease associations." *Human Genetics* 78:299–312.

Cooper DN, Schmidtke J (1991). "Diagnosis of genetic diseases using recombinant DNA." *Human Genetics* 87:519–560.

Cooper DN, Smith BA, Booke HJ, Niemann S, Smidtke J (1985). "An estimate of unique DNA sequence heterozygosity in the human genome." *Human Genetics* 69:201–205.

Cordero JF (1992). "Registries of birth defects and genetic diseases." *Pediatric Clinics of North America* 39:65–77.

Costa T, Scriver CR, Childs B (1985). "The effect of mendelian disease on human health: A measurement." *American Journal of Medical Genetics* 21:231–242.

Cotch MF, Beaty TH, Cohen BH (1990). "Path analysis of familial resemblance of pulmonary function and cigarette smoking." *American Review of Respiratory Disease* 142:1337–1343.

Cox DW, Woo SLC, Mansfield T (1985). "DNA restriction fragments associated with alpha-1-antitrypsin indicate a single origin for the deficiency allele." *Nature* 316:79–81.

Crow JF (1963). "The concept of genetic load: A reply." *American Journal of Human Genetics* 15:310–315.

Crow JF (1986). *Basic Concepts in Population, Quantitative and Evolutionary Genetics*. New York, WH Freeman.

Crow JF, Denniston C (1981). "The mutation component of genetic damage." *Science* 212:888–893.

Curnow RN, Smith C (1975). "Multifactorial models for familial disease in man." *Journal of the Royal Statistical Society A* 138:131–169.

Dadone MM, Kushner JP, Edwards CQ, et al (1982). "Hereditary hemochromatosis: analysis of the laboratory expression of the disease by genotype in 18 pedigrees." *American Journal of Clinical Pathology* 78:196–207.

Dausset J, Svejggard A (eds). (1977). "HLA and disease." Copenhagen, Munksgaard.

Davies AM (1979). "The 'singles' method for segregation analysis under incomplete ascertainment." *Annals of Human Genetics* 41:507–512.

Dawber TR (1980). "The Framingham study. The epidemiology of atherosclerotic heart disease." Cambridge, MA, Harvard University Press.

Delehanty J, White RL, Mendelshon ML (1986). "Approaches to determining mutation rates in human DNA." *Mutation Research* 167:215–232.

del Junco D, Luthra HS, Annegers JF, Worthington JW, Kurland LT (1984). "The familial aggregation of rheumatoid arthritis and its relationship to the HLA-DR4 association." *American Journal of Epidemiology* 119:813–829.

Demenais F (1991). "Regressive logistic models for familial disease: A formulation assuming an underlying liability model." *American Journal of Human Genetics* 49:772–785.

Demenais FM, Bonney GE (1989). "Equivalence of the mixed and regressive models for genetic analysis. I. Continuous traits." *Genetic Epidemiology* 6:597–618.

Demenais F, Lathrop M, Lalouel JM (1986). "Robustness and power of the unified model in the analysis of quantitative measurements." *American Journal of Human Genetics* 38:228–234.

Detels R, Breslow L (1984). "Current scope." In Holland WW, Detels R, Knox G (eds), *Oxford Textbook of Public Health*, Vol. I: *History, Determinants, Scope and Strategies*. New York, Oxford University Press, pp 20–32.

DeWals P, Weatherall JAC, LeChat MF (1985). *Registration of Congenital Anomalies in EUROCAT Centres, 1979–1983*. Louvain-La-Neuve, Belgium, pp. 4–144.

DiLella AG, Marvit J, Lidsky AS, Guttler F, Woo SL (1986). Tight linkage between a splicing mutation and a specific DNA haplotype in phenylketonuria." *Nature* 322:799–803.

Donner A, Koval JJ (1981). "A multivariate analysis of family data." *American Journal of Epidemiology* 114:149–154.

Dorman JS, Trucco M, LaPorte RE, et al (1988). "Family studies: The key to understanding the genetic and environmental etiology of chronic disease?" [Invited Editorial]. *Genetic Epidemiology* 5:305–310.

Dulbecco R (1986). "A turning point in cancer research: Sequencing the human genome." *Science* 231:1055–1056.

East EM (1916). "Studies on size inheritance in *Nicotiana*." *Genetics* 1:164–176.

Edmonds LD, Layde PM, James LM, Flynt JW Jr, Erickson JD, Oakley GP (1981).

"Congenital malformations surveillance: Two American systems." *International Journal of Epidemiology* 10:247–252.

Edwards AWF (1978). *Likelihood: An Account of the Statistical Concept of Likelihood and its Application to Scientific Inference* 2nd Ed. London, Cambridge University Press.

Edwards CQ, Griffen LM, Goldgar D, et al (1988). Prevalence of hemochromatosis among 11,065 presumably healthy blood donors." *New England Journal of Medicine* 318:1355–1362.

Edwards CQ, Dadone MM, Skolnick MH, Kushner JP (1982). "Hereditary hemochromatosis." *Clinics in Haematology* 11:411–435.

Edwards JH (1960). "The simulation of mendelism." *Acta Geneticae Medicae et Gemellogiae (Roma)* 10:63–70.

Edwards JH (1989). "Familiarity, recessivity, and germline mosaicism." *Annals of Human Genetics* 53:33–47.

Edwards JH (1981). "Vitamin supplementation and neural tube defects." *Lancet* 1:275–276.

Elandt-Johnson RC (1970). "Segregation analysis for complex modes of inheritance." *American Journal of Human Genetics* 22:129–144.

Elandt-Johnson RC (1971). *Probability Models and Statistical Methods in Genetics.* New York, Wiley.

Elandt-Johnson RC (1975). "Definition of rates: Some remarks on their use and misuse." *American Journal of Epidemiology* 102:267–271.

Elford J, Phillips AN, Thomson AG, Shaper AG (1989). "Migration and geographic variations in ischemic heart disease in Great Britain." *Lancet* 1:343–346.

Elston RC (1971). "The estimation of admixture in racial hybrids." *Annals of Human Genetics* 35:9–17.

Elston RC (1975). "On the correlation between correlations." *Biometrika* 62:133–140.

Elston RC (1981). "Segregation analysis." *Advances in Human Genetics* 11:63–120.

Elston RC (1988). "The use of polymorphic markers to detect genetic variability." In Woodhead AD, Bender, MA. Leonard RC (eds), *Phenotypic Variation in Populations: Relevance to Risk Assessment.* New York, Plenum Press, pp 105–112.

Elston RC (1990). "A general method for the detection of major genes." In Giannola D, Hammond K (eds), *Advances in Statistical Methods for Genetic Livestock.* New York, Springer-Verlag.

Elston RC, Sobel E (1979). "Sampling considerations in the gathering and analysis of pedigree data." *American Journal of Human Genetics* 31:62–69.

Elston RC, Stewart J (1971). "A general model for the genetic analysis of pedigrees." *Human Heredity* 21:523–542.

Elwood JM, Elwood JH (1980). *Epidemiology of Anencephalus and Spina Bifida.* Oxford, Oxford University Press.

Emery AEH, Rimoin DL (eds) (1983). *Principles and Practice of Medical Genetics,* Vol. II, Sect. 4: *Applied Genetics.* Edinburgh, Churchill-Livingstone, pp 1427–1502.

Epstein FH (1989). "The relationship of lifestyle to international trends in CHD." *International Journal of Epidemiology* 18:S203–S209.

Erbe RW, Boss GR (1983). "Newborn genetic screening." In Emery AEH, Rimoin DL (eds), *Principles and Practice of Medical Genetics,* Vol. II. Edinburgh, Churchill Livingstone, pp 1437–1450.

Erickson JD (1978). "Down syndrome, paternal age, maternal age and birth order." *Annals of Human Genetics* 41:289–298.

Erickson JD, Mulinare J, McClain PW, et al (1984). *Vietnam Veteran's Risks for Fathering Babies with Birth Defects*. Atlanta, GA, Centers for Disease Control.

Ericson A, Kallen B, Westenholen P (1979). "Cigarette smoking as an etiologic factor in cleft lip and palate." *American Journal of Obstetrics and Gynecology* 135:348–351.

The EUROCAT Working Group (1988). "Preliminary evaluation of the impact of the Chernobyl radiological contamination on the frequency of central nervous system malformations in 18 regions of Europe." *Paediatric and Perinatal Epidemiology* 2:253–264.

Evans AS (1987). "Subclinical epidemiology: The first Harry A. Feldman Memorial Lecture." *American Journal of Epidemiology* 125:545–555.

Evans AS, Brachman PS (1986). "Emerging issues in infectious disease epidemiology." *Journal of Chronic Disease* 39:1105–1124.

Evans DAP (1983). "Pharmacogenetics." In Emery AEH, Rimoin DL (eds), *Principles and Practice of Medical Genetics*, Vol. 2. London, Churchill-Livingstone, pp 1389–1400.

Evans DAP (1984). "Survey of the human acetylator phenotype in spontaneous disorders." *Journal of Medical Genetics* 21:243–253.

Evans HJ (1988). "Mutation cytogenetics: Past, present and future." *Mutation Research* 204:355–363.

Ewens WJ (1978). "Tay-Sachs disease and theoretical population genetics." [Editorial]. *American Journal of Human Genetics* 30:328–329.

Ewens WJ, Shute NE (1986). "A resolution of the ascertainment sampling problem. I. Theory." *Theoretical Population Biology* 30:388–412.

Falconer DS (1960). *Introduction to Quantitative Genetics*. New York, Ronald Press.

Falconer DS (1965). "The inheritance of liability to certain diseases estimated from the incidence among relatives." *Annals of Human Genetics* 29:51–76.

Farr W (1975). Vital Statistics: A memorial volume of selections from the reports and writings of William Farr." Metuchen, NJ, New York Academy of Medicine.

Falconer DS (1981). *Introduction to Quantitatitve Genetics*, 2nd Ed. Essex, England, Longman Scientific & Technical.

Feinleib M (1984). "History of the genetic epidemiology of coronary heart disease." *Progress in Clinical Biology Research* 147:1–10.

Feinleib M, Garrison RJ, Fabsitz R, et al (1977). "The NHLBI twin study of cardiovascular disease risk factors: Methodology and summary of results." *American Journal of Epidemiology* 106:284–295.

Ferns GAA, Stocks J, Galton DJ (1986). "C-III DNA restriction fragment length polymorphism and myocardial infarction." *Lancet* 1:94.

Field LL (1988). "Insulin-dependent diabetes mellitus: A model for the study of multifactorial disorders." [Invited Editorial]. *American Journal of Human Genetics* 43:793–798.

Fielding JE (1986). "Smoking: Health effects and control." In Last JM (ed), *Maxcy-Rosenau Public Health and Preventive Medicine*, 12th Ed. Norwalk, CT, Appleton & Lange, pp 999–1038.

Fineman RM, Jorde LB (1980). "Establishment of a birth defects registry with the aid of a genealogical data base." In Cairns L, Lyon JL, Skolnick M (eds), *Banbury Report No. 4*. New York, Cold Spring Harbor Laboratory, 319–332.

Fisher RA (1918). "The correlation between relatives on the supposition of Mendelian inheritance." *Transactions of the Royal Society Edinburgh* 52:399–433.

Flanders WD, Khoury MJ (1990). "Indirect assessment of confounding: Graphical description and limits on effect of adjusting for covariates." *Epidemiology* 1:239–246.

Flegal KM, Brownie C, Haas JD, et al (1986). "The effects of exposure misclassification on estimates of relative risk." *American Journal of Epidemiology* 123:736–751.

Fleiss JJ (1981). *Statistical Methods for Rates and Proportions*, 2nd Ed. New York, Wiley.

Fletcher RH, Fletcher SW, Wagner EH (1982). *Clinical Epidemiology: The Essentials.* Baltimore, MD, Williams & Williams, p 53.

Flynt JW, Norris CK, Zaro S, et al (1987). *State Surveillance of Birth Defects and Other Reproductive Outcomes. Final Report to Office of Assistant Secretary for Planning and Evaluation.* Washington, DC, Department of Health and Human Services; Atlanta, GA, Centers for Disease Control.

Fost N (1992). "Ethical issues in genetics." *Pediatric Clinics of North America* 39:79–89.

Frank AL, Slesis I (1986). "Nonionizing radiation." In Last JM (ed), *Maxcy-Rosenau Public Health and Preventive Medicine*, 12th Ed., Norwalk, CT, Appleton & Lange, pp 714–726.

Fraser FC, Nora JJ (1975). *Genetics of Man.* Philadelphia, PA, Lea & Febiger, pp. 14–15.

Freire-Maia N (1990). "Five landmarks in inbreeding studies." *American Journal of Medical Genetics* 35:118–120.

Freire-Maia N, Elisbao T (1984). "Inbreeding effects on morbidity. III. A review of the world literature." *American Journal of Medical Genetics* 18:401–406.

Friedman T (1989). "Progress toward human gene therapy." *Science* 244:1275–1281.

Frost WH (1941). "Epidemiology." In *Papers of Wade Hampton Frost M.D.* New York, The Commonwealth Fund, 493–542.

Galton F (1865). "Hereditary talent and character." *Mcmillan's Magazine* 12:157.

Galton F (1887). *Natural Inheritance.* London, Macmillan.

Gantt RC, Lincoln JE (1988). "Effects of passive smoking in the multiple risk factor intervention trial." [Letter]. *American Journal of Epidemiology* 128:242.

Garrod AE (1902). "The incidence of alcaptonuria: A study in chemical individuality." *Lancet* 2:1616–1620.

Gelehrter TD, Collins FS (1990). *Principles of Medical Genetics.* Baltimore, Williams & Wilkins.

George NT, Elston RC (1987). "Testing associations between polymorphic markers and quantitative traits in pedigrees." *Genetic Epidemiology* 4:193–201.

Gibbs RA, Caskey CT (1989). "The application of recombinant DNA technology for genetic probing in epidemiology." *Annual Review of Public Health* 10:27–48.

Giblett ER (1977). "Genetic polymorphisms in human blood." *Annual Review of Genetics* 11:13–28.

Go RCP, Elston RC, Kaplan EB (1978). "Efficiency and robustness of pedigree segregation analysis." *American Journal of Human Genetics* 30:28–37.

Go RC, King MC, Bailey-Wilson J, et al (1983). "Genetic epidemiology of breast cancer and associated cancers in high risk families. I. Segregation analysis." *Journal of the National Cancer Institute* 71:455–461.

Goldberg MF, Edmonds LD, Oakley GP (1979). "Reducing birth defect risk in advanced maternal age." *Journal of the American Medical Association* 242:2292–2294.

Goldring JM, Lucier GW (1990). "Protein and DNA adducts." In Hulka BS, Wilcosky

TC, Griffith JD (eds), *Biological Markers in Epidemiology*. New York, Oxford University Press, pp 78–104.

Goldstein AM, Haile RWC, Hodge SE, Paganini-Hill A, Spence MA (1988). "Possible heterogeneity in the segregation pattern of breast cancer in families with bilateral breast cancer." *Genetic Epidemiology* 5:121–133.

Goldstein AM, Hodge SE, Haile RWC (1990). "Selection bias in case-control studies using relatives as the controls." *International Journal of Epidemiology* 18:985–989

Goldstein JL, Brown MS (1989). "Familial hypercholesterolemia." In Scriver CR, Beaudet AL, Sly WS, Valle D (eds), 6th Ed. *The Metabolic Basis of Inherited Disease*, New York, McGraw-Hill, pp 1215–1250.

Gonzalez FJ, Jaiswal AK, Nebert DW (1986). "*P450* genes: Evolution, regulation, and relationship to human cancer and pharmacogenetics." *Cold Spring Harbor Symposia on Quantitative Biology* LI:879–890.

Gonzalez FJ, Skoda RC, Kimura S, et al (1988). "Characterization of the common genetic defect in humans deficient in debrisoquine metabolism." *Nature* 331:442–446.

Goodwin DW, Schulsinger F, Hermansen L, Guze SB, Winokur G (1973). "Alcohol problems in adoptees raised apart from biological parents." *Archives of General Psychiatry* 28:238–243.

Gordis L (1988a). "Estimating risk and inferring causality in epidemiology." In Gordis L (ed), *Epidemiology and Health Risk Assessment*. New York, Oxford University Press, pp 51–60.

Gordis L (1988b). "Challenges to epidemiology in the next decade." *American Journal of Epidemiology* 128:1–9.

Gordis L (ed) (1988c). *Epidemiology and Health Risk Assessment*. New York, Oxford University Press.

Gottesman II, Shields J (1976). "A critical review of recent adoption, twin and family studies." *Schizophrenia Bulletin* 2:360–400.

Green A (1982a). "Epidemiologic considerations on studies of HLA and disease associations. I. The basic measures, concepts and estimation procedures." *Tissue Antigens* 19:245–258.

Green A (1982b). "The epidemiologic approach to studies of association between HLA and disease. II. Estimation of absolute risks, etiologic and preventive fraction." *Tissue Antigens* 19:259–268.

Greenberg DA (1986). "The effect of proband designation on segregation analysis." *American Journal of Human Genetics* 39:329–339.

Greenberg DA, Hodge SE (1985). "The heterogeneity problem. I. Separating genetic from environmental forms of the same disease." *American Journal of Medical Genetics* 21:357–371.

Greenberg F, Elder FFB, Haffner P, et al (1988). "Cytogenetic findings in a prospective series of patients with DiGeorge anomaly." *American Journal of Human Genetics* 43:605–611.

Greenberg F, James LM, Oakley GP (1983). "Estimates of birth prevalence rates of spina bifida in the United States from computer-generated maps." *American Journal of Obstetrics and Gynecology* 145:570–573.

Greenland S (1987a). "Interpretation and choice of effect measures in epidemiologic studies." *American Journal of Epidemiology* 125:761–768.

Greenland S (ed) (1987b). *Evolution of Epidemiologic Ideas. Annotated Readings on Concepts and Methods*. Chestnut Hill, MA, Epidemiology Resources.

Greenland S, Robins JM (1988). "Conceptual problems in the definition and interpretation of attributable fractions." *American Journal of Epidemiology* 128:1185–1197.

Gusella JF, Wexler NS, Conneally PM, et al (1983). "A polymorphic DNA marker genetically linked to Huntington disease." *Nature* 308:234–238.

Gustavson KH, Blomquist HK, Holmgren G (1986). "Prevalence of the fragile X syndrome in mentally retarded boys in a Swedish county." *American Journal of Medical Genetics* 23:581–587.

Guttler F, Woo SLC (1986). "Molecular genetics of PKU." *Journal of Inherited Disease, Supplement 1* 9:58–68.

Haenzel W (ed) (1970). "Symposium on cancer in migratory populations." Journal of Chronic Diseases 23:289–448.

Haenzel W, Kurihara M (1968). "Studies of Japanese migrants. I. Mortality from cancer and other diseases among Japanese of the United States." *Journal of the National Cancer Institute* 40:43–68.

Hakama M, Saxen EA (1967). "Cereal consumption and gastric cancer." *International Journal of Cancer* 2:265–268.

Haldane JBS (1919). "The combination of linkage values and the calculation of distance between the loci of linked factors." *Journal of Genetics* 8:299–309.

Haldane JBS (1946). "The interaction of nature and nurture." *Annals of Eugenics* 13:197–205.

Haldane JBS (1961). "Natural selection in man." *Progress in Medical Genetics* 1:27–37.

Haldane JBS, Smith CAB (1947). "A new estimate of the linkage between the genes for colour-blindness and haemophilia in man." *Annals of Eugenics* 14:10–31.

Hall JG (1988a). "The value of the study of the natural history in genetic disorders and congenital anomaly syndromes." *Journal of Medical Genetics* 25:434–444.

Hall JG (1988b). "Somatic mosaicism: Observations related to clinical genetics." *American Journal of Human Genetics* 43:355–363.

Hall JH, Powers EK, MiClvaine RT, Ean VH (1978). "The frequency and financial burden of genetic disease in a pediatric hospital." *American Journal of Medical Genetics* 1:417–436.

Hall JM, Lee MK, Newman B, et al (1990). "Linkage of early-onset familial breast cancer to chromsome 17q21." *Science* 250:1684–1689.

Hanis CL, Chakraborty R, Ferrell RE, Schull WJ (1986). "Individual admixture estimates: Disease associations and individual risk of diabetes and gall bladder disease among Mexican-Americans in Starr County, Texas." *American Journal of Physical Anthropology* 70:433–441.

Hanis CL, Sing CF, Clarke WR, Schrott HG (1983). "Multivariate models for human genetic analysis: Aggregation, coaggregation, and tracking of systolic blood pressure and weight." *American Journal of Human Genetics* 35:1196–1210.

Harburg E, Schull WJ, Erfurt JC, Schork MA (1970). "A family set method for estimating heredity and stress. I. A pilot survey of blood pressure among Negroes in high and low stress areas, Detroit, 1966–1967." *Journal of Chronic Diseases* 23:69–81.

Hardy GH (1908). "Mendelian proportions in a mixed population." *Science* 28:49–50.

Harper AE (1988). "Potential contributions of genetic epidemiology." [Invited commentary]. *Genetic Epidemiology* 5:203–206.

Harris H (1969). "Enzyme and protein polymorphisms in human populations." *British Medical Bulletin* 25:5.

Harris H (1980). *Principles of Human Biochemical Genetics*, 3rd Ed. Amsterdam, North-Holland.

Hartl DL (1980). *Principles of Population Genetics*. Sunderland, MA, Sinauer Associates.

Hartl DL (1983). *Human Genetics*. New York, Harper & Row.

Hartl DL, Clark AG (1989). *Principles of Population Genetics*, 2nd Ed. Sunderland, MA, Sinauer Associates.

Haseman JK, Elston RC (1972). "The investigation of linkage between a quantitative trait and marker locus." *Behavior Genetics* 2:3–19.

Hassold T, Jacobs P (1984). "Trisomy in man." *Annual Review of Genetics* 18:69–97.

Hassold T, Jacobs PA, Pettay D (1987). "Analysis of nucleolar organizer regions in parents of trisomic spontaneous abortions." *Human Genetics* 76:381–384.

Hasstedt SJ (1982). "A mixed model likelihood approximation on large pedigrees." *Computers and Biomedical Research* 15:295–307.

Hasstedt SJ (1991). "A variance components/major locus likelihood approximation on quantitative data." *Genetic Epidemiology* 8:113–125.

Hasstedt SJ, Cartwright P (1981). *PAP: Pedigree Analysis Program*. Technical Report 13, Department of Medical Computing and Biophysics, University of Utah. Salt Lake City, University of Utah Press.

Hasstedt SJ, Kuida H, Ash KO, Williams WR (1985). "Effects of household sharing on high-density lipoprotein and its subfractions." *Genetic Epidemiology* 2:339–348.

Hastrup JL, Hotchkiss AP, Johnson CA (1985). "Accuracy of knowledge of family history of cardiovascular disorders." *Health Psychology* 4:291–306.

Hauge M (1980). "The Danish twin register." In Mednick SA, Baert AE (eds), *An Empirical Basis for Primary Prevention: Prospective Longitudinal Research in Europe*. Oxford, Oxford University Press, pp 217–221.

Hayden MR, Robbins C, Allard D, et al (1988). "Improved predictive testing for Huntington disease by using three linked DNA markers." *American Journal of Human Genetics* 43:689–694.

Hayes A, Costa T, Scriver CR, Childs B (1985). "The effect of mendelian disease on human health. II. Response to treatment." *American Journal of Medical Genetics* 21:243–255.

Hecht NB (1987). "Detecting the effects of toxic agents on spermatogenesis using DNA probes." *Environmental Health Perspectives* 74:31–40.

Heinonen OP, Slone D, Shapiro S (1977). *Birth Defects and Drugs in Pregnancy*. Littleton, MA, Publishing Group.

Helena M, Franco LP, Weimer TA, Salzano FM (1982). "Blood polymorphisms and racial admixture in two Brazilian populations." *American Journal of Physical Anthropology* 58:127–132.

Heston LL (1966). "Psychiatric disorders in foster-home–reared children of schizophrenic mothers." *British Journal of Psychiatry* 112:819–825.

Hewson D, Bennet A (1987). "Childbirth research data: Medical records or women's reports." *American Journal of Epidemiology* 125:484–491.

Hill AB (1965). "The environment and disease: Association or causation?" *Proceedings of the Royal Society of Medicine* 58:295–300.

Hill AVS, Wainscoat JS. 1986. "The evolution of the alpha and beta gene clusters in human populations." *Human Heridity* 74:16–23.

Hodge SE (1988). "Conditioning on subsets of the data: Applications to ascertainment and other genetic problems." *American Journal of Human Genetics* 43:364–373.

Hogue CJR, Brewster MA (1988). "Developmental risks: Epidemiologic advances in health assessment." In Gordis L (ed), *Epidemiology and Health Risk Assessment*. New York, Oxford University Press, pp. 61–81.

Holland WW, Detels R, Knox G (eds) (1984). *Oxford Textbook of Public Health*, Vol. I: *History, Determinants, Scope and Strategies*. New York, Oxford University Press.

Holmes LB, Driscoll S, Atkins L (1976). "Etiologic heterogeneity of neural tube defects." *New England Journal of Medicine* 294:365–369.

Holmes LB, Vincent SE, Cook C, Cote KR (1981). "Surveillance of newborn infants for malformations due to spontaneous germinal mutations." In Hook EB, Porter IH (eds), *Population and Biological Aspects of Human Mutation* New York, Academic Press, pp 351–360.

Holmes-Snedle M, Lindenbaum RH, Galliard A (1982). "Vitamin supplementation and neural tube defects." *Lancet* 1:276.

Holtzman NA (1978). "Genetic screening for phenylketonuria and its effectiveness." In Cohen BH, Lilienfeld AM, Huang PC (eds), *Genetic Issues in Public Health and Medicine*. Springfield, IL, CC Thomas, pp 193–205.

Holtzman NA (1989). *Proceed with Caution: Predicting Genetic Risks in the Recombinant DNA Era*. Baltimore, MD, Johns Hopkins University Press.

Holtzman NA, Khoury MJ (1986). Monitoring for congenital malformations. *Annual Reviews of Public Health* 7:237–266.

Hook EB (1982). "Contributions of chromosomal abnormalities to human morbidity and mortality and some comments upon surveillance of chromosome mutation rates." *Progress in Mutation Research* 3:9–38.

Hook EB, Cross PK (1988). "Maternal cigarette smoking, Down syndrome in live births, and infant race." *American Journal of Human Genetics* 42:482–489.

Hook EB, Cross PK, Schreinemachers D (1981). "The evolution of the New York State Chromosome Registry." In Hook EB, Cross PK (eds), *Population and Biological Aspects of Human Mutation*. New York, Academic Press, pp 389–428.

Hook EB, Lamson SH (1980). "Rates of Down syndrome at the upper extreme of maternal age—absence of a levelling effect and evidence for artifacts resulting from analyses of rates by five-year maternal age intervals." *American Journal of Epidemiology* 112:75–80.

Hook EB, Porter IH (eds) (1981). *Population and Biological Aspects of Human Mutation*. New York, Academic Press.

Hopper JL (1986). "On analysis of path models by multivariate normal model for pedigree analysis." *Genetic Epidemiology* 3:279–281.

Hopper JL, Derrick PL (1986). "A log linear model for binary pedigree data." *Genetic Epidemiology, Supplement* 1:73–82.

Hopper JL, Hannah MC, Mathews JD (1984). "Genetic analysis workshop II: Pedigree analysis of a binary trait without assuming an underlying liability." *Genetic Epidemiology* 1:184–188.

Hopper JL, Judd FK, Derrick PL, Macaskill GT, Burrows GD (1990). "A family study of panic disorder: Reanalysis using a regressive logistic model that incorporates sibship environment." *Genetic Epidemiology* 7:151–161.

Hopper JL, Mathews JD (1982). "Extensions to multivariate normal models for pedigree analysis." *Annals of Human Genetics* 39:485–491.

Hopper JL, Mathews JD (1983.) "Extensions to multivariate normal models for pedigree analysis. II. Modeling the effect of shared environment in the analysis of variation in blood lead levels." *American Journal of Epidemiology* 117:344–355.

Horn N, Morton NE (1986). Genetic epidemiology of Menkes disease." *Genetic Epidemiology* 3:225–230.

Howson CP, Hiyama T, Wynder EL (1986). "The decline in gastric cancer: Epidemiology of an unplanned triumph." *Epidemiologic Reviews* 8:1–27.

Hrubec Z, Neel JV (1978). "The National Academy of Sciences–National Research Council Twin Registry: 10 years of operation." *Progress in Clinical and Biological Research* 24B:153–172.

Hrubec Z, Robinette CD (1984). "The study of human twins in medical research." *New England Journal of Medicine* 310:435–441.

Huggins M, Bloch M, Kanani S, et al (1990). "Ethical and legal dilemmas arising during predictive testing for adult-onset disease: The experience of Huntington disease." *American Journal of Human Genetics* 47:4–12.

Hulka BS, Hogue CJR, Greenberg BG (1978). "Methodologic issues in epidemiologic studies of endometrial cancer and exogenous estrogens." *American Journal of Epidemiology* 107:267–276.

Hulka BS, Wilcosky T (1988). "Markers in epidemiologic research." *Archives of Environmental Health* 43:83–89.

Humphries P, Kenna P, Farrer GJ (1992). "On the molecular genetics of retinitis pigmentosa." *Science* 256:805–808.

Hunt SC, Hasstedt SJ, William RR (1986). "Testing for familial aggregation of a dichotomous trait." *Genetic Epidemiology* 3:299–312.

Hutchinson GB (1980). "Prevalence, incidence and duration." *American Journal of Epidemiology* 112:707–723.

Hutchinson TP (1980). "An easy method of calculating approximate recurrence risks using a multifactorial model of disease transmission." *Annals of Human Genetics* 43:285–293.

International Clearinghouse for Birth Defects Monitoring Systems (1985). *Annual Report.*

International Clearinghouse for Birth Defects Monitoring Systems (1987). "Epidemiology of bladder extrophy and epispadias." *TERATOLOGY* 36:221–228.

Jackson-Cook CK, Flannery DB, Corey LA, Nance WE, Brown JA (1985). "Nucleolar organizer region variants as a risk factor for Down syndrome." *American Journal of Human Genetics* 37:1049–1061.

Jacquard A (1974). *The Genetic Structure of Populations.* New York, Springer-Verlag.

Jacquard A (1983). "Heritability: One word, three concepts." *Biometrics* 39:465–477.

Janerich DT, Bracken MB (1986). "Epidemiology of trisomy 21: A review and theoretical analysis." *Journal of Chronic Diseases* 39:1079–1093.

Jeffreys AJ, Royle NJ, Wilson V, Wong Z (1988). "Spontaneous mutation rates to new length alleles at tandem-repetitive hypervariable loci in human DNA." *Nature* 332:278–281.

Jenkins JB, Conneally PM (1989). "The paradigm of Huntington disease." *American Journal of Human Genetics* 45:169–175.

Jones KL (1988). *Smith's Recognizable Patterns of Human Malformations*, 4th Ed. Philadelphia, PA, WB Saunders.

Jones ME (1980). Pyrimidine nucleotide biosynthesis in animals: Genes, enzymes and regulation of UMP biosynthesis." *Annual Review of Biochemistry* 49:253–.

Jorde LB, Fineman RM, Martin RA (1983). "Epidemiology and genetics of neural tube defects: An application of the Utah genealogic data base." *American Journal of Physical Anthropolgy* 62:32–51.

Kaback M (1981). "Heterozygote screening and prenatal diagnosis in Tay-Sachs disease: A worldwide update." In Callhan J, Lowden J (eds), *Lysomes and Lyso-somal Storage Diseases*. New York, Raven Press, p 331.

Kaback MM (1983). "Heterozygote screening." In Emery AEH, Rimoin DL (eds), *Principles and Practice of Medical Genetics*, Vol. II. Edinburgh, Churchill Livingstone, pp 1451–1457.

Kahkonen M, Alitalo T, Airaksinen E, et al (1987). "Prevalence of the fragile X syndrome in four birth cohorts of children of school age." Human Genetics 77:85–87.

Kahn H (1983). *An Introduction to Epidemiologic Methods*. New York, Oxford University Press.

Kahn HA, Sempos CT (1989). *Statistical Methods in Epidemiology*. New York, Oxford University Press.

Kallen B (1988). *Epidemiology of Human Reproduction*. Boca Raton, CRC Press.

Kallen B, Hay S, Klinberg M (1984.) "Birth defects monitoring systems: accomplishments and goals." In Kalter H (ed), *Issues and Reviews in Teratology*, Vol. 2. New York, Plenum Press, pp 1–22.

Kallen B, Knudsen LB (1989). "Effect of maternal age distribution and prenatal diagnosis on the population rates of Down syndrome: A comparative study of nineteen populations." *Hereditas* 110:55–60.

Kaprio J, Sarna S, Koskenvuo M, Rantasalo I (1978). "The Finnish Twin Registry: Formation and compilation, questionnaire study, zygosity determination procedures, and research programs." *Progress in Clinical and Biological Research* 24B: 179–184.

Kark JA, Posey DM, Schumacher HR, Ruehle CJ (1987). "Sickle cell trait as a risk factor for sudden death in physical training." New England Journal of Medicine 317:781–787.

Kaslow RA, Shaw S (1981). "The role of histocompatibility antigens (HLA) in infection." *Epidemiologic Reviews* 3:90–114.

Kato H, Tillotson J, Nichaman MZ, et al (1973). "Epidemiologic studies of coronary heart disease and stroke in Japanese men living in Japan, Hawaii, and California." *American Journal of Epidemiology* 97:372–385.

Kazazian HH (1978). "Genetic screening: Prerequisites and further considerations." In Cohen BH, Lilienfeld AM, Huang PC (eds), *Genetic Issues in Public Health and Medicine* Springfield, IL, CC Thomas, pp 193–205.

Kellerman G, Shaw CR, Luyten-Kellerman M (1973). "Aryl hydrocarbon hydroxylase inducibility and bronchogenic carcinoma." *New England Journal of Medicine* 289:934–937.

Kelsey JL (1979). "A review of the epidemiology of human breast cancer. *Epidemiologic Reviews* 1:74–109.

Kelsey JL, Thompson WD, Evans AS (1986). *Methods in Observational Epidemiology*. New York, Oxford University Press.

Kessler S (1976). "Progress and regress in the research of the genetics of schizophrenia." *Schizophrenia Bulletin* 2:434–438.

Khlat M, Khoury MJ (1991). "Inbreeding and diseases: Demographic, genetic and epidemiologic perspectives." *Epidemiologic Reviews* 13:28–41.

Khoury MJ (1985). "A genealogic study of inbreeding and prereproductive mortality in the Old Order Amish." PhD Thesis, The Johns Hopkins University, Baltimore, MD.

Khoury MJ, Adams MJ, Flanders WD (1988a). "An epidemiologic approach to eco-genetics." *American Journal of Human Genetics* 42:89–95.

Khoury MJ, Beaty TH, Flanders WD (1990). "Epidemiologic approaches to the use of DNA markers in the search for disease susceptibility genes." *Epidemiologic Reviews* 12:41–55.

Khoury MJ, Beaty TH, Liang KY (1988b). "Can familial aggregation of disease be explained by familial aggregation of environmental risk factors?" *American Journal of Epidemiology* 127:674–683.

Khoury MJ, Beaty TH, Newill CA, Bryant S, Cohen BH (1986). "Genetic-environmental interaction in chronic obstructive pulmonary disease." *International Journal of Epidemiology* 15:64–71.

Khoury MJ, Beaty TH, Tockman MS, Self SG, Cohen BH (1985a). "Familial aggregation in chronic obstructive pulmonary disease: Use of the loglinear model to analyze intermediate genetic and environmental risk factors." *Genetic Epidemiology* 2:155–166.

Khoury MJ, Becerra JE, d'Almada P (1989a). "Maternal thyroid disease and the risk of birth defects in offspring: A population-based case-control study." *Paediatric and Perinatal Epidemiology* 3:420–439.

Khoury MJ, Cohen BH (1988). "Concepts and terms in genetic epidemiology: Some similarities to infectious disease epidemiology." *Journal of Clinical Epidemiology* 41:1181–1187.

Khoury MJ, Cohen BH, Chase GA, Diamond EL (1987a). "An epidemiologic approach to the evaluation of the effect of inbreeding on prereproductive mortality." *American Journal of Epidemiology* 125:251–262.

Khoury MJ, Cohen BH, Diamond EL, Chase GA, McKusick VA (1987b) "Inbreeding and prereproductive mortality in the Old Order Amish. I. Genealogic epidemiology of inbreeding." *American Journal of Epidemiology* 125:453–461.

Khoury MJ, Erickson JD (1983a). "Maternal factors in dizygotic twinning: Evidence from interracial crosses." *Annals of Human Biology* 10:409–415.

Khoury MJ, Erickson JD, James LM (1983b). "Maternal factors in cleft lip with or without cleft palate: Evidence from interracial crosses in the United States." *Teratology* 27:351–357.

Khoury MJ, Erickson JD, James LM (1982a). "Etiologic heterogeneity of neural tube defects: Clues from epidemiology." *American Journal of Epidemiology* 115:538–548.

Khoury MJ, Erickson JD, James LM (1982b). "Etiologic heterogeneity of neural tube defects. II. Clues from family studies." *American Journal of Human Genetics* 34:980–987.

Khoury MJ, Erickson JD, James LM (1984). "Paternal effects on the secondary sex ratio: Evidence from interracial crosses in the United States." *American Journal of Human Genetics* 36:1103–1111.

Khoury MJ, Farias MG, Mulinare J (1989b). "Does maternal cigarette smoking during pregnancy cause cleft lip and palate in offspring?" *American Journal of Diseases of Children* 143:333–337.

Khoury MJ, Flanders WD (1989). "On the measurement of susceptibility to genetic factors." *Genetic Epidemiology* 6:699–711.

Khoury MJ, Flanders WD, Adams MJ, Greenland S (1989c). "On the measurement of susceptibility in epidemiologic studies." *American Journal of Epidemiology* 129:183–190.

Khoury MJ, Flanders WD, Beaty TH (1988c). "Penetrance in the presence of genetic susceptibility to environmental factors." *American Journal of Medical Genetics* 29:397–404.

Khoury MJ, Flanders WD, James LM, Erickson JD (1989d). "Human teratogens, prenatal mortality, and selection bias." *American Journal of Epidemiology* 130:361–370.

Khoury MJ, Holtzman NA (1987). "On the ability of birth defects monitoring to detect new teratogens." *American Journal of Epidemiology* 126:136–143.

Khoury MJ, Newill CA, Chase GA (1985b). "Epidemiologic evaluation of screening for risk factors: Application to genetic screening." *American Journal of Public Health* 75:1204–1208.

Khoury MJ, Stewart W, Beaty TH (1987c). "The effect of genetic susceptibility on causal inference in epidemiologic studies." *American Journal of Epidemiology* 126:561–567.

Khoury MJ, Stewart W, Weinstein A, Panny S, Lindsay P, Eisenberg M (1988d). "Residential mobility during pregnancy: Implications for environmental teratogenesis." *Journal of Clinical Epidemiology* 41:15–20.

Kimbel P (1988). "Proteolytic damage and emphysema pathogenesis." In Petty TL (ed), *Chronic Obstructive Pulmonary Disease.* 2nd Ed. New York, Marcel Dekker, pp 105–128.

King H, Jun-Yao L, Locke FB, et al (1985). "Patterns of age-specific displacement in cancer mortality among migrants: The Chinese in the United States." *American Journal of Public Health* 75:237–242.

King JL, Jukes TH (1969). "Non-darwinian evolution." *Science* 164:788–798.

King MC (1984). "Genetic and epidemiologic approaches to detecting genetic susceptibility to chemical exposure. Genetic variability in responses to chemical exposure." *Banbury Report* 16:377–392.

King MC, Go RC, Lynch HT, et al (1983). "Genetic epidemiology of breast cancer and associated cancers in high-risk families. II. Linkage analysis." *Journal of the National Cancer Institute* 71:463–467.

King MC, Lee GM, Spinner NB, Thomson G, Wrensch MR (1984). "Genetic epidemiology." *American Review of Public Health* 5:1–52.

Klemetti A, Saxen L (1967). "Prospective versus retrospective approach in the search for environmental causes of malformations." *American Journal of Public Health* 57:2071–2075.

Klinberg MA, Papier CM, Hart J (1983). "Birth defects monitoring." *American Journal of Industrial Medicine* 4:309–338.

Kline J, Stein Z, Susser M (1989). *Conception to Birth: Epidemiology of Prenatal Development.* New York, Oxford University Press.

Knowler WC, Williams RC, Pettitt DJ, Steinberg AG (1988). "Gm 3;5,13,14 and type 2 diabetes mellitus: An association in American Indians with genetic admixture." *American Journal of Human Genetics* 43:520–526.

Knudson AG, Wayne L, Hallet WY (1967). "On the selective advantages of cystic fibrosis heterozygotes." *American Journal of Human Genetics* 19:388–392.

Konecki DS, Lichter-Konecki UL. (1991). "The phenylketonuria locus: Current knowledge about alleles and mutations of the phenylalanine hydroxylase gene in various populations." *Human Genetics* 83:377–388.

Konigsberg LW, Blangero J, Kammerer CM, Mott GE (1991). "Mixed model segregation analysis of LDL-C concentration with genotype-covariate interaction." *Genetic Epidemiology* 8:69–80.

Kosambi DD (1944). "The estimation of map distances from recombination values." *Annals of Eugenics* 12:172–175.

Kovacs BW, Shahbahrami B, Comings DE (1989). "Studies of human germinal mutations by deoxyribonucleic acid hybridization." *American Journal of Obstetrics and Gynecology* 160:798–804.

Kravitz K, Skolnick M, Cannings C, et al (1979). "Genetic linkage between hereditary hemochromatosis and HLA." *American Journal of Human Genetics* 31:601.

Krieger H, Morton NE, Mi MP, Azevedo E, Freire-Maia A, Yasuda N (1965). "Racial admixture in north-east Brazil." *Annals of Human Genetics* 29:113–125.

Kristensen P (1992). Bias from nondifferential but dependent misclassification of exposure and outcome. *Epidemiology* 3:210–215.

Krolewski AS, Warram JH, Rand LI, Kahn CR (1987). "Epidemiologic approach to the etiology of type I diabetes mellitus and its complications." *New England Journal of Medicine* 317:1390–1398.

Kueppers F (1978). "Inherited differences in alpha 1-antitrypsin." In Litwin SD (ed), *Genetic Determinants of Pulmonary Disease*. New York, Marcel Dekker, pp 23–74.

Kunkel LM (1986). "Analysis of deletions in DNA from patients with Becker and Duchenne muscular dystrophy." *Nature* 322:73–77.

Kurland LT, Molgaard CA (1981). "The patient record in epidemiology." *Scientific American* 245:54–63.

Kwon JM, Boehnke M, Burns TL, Moll PP 1990. "Commingling and segregation analyses: Comparison of results from a simulation study of a quantitative trait." *Genetic Epidemiology* 7:57–68.

Lalouel JM, Morton NE (1981). "Complex segregation analysis with pointers." *Human Heredity* 31:312–321.

Lalouel JM, Rao DC, Morton NE, Elston RC (1983). "A unified model for complex segregation analysis." *American Journal of Human Genetics* 35:816–826.

Lander ES, Botstein D (1987). "Homozygosity mapping: A way to map human recessive traits with the DNA of inbred children." *Science* 236:1567–1570.

Lange K (1978). "Central limit theorems for pedigrees." *Journal of Mathematical Biology* 6:59–66.

Lange K, Boehnke M (1983). "Extensions to pedigree analysis. IV. Covariance components models for multivariate traits." *American Journal of Medical Genetics* 14:513–524.

Lange K, Elston RC (1975). "Extensions to pedigree analysis: Likelihood computations for simple and complex pedigrees." *Human Heredity* 25:95–105.

Lange K, Westlake J, Spence MA (1976). "Extensions to pedigree analysis. III. Variance components by the scoring method." *Annals of Human Genetics* 39:485–491.

LaPorte RE, Tajima N, Akerblom HK, et al (1985). "Geographic differences in the risk for insulin dependent diabetes mellitus: The importance of registries." *Diabetes Care, Supplement 1* 8:101–end.

Lappe MA (1986). "Ethical concerns in occupational screening programs." *Journal of Medicine* 28:930–934.

Last JM (1986a). "Epidemiology and health information." In Last JM (ed), *Maxcy-Rosenau Public Health and Preventive Medicine*, 12th Ed. Norwalk, CT, Appleton & Lange, pp 9–74.

Last JM (1986b). In Last, JM (ed), *Maxcy-Rosenau Public Health and Preventive Medicine*, 12th Ed. Norwalk, CT, Appleton & Lange, pp 3–7.

Lathrop GM, Lalouel JM, Julier C, Ott J (1984). "Strategies for multilocus linkage analysis in humans." *Proceedings of the National Academy of Sciences of the United States of America* 81:3443–3446.

Lathrop GM, Lalouel JM, Julier C, Ott J (1985). "Multilocus linkage analysis in humans: Detection of linkage and estimation of recombination." *American Journal of Human Genetics* 37:482–498.

Lathrop GM, Lalouel JM, White NW (1986). "Construction of human linkage maps: Likelihood calculations for multilocus linkage analysis." *Genetic Epidemiology* 3:39–52.

Laurence KM, James N, Miller MH et al (1981). "Double blind randomized controlled clinical trial of folate treatment before conception to prevent the recurrence of neural tube defects." *British Medical Journal* 282:1509–1511.

Lebel RR (1983). "Consanguinity studies in Wisconsin. I. Secular trends in consanguineous marriages, 1843–1981." *American Journal of Medical Genetics* 15:543–560.

Ledbetter DH, Cassidy SB (1988). "Etiology of Prader-Willi syndrome." In Caldwell ML, Taylor FL (eds), *Prader-Willi Syndrome: Selected Research and Management Issues*. New York, Springer-Verlag, pp 13–28.

Lemma W, Feldman GL, Kerem B, et al (1990). "Mutation analysis for heterozygote detection and prenatal diagnosis of cystic fibrosis." *New England Journal of Medicine* 322:291–296.

Lenke RR, Levy HL (1980). "Maternal phenylketonuria and hyperphenylalaninemia." *New England Journal of Medicine* 303:1202–1208.

Lennard L, Lilleyman JS, Van Loon J, Weinshilboum RM (1990). "Genetic variation in response to 6-mercaptopurine for childhood acute lymphoblastic leukemia." *Lancet* 336:225–229.

Levin ML (1953). "The occurrence of lung cancer in man." *Acta Unio International Contra Cancrum* 9:531–541.

Levitan M (1988). *Textbook of Human Genetics*. New York, Oxford University Press.

Leviton A (1973). "Definitions of attributable risk." *American Journal of Epidemiology* 98:231.

Li CC (1961). *Human Genetics: Principles and Methods*. New York, McGraw-Hill, pp 131–141.

Li CC (1963). "The way the load works." *American Journal of Human Genetics* 15:316–321.

Li CC (1975). *Path Analysis—A Primer*. Pacific Grove, CA, Boxwood Press.

Li CC (1987). "A genetical model for emergenesis: In memory of Laurence H. Snyder 1901–86." *American Journal of Human Genetics* 41:517–523.

Li CC, Chakravarti A, Halloran SL (1987). "Estimation of segregation and ascertainment probabilities by discarding the single probands." *Genetic Epidemiology* 4:185–191.

Li CC, Mantel N (1968). "A simple method of estimating the segregation ratio under complete ascertainment." *American Journal of Human Genetics* 20:61–81.

Li CC, Sacks L (1954). "The derivation of joint distribution and correlation between relatives by the use of stochastic matrices." *Biometrics* 10:347–360.

Liang KY (1987). "Extended Mantel-Haenszel estimating procedure for multivariate logistic regression models." *Biometrics* 43:289–299.

Liang KY, Beaty TH (1991). "Measuring familial aggregation using odds ratio regression models." *Genetic Epidemiology* 8:361–370.

Liang KY, Beaty TH, Cohen BH (1986). "Application of odds ratio regression models for assessing familial aggregation from case-control studies." *American Journal of Epidemiology* 124:678–683.

Liang KY, Zeger SL (1985). "Longitudinal data analysis using generalized linear model." *Biometrika* 73:13–22.

Liang KY, Zeger SL, Qaqish B (1992). "Multivariate regression analyses for categorical data." *Journal of the Royal Statistical Society, Series B* 54:3–40.

Liberatos P, Link BG, Kelsey JL (1988). "The measurement of social class in epidemiology." *Epidemiologic Reviews* 10:87–121.

Lilienfeld AM (1959). "A methodological problem in testing a recessive genetic hypothesis in human disease." *American Journal of Public Health* 49:199–204.

Lilienfeld AM (1961). "Problems and areas in genetic-epidemiological field studies." *New York Academy of Science* 91:797–805.

Lilienfeld AM (1965). "Formal discussion of the role of genetic factors in the etiology of cancer: An epidemiologic view." *Cancer Research* 25:1330–1335.

Lilienfeld AM (1969). *Epidemiology of Mongolism*. Baltimore, The Johns Hopkins University Press.

Lilienfeld AM (1973). "Epidemiology in infectious and non-infectious disease: Some comparisons." *American Journal of Epidemiology* 97:135–147.

Lilienfeld AM, Lilienfeld DE (1980). *Foundations of Epidemiology*, 2nd Ed. New York, Oxford University Press.

Lin HJ, Conte WJ, Rotter JI (1985). "Disease risk estimates from marker association data: Application to individuals at risk for hemochromatosis." *Clinical Genetics* 27:127–133.

Lindgren BE (1976). *Statistical Theory*. 3rd Ed. New York, Macmillan, p 130.

Linet MS, Van Natta ML, Brookmeyer R, et al (1989). "Familial cancer history and chronic lymphocytic leukemia: A case-control study." *American Journal of Epidemiology* 130:655–664.

Lipton R, LaPorte RE (1989). "Epidemiology of islet cell antibodies." *Epidemiologic Reviews* 11:182–203.

Littlefield JW (1984). "Genes, chromosomes and cancer." *Journal of Pediatrics* 104:489–494.

Loomis D, Wing S (1990). "Is molecular epidemiology a germ theory for the end of the twentieth century?" *International Journal of Epidemiology* 19:1–3.

Lubin JH, Bale SJ (1987). "On the detection of excess disease risk in family data." *Genetic Epidemiology* 4:447–456.

Lyon MF (1985). "Measuring mutation in man." *Nature* 318:315–316.

MacKenzie SG, Lippman A (1989). "An investigation of report bias in a case-control study of pregnancy outcome." *American Journal of Epidemiology* 129:65–75.

MacLaughlin JK, Blot WJ, Mehl ES, et al (1985). "Problems in the use of dead controls in case-control studies. I. General results." *American Journal of Epidemiology* 121:131–139.

MacLean CJ, Morton NE, Lew R (1975). "Analysis of family resemblance. IV. Operational characteristics of segregation analysis." *American Journal of Human Genetics* 27:365–384.

MacMahon B (1978). "Epidemiologic approaches to family resemblance." In Morton NE, Chung CS (eds), *Genetic Epidemiology*. New York, Academic Press, pp 3–11.

MacMahon B, Pugh TF (1970). *Epidemiology: Principles and Methods*. Boston, Little, Brown.

Maestri NE, Beaty TH, Liang KY, Boughman JA, Ferencz C (1988). "Assessing familial aggregation of congenital cardiovascular malformations in case-control studies." *Genetic Epidemiology* 5:343–354.

Magenis RE (1988). "On the origin of chromosomal anomaly." *American Journal of Human Genetics* [Invited Editorial]. 42:529–533.

Mahler H (1988). "Present status of WHO's initiative, 'Health for All by the year 2000'." *Annual Review of Public Health* 9:71–97.

Mahley RW (1988). "Apolipoprotein E: Cholesterol transport protein with expanding role in cell biology." *Science* 240:622–624.

Majumder P, Chakraborty R, Weiss KM, Smouse PE (1983). "Relative risks of diseases in the presence of incomplete penetrance and sporadics." *Statistics in Medicine* 2:13–24.

Mange AP, Mange EJ (1990). *Genetics: Human Aspects*. 2nd Ed. Sunderland, MA, Sinauer Associates.

Mantel H, Haenszel W (1959). "Statistical aspects of the analysis of data from retrospective studies." *Journal of the National Cancer Institute* 22:719–748.

Mantel N (1963). "Chi-square tests with one degree of freedom: Extensions of the Mantel-Haenzel procedure." *Journal of the American Statistical Association* 58:690–700.

Marayuma T, Yasuda N (1970). "Use of graph theory in computation of inbreeding and kinship coefficients." *Biometrics* 26:209–219.

Marmot MG (1989). "Socioeconomic determinants of CHD mortality." *International Journal of Epidemiology* 18:S196–S202.

Marmot MG, Kogevinas M, Elston MA (1987). "Social/economic status and disease." *Annual Review of Public Health* 8:111–135.

Mather K (1949). *Biometrical Genetics*. New York, Dover Publishers.

Mattei JF, Mattei MG, Giraud F (1985). "Prader-Willi syndrome and chromosome 15: A clinical discussion of 20 cases." *Human Genetics* 64:356–362.

Mattson ME, Pollack ES, Cullen JW (1987). "What are the odds that smoking will kill you?" *American Journal of Public Health* 77:425–431.

Mausner JS, Kramer S (1985). *Epidemiology: An Introductory Text*, 2nd Ed. Philadelphia, PA, WB Saunders.

McGinnis JM, Shopland D (1987). "Tobacco and health: Trends in smoking and smokeless tobacco consumption in the United States." *Annual Review of Public Health* 8:441–467.

McGue M, Wette R, Rao DC (1984). "Evaluation of path analysis through computer simulation: Effect of incorrectly assuming independent distribution of familial correlations." *Genetic Epidemiology* 1:255–270.

McGuffin P, Huckle P (1990). "Simulation of Mendelism revisited: The recessive gene for attending medical school." *American Journal of Human Genetics* 46:994–999.

McKusick VA (1978). *Medical Genetic Studies of the Amish: Selected Papers*. Baltimore, MD, Johns Hopkins University Press.

McKusick VA (1986). *Mendelian Inheritance in Man: Catalogs of Autosomal Dominant, Autosomal Recessive, and X-Linked Phenotypes*, 7th Ed. Baltimore, MD, Johns Hopkins University Press.

McKusick VA (1988a). *Mendelian Inheritance in Man: Catalogs of Autosomal Dominant, Autosomal Recessive, and X-Linked Phenotypes*, 8th Ed. Baltimore, MD, Johns Hopkins University Press.

McKusick VA (1988b). *The Morbid Anatomy of the Human Genome: A Review of Gene Mapping in Clinical Medicine*. Howard Hughes Medical Institute.

McKusick VA (1989). "Mapping and sequencing the human genome." *New England Journal of Medicine* 320:910–915.

McKusick VA (1990). *Mendelian Inheritance in Man*, 9th Ed. Baltimore, MD, Johns Hopkins University Press.

McMichael AJ, Bonnett A, Roder D (1989). "Cancer incidence among migrant populations in South Australia." *Medical Journal of Australia* 150:417–420.

McMichael AJ, McCall MG, Hartshorne JM, et al (1980). "Patterns of gastrointestinal cancer in European migrants to Australia: The role of dietary change." *International Journal of Cancer* 25:431–437.

Meade MS (1986). "Geographic analysis of disease and care." *Annual Review of Public Health* 7:313–335.

Medical Research Council Vitamin Study Research Group (1991). "Prevention of neural tube defects: Results of the Medical Research Council Vitamin study." *Lancet* 338:131–137.

Meinert CL (1986). *Clinical Trials: Design, Conduct and Analysis*. New York, Oxford University Press.

Meissen GJ, Myers RH, Mastromauro CA, et al (1988). "Predictive testing of Huntington disease with use of a linked DNA marker." *New England Journal of Medicine* 318:535–542.

Mendelsohn ML (1987). "Biomarkers in the detection of human heritable and germinal mutations." *Environmental Health Perspectives* 74:49–53.

Menkes HA, Cohen BH, Beaty TH, Newill CA, Khoury MJ (1984). "Risk factors, pulmonary function and mortality." *Progress in Clinical and Biological Research* 147:501–521.

Meyers DA, Beaty TH, Colyer CR, Francomano CA (1989). "Methods for genetic mapping in an inbred population isolate." *American Journal of Human Genetics* 45.A152.

Miettinen OS (1974). "Proportion of disease caused or prevented by a given exposure, trait or intervention." *American Journal of Epidemiology* 99:325–332.

Miettinen OS, Cook EF (1981). "Confounding: Essence and detection." *American Journal of Epidemiology* 114:593–603.

Mili F, Khoury MJ, Flanders WD, Greenberg R (199). "The risk of childhood cancer in infants with birth defects: A record-linkage study." [Abstract]. *American Journal of Epidemiology* 132:764–765.

Miller JR (1983). "Perspectives in mutation epidemiology. 4. General principles and considerations." *Mutation Research* 114:425–447.

Miller RC (1988). "Epidemiologic evidence for genetic variability in the frequency of cancer: Ethnic differences." In Woodhead AD, Bender MA, Leonard RC (eds), *Phenotypic Variation in Populations: Relevance to Risk Assessment*. New York, Plenum Press, pp 65–70.

Miller RW (1968). "Relation between cancer and congenital defects in man." *New England Journal of Medicine* 275:87–93.

Miller RW (1969). "Childhood cancer and congenital defects. A study of U.S. death certificates during the period 1960–1966." *Pediatric Research* 3:389–397.

Mills JL, Rhoads GG, Simpson JL, et al (1989). "The absence of a relation between the periconceptional use of vitamins and neural tube defects." *New England Journal of Medicine* 321:430–435.

Milunsky A, Jick H, Jick S, et al (1989). "Multivitamin/folic acid supplementation in early pregnancy reduces the prevalence of neural tube defects." *Journal of the American Medical Association* 262:2847–2852.

Mitchell AA, Cottler LB, Shapiro S, et al (1986). "Effect of questionnaire design on recall of drug exposure in pregnancy." *American Journal of Epidemiology* 123:670–676.

Modan B (1980). "Role of migrant studies in understanding the etiology of cancer." *American Journal of Epidemiology* 112:289–295.

Moldin SO, Rice JP, Van Eerdewegh P, Grottesman II, Erlenmeyer-Kimling L (1990). "Estimation of disease risk under bivariate models of multifactorial inheritance." *Genetic Epidemiology* 7:371–386.

Moll PP (1984). "The Tecumseh community health study." [Discussion]. In Rao DC, Elston RC, Kuller LH, Feinleib M, Carter C, Havlik R (eds), *Genetic Epidemiology of Coronary Heart Disease: Past, Present and Future*. New York, Alan R Liss, pp 37–42.

Moll PP, Berty TD, Weidman WH, Ellefson R, Gordon H, Kottke B (1984a). "Detection of genetic heterogeneity among pedigrees through complex segregation analysis: An application to hypercholesterolemia." *American Journal of Human Genetics* 36:197–211.

Moll PP, Harburg E, Burns TL, Schork MA, Ozgoren F (1983). "Heredity, stress and blood pressure; a family set approach: The Detroit project revisited." *Journal of Chronic Diseases* 36:317–328.

Moll PP, Michels VV, Weidman WH, Kottke BA (1989). "Genetic determination of plasma apolipoprotein A_1 in a population-based sample." *American Journal of Human Genetics* 44:124–139.

Moll PP, Sing CF, Lussier-Cacan S, Davignon J (1984b). "An application of a model for a genotype-dependent relationship between a concomitant (age) and a quantitative trait (LDL cholesterol) in pedigree data." *Genetic Epidemiology* 1:301–314.

Moody PA (1975). *Genetics of Man*. 2nd Ed. New York, WW Norton, pp 25, 297.

Morel PA, Dorman JS, Todd JA, McDevitt HO, Trucco M (1988). "Aspartic acid at position 57 of the HLA-DQ beta chain protects against type I diabetes: A family study." *Proceedings of the National Academy of Sciences of the United States of America* 85:8111–8115.

Morgenstern H (1982). "Uses of ecologic analysis in epidemiologic research." *American Journal of Public Health* 72:1336–1344.

Morton NE (1955). "Sequential tests for the detection of linkage." *American Journal of Human Genetics* 7:277–318.

Morton NE (1956). "The detection and estimation of linkage between the genes for elliptocytosis and the Rh blood type." *American Journal of Human Genetics* 8:80–91.

Morton NE (1964). "Genetic studies of North-East Brazil." *Cold Spring Harbor Symposia on Quantitative Biology* 29:69–79.

Morton NE (1981). "Mutation rates in human autosomal recessives." In Hook EB, Porter IH (eds), *Population and Biological Aspects of Human Mutation*. New York, Academic Press, pp 65–89.

Morton NE (1982). *Outline of Genetic Epidemiology* Basel, S Karger.

Morton NE (1984). "Linkage and association." In Rao DC, Elston RC, Kuller LH, Feinleib M, Carter C, Havlik R (eds), *Genetic Epidemiology of Coronary Heart Disease: Past, Present, and Future*. New York, Alan R Liss, pp 245–265.

Morton NE (1986). "Foundations of genetic epidemiology." *Journal of Genetics* 65:205–212.

Morton NE, Chin S, Chung CS, Mi PI (1967). "Genetics of interracial crosses in Hawaii." *Progress in Medical Genetics* 5:1–158.

Morton NE, Chung CS (eds) (1978). *Genetic Epidemiology*. New York: Academic Press, pp 3–11.

Morton NE, Crow JF, Muller HJ (1956). "An estimate of the mutational damage in man from data on consanguineous marriages." *Proceedings of the National Academy of Sciences of the United States of America* 42:855–863.

Morton NE, Jacobs PA, Hassold T, Wu D (1988). "Maternal age in trisomy." *Annals of Human Genetics* 52:227–235.

Morton NE, MacLean CJ (1974). "Analysis of family resemblance. III. Complex segregation analysis of quantitative traits." *American Journal of Human Genetics* 26:489–503.

Motulsky AG, Campbell-Krant JM (1962). "Population genetics of glucose-6-phosphate dehydrogenase deficiency of the red cell." In *Proceedings of the Conference on Genetic Polymorphisms and Geographic Variation in Disease*. New York, Grune and Stratton, pp 159–191.

Motulsky AG (1978). "Pharmacogenetics and ecogenetics: The problem and its scope." *Human Genetics, Supplement* 1:1–3.

Motulsky AG (1984). [Editorial]. *Genetic Epidemiology* 1:143–144.

Motulsky AG (1991). "Pharmacogenetics and ecogenetics in 1991." [Invited commentary]. *Pharmacogenetics* 1:2 3.

Mourant AE, Kopec AC, Domaniewska-Sobezak L (1978). *Blood Groups and Diseases*. London, Oxford University Press.

Moy CS, LaPorte RE, Dorman JS, Dokheel T, Fourmier H (1989). "Heritage research: The next generation of migrant studies." *American Journal of Epidemiology* 130:819–820.

Mueller RF, Hornung S, Furlong CE, et al (1983). "Plasma paraoxonase polymorphism: A new enzyme assay, population, family, biochemical and linkage studies." *American Journal of Human Genetics* 35:393–408.

Mulinare J, Cordero JF, Erickson JD, Berry RJ (1988). "Periconceptional use of multivitamins and the occurrence of neural tube defects." *Journal of the American Medical Association* 260:3141–3145.

Mulinare J, Cordero JF, Erickson JD, Berry RJ (1989). "Does maternal recall bias account for the apparent protective effect of periconceptional vitamin use on the occurrence of neural tube defects?" *American Journal of Epidemiology* 130:805.

Mulvihill JJ (1984). "Clinical ecogenetics of cancer in humans." In *Genes and Cancer*. New York, Alan R Liss, pp 19–36.

Mulvihill JJ, Czeizel A (1983). "Perspectives in mutation epidemiology. 6. A 1983 view of sentinel phenotypes." *Mutation Research* 123:345–361.

Murphy EA (1978). "Epidemiological strategies and genetic factors." *International Journal of Epidemiology* 7:7–14

Murphy EA (1989). "The basis for interpreting family history." [Editorial]. *American Journal of Epidemiology* 129:19–22.

Murphy EA, Chase GA (1974). *Principles of Genetic Counselling*. Chicago, IL, Year Book Medical Publishers.

Murray RF (1986). "Tests of so-called genetic susceptibility." *Journal of Medicine* 28:1103–1107.

Nance WE (1984). "The relevance of twin studies to cardiovascular research." In Rao DC, Elston RC, Kuller LH, Feinlieb M, Carter C, Havlik R (eds), *Genetic Epidemiology of Coronary Heart Disease: Past, Present, and Future*. New York, Alan R Liss, pp 325–348.

Nance WE, Corey LA, Boughman JA (1978). "Monozygotic twin kinships: A new design for genetic-epidemiologic research." In Morton NE, Chung CS (eds), *Genetic Epidemiology*. New York, Academic Press, pp 87–132.

Nance WE, Kramer AA, Corey LA, Winter PM, Eaves LJ (1983). "A causal analysis of birth weight in the offspring of monozygotic twins." *American Journal of Human Genetics* 35:1211–1223.

Napier JA, Metzner H, Johnson BC (1972). "Limitations of morbidity and mortality data obtained from family histories: A report from the Tecumseh Community health study." *American Journal of Public Health* 62:30–35.

National Academy of Sciences, Committee for the Study of Inborn Errors of Metabolism (1975). *Genetic Screening: Program, Principles and Research*. Washington, DC, National Academy of Sciences.

National Research Council, Committee on Mapping and Sequencing the Human Genome (1988). *Mapping and Sequencing the Human Genome*. Washington, DC, National Academy Press.

National Research Council (1989). *Biologic Markers in Reproductive Toxicology*. Washington, DC, National Academy Press.

Neel JV, Mohrenweiser HW, Gershowitz H (1988a). "A pilot study of the use of placental cord blood samples in monitoring for mutational events." *Mutation Research* 204:365–377.

Neel JV, Mohrenweiser HW, Hanash S, et al (1983). "Biochemical approaches to monitoring human populations for germinal mutation rates. I. Electrophoresis." In Sheridan W, de Serres JF (eds), *Utilization of Mammalian Specific Locus Studies in Hazard Evaluation and Estimation of Genetic Risk*. New York, Plenum Press, pp 71–93.

Neel JV, Satoh K, Goriki M, et al (1986). "The rate with which spontaneous mutation alters the electrophoretic mobility of polypeptides." *Proceedings of the National Academy of Sciences of the United States of America* 83:389–393.

Neel JV, Satoh C, Goriki K, et al (1988b). "Search for mutations altering protein charge and/or function in children of atomic bomb survivors: Final report." *American Journal of Human Genetics* 42:663–676.

Neel JV, Schull WJ (1954). *Human Heredity*. Chicago, The University of Chicago Press, pp 283–306.

Neet JV, Shaw MW, Schull WJ (1965). *Genetics and the Epidemiology of Chronic Diseases*. Washington, DC, USPHS Publication No. 1163.

Nelkin D (1989). "Communicating technological risk: The social construction of risk perception." *Annual Review of Public Health* 10:95–113.

Nelson K, Holmes LB (1989). "Malformations due to presumed spontaneous mutations in newborn infants." *New England Journal of Medicine* 320:19–23.

Newill CA, Khoury MJ, Chase GA (1986). "An epidemiologic approach to the evaluation of genetic screening in the workplace." *Journal of Medicine* 28:1108–1111.

Newman B, Austin MA, Lee M, King MC (1988). "Inheritance of human breast cancer evidence for autosomal dominant transmission in high risk families." *Proceedings of the National Academy of Sciences of the United States of America* 85:3044–3048.

Nielsen HE, Haase P, Blaabjerg J, Stryhn H, Hilden J (1987). "Risk factors and sib correlation in physiological neonatal jaundice." *Acta Paediatrica Scandinavica* 76:504–511.

Niswander KR, Gordon M (eds) (1972). *The Women and Their Pregnancies*. Philadelphia, PA, WB Saunders.

O'Connell P, Lathrop GM, Nakamura Y, Leppert ML, Lalouel J-M, White R (1989). "Twenty loci form a continuous linkage map of markers for human chromosome 2." *Genomics* 5:738–745.

Omenn GS (1983). "Environmental risk assessment: Relation to mutagenesis, teratogenesis, and reproductive effects." *Journal of the American College of Toxicology* 2:113–25.

Office of Technology and Assessment (1983). *The Role of Genetic Testing in the Prevention of Occupational Disease*. Washington, DC,

Olshan AF, Baird PA, Tesckle K (1989). "Paternal occupational exposures and the risk of Down syndrome." *American Journal of Human Genetics* 44:646–651.

Omenn GS (1982). "Predictive identification of hypersusceptible individuals." *Journal of Medicine* 24:369–374.

Omenn GS (1988). "Genetic susceptibility and the estimation of risk." In Gordis L (ed), *Epidemiology and Health Risk Assessment*. New York, Oxford University Press, pp 92–104.

Omenn GS, Motulsky AG (1978). "Ecogenetics: Genetic variation in susceptibility to environmental agents." In Cohen BH, Lilienfeld AM, Huang PC (eds), *Genetic Issues in Public Health and Medicine*. Springfield, IL, CC Thomas, pp 83–111.

Orchard TJ, Dorman JS, LaPorte RE, Ferrell RE, Drash AL (1986). Host and environmental interaction in diabetes mellitus." *Journal of Chronic Diseases* 39:979–999.

Orkin SH (1986). "Reverse genetics and human disease." *Cell* 47:845–850.

Orkin SH, Kazazian HH (1984). "The mutation and polymorphism of the human β-globin gene and its surrounding DNA." *Annual Review of Genetics* 18:131–171.

Ostrer H, Hejtmancik JF (1988). "Prenatal diagnosis and carrier detection of genetic diseases by analysis of deoxyribonucleic acid." *Journal of Pediatrics* 112:679–687.

Ott J (1974). "Estimation of the recombination fraction in human pedigrees: Efficient computation of the likelihood for human linkage studies." *American Journal of Human Genetics* 26:588–597.

Ott J (1977). "Counting methods (EM algorithm) in human pedigree analysis: Linkage and segregation analysis." *Annals of Human Genetics* 40:443–454.

Ott J (1985). *Analysis of Human Genetic Linkage*. Baltimore, MD, Johns Hopkins University Press.

Ottman R (1990). "An epidemiologic approach to gene-environment interaction." *Genetic Epidemiology* 7:177–185.

Page DC, Mosher R, Simpson EM, et al (1987). "The sex determining region of the human Y chromosome encodes a finger protein." *Cell* 51:1091–1104.

Patrick SL, LaPorte RE, Khoury MJ (1992). "Insight into the magnitude of etiologic co-factors producing ankylosing spondylitis." (submitted).

Payami H, Joe S, Farid NR, Stenszky V, Chan SH, Yeo PPB, Cheah JS, Thomson G (1989). "Relative predispositional effects (RPEs) of marker alleles with disease: HLA-DR alleles and Graves disease." *American Journal of Human Genetics* 45:541–546.

Pearson K (1901). "I. Mathematical contributions to the theory of evolution. VII. On the correlation of characters not quantitatively measurable." *Philosophical Transactions of the Royal Society of London, Series A* 195:1–47.

Penrose LS (1935). "The detection of autosomal linkage in data which consist of pairs of brothers and sisters of unspecified parentage." *Annals of Eugenics* 5:133–148.

Penrose LS (1938). "Genetic linkage in graded human characters." *Annals of Eugenics* 8:233–237.

Penrose LS (1953). "The general sib-pair linkage test." *Annals of Eugenics* 18:120–144.

Perkins KA (1986). "Family history of coronary heart disease: Is it an independent risk factor?" *American Journal of Epidemiology* 124:182–194.

Perusse L, Moll PP, Sing CF (1991). "Evidence that a single locus with gender and age-dependent effects influences systolic blood pressure determination in a population-based sample." *American Journal of Human Genetics* 49:94–105.

Philippe P (1982). "L'epidemiologie genetique, fondement d'une veritable prevention: L'approache et ses resultats." *Canadian Journal of Public Health* 73:350–357.

Phillips JA, Kazazian HH (1983). "Hemoglobinopathies and thalassemias." In Emery

AEH, Rimoin DL (eds), *Principles and Practice of Medical Genetics*. Edinburgh, Churchill-Livingstone, pp 1019–1043.

Phillips PH, Linet MS, Harris EL (1991). "Assessment of family history information in case-control cancer studies." *American Journal of Epidemiology* 133:757–765.

Ploughman LM, Boehnke M (1989). "Estimating the power of a proposed linkage study for a complex genetic trait." *American Journal of Human Genetics* 44:543–551.

Polednak AP (1987). *Host Factors in Disease: Age, Sex, Racial and Ethnic Group, and Body Build*. Springfield, IL, CC Thomas.

Poole C (1986). "Exposure opportunity in case-control studies." *American Journal of Epidemiology* 123:352–358.

Porter IH (1982). "Control of hereditary disorders." *Annual Review of Public Health* 3:277–319.

Porter IH (1986). "Genetic aspects of preventive medicine." In Last JM (ed), *Maxcy-Rosenau Public Health and Preventive Medicine*, 12th Ed. Norwalk, CT, Appleton & Lange, pp 1427–1472.

Pratt JH, Jones JJ, Miller JZ, Wagner MA, Fineberg NS (1989). "Racial differences in aldosterone excretion and plasma aldosterone concentrations in children." *New England Journal of Medicine* 321:1152–1157.

Prentice RL, Farewell VT (1986). Relative risk and odds ratio regression. *Annual Review of Public Health* 7:35–58.

Prentice RL, Sheppard L (1989). "Validity of international, time trend. and migrant studies of dietary factors and disease risk." *Preventive Medicine* 18:167–179.

Price B (1950). "Primary biases in twin studies: A review of prenatal and natal difference-producing factors in monozygotic pairs." *American Journal of Human Genetics* 2:293–352.

Price-Evans DA (1983). "Pharmacogenetics." In Emery AEH, Rimoin DL (eds), *Principles and Practice of Medical Genetics*, Volume 2. Edinburgh, Churchill-Livingstone, pp 1389–1400.

Qaqish B, Liang KY (1992). Marginal models for correlated binary responses with multiple classes and multiple levels of nesting. *Biometrics* (in press).

Radiation Effects Research Foundation (1987). "US–Japan joint reassessment of atomic bomb radiation dosimetry in Hiroshima and Nagasaki: Final report." In Roesch WC (ed), *Hiroshima: Radiation Effects Research Foundation*. Hiroshima, Radiation Effects Research Foundation.

Rao DC (1984). Editorial Comment. *Genetic Epidemiology* 1:5–6.

Rao DC (1985). "Application of path analysis in human genetics." In Krishnaiah PR (ed), *Multivariate Analysis VI*. pp 467–484.

Rao DC (1990). "Environmental index in genetic epidemiology: An investigation of its role, adequacy and limitations." *American Journal of Human Genetics* 46:168–178.

Rao DC, Keats BJB, Lalouel JM, Morton NE, Yee S (1979). "A maximum likelihood map of chromosome 1." *American Journal of Human Genetics* 31:680–696.

Rao DC, Keats BJB, Morton NE, Yee S, Lew R (1978). "Variability of human linkage data." *American Journal of Human Genetics* 30:516–529.

Rao DC, Morton NE, Lindsten J, Hulten M, Yee S (1977). "A mapping function for man." *Human Heredity* 27:99–104.

Rao DC, Morton NE, Yee S (1974). "Analysis of family resemblance. II. A linear model for familial correlations." *American Journal of Human Genetics* 26:331–359.

Rao DC, Province MA, Wette R, Glueck CJ (1984). "The role of path analysis in coronary heart disease research." In Rao DC, Elston RC, Kuller LH, Feinleib M, Carter C, Havlik R (eds), *Genetic Epidemiology of Coronary Heart Disease: Past, Present, and Future.* New York, Alan R Liss, pp 193–212.

Rao DC, Vogler GP, Borecki IB, Province MA, Russell JM (1987). "Robustness of path analysis of family resemblance against deviations from multivariate normality." *Human Heredity* 37:107–112.

Rao DC, Wette R (1987). "Non-random sampling in genetic epidemiology: Maximum likelihood methods for truncate selection." *Genetic Epidemiology* 4:357–376.

Rao DC, Williams WR, McGue M, et al (1983). "Cultural and biological inheritance of plasma lipids." *American Journal of Physical Anthropology* 62:33–49.

Ray PN, Bellfall B, Duff C, et al (1985). "Cloning of the breakpoint of an X;21 translocation associated with Duchenne muscular dystrophy." *Nature* 318:672–675.

Reed T, Fabsitz RR, Quiroga J (1990). "Family history of ischemic heart disease with respect to mean twin-pair cholesterol and subsequent ischemic heart disease in the NHLBI twin study." *Genetic Epidemiology* 7:335–347.

Reed T, Wagener DK, Donahue RP, Kuller LH (1986). "Young adult cholesterol as a predictor of familial ischemic heart disease." *Preventive Medicine* 15:292–303.

Reid DD (1966). "Studies of disease among migrant and native populations in Great Britain, Norway, and the United States. I. Background and design." *National Cancer Institute Monograph* 19:287–299.

Reitnauer PJ, Go RCP, Acton RT, et al (1982). "Evidence for genetic admixture as a determinant in the occurrence of insulin-dependent diabetes mellitus in U.S. blacks." *Diabetes* 31:532–537.

Renwick JH (1971). "The mapping of human chromosomes." *Annual Review of Genetics* 5:81–120.

Rice JP (1986). "Genetic epidemiology: Models of multifactorial inheritance and path analysis applied to qualitative traits." In Moulgavkar SK, Prentice RL (eds), *Modern Statistical Methods in Chronic Disease Epidemiology.* New York, Wiley.

Rice JP, Nichols PL, Gottesman II (1981). "Assessment of sex differences for multifactorial traits using path analysis: Application to learning difficulties." *Psychiatry Research* 4:301–312.

Rice JP, Reich T (1985). "Familial analysis of qualitative traits under multifactorial models." *Genetic Epidemiology* 2:301–315.

Rice TR, Vogler GP, Perry TS, Laskarzewski PM, Rao DC (1991). "Familial aggregation of lipids and lipoproteins in families ascertained through random and nonrandom probands in the Iowa Lipid Research Clinics Family Study." *Human Heredity* 41:107–121.

Riordan JR, Rommens JM, Kerme B, et al (1989). "Identification of the cystic fibrosis gene: Cloning and characterization of complementary DNA." *Science* 245:1066–1073.

Risch N (1988). "A new statistical test for linkage heterogeneity." *American Journal of Human Genetics* 42:353–364.

Risch N (1990a). "Genetic linkage and complex diseases, with special reference to psychiatric disorders." *Genetic Epidemiology* 7:3–16.

Risch N (1990b). "Linkage strategies for genetically complex traits. II. The power of affected relative pairs." *American Journal of Human Genetics* 46:229–241.

Risch N (1990c). "Linkage strategies for genetically complex traits. III. The effects of marker polymorphism on analysis of affected relative pairs." *American Journal of Human Genetics* 46:242–253.

Risch N, Baron M (1982). "X-linkage and genetic heterogeneity in bipolar-related major affective illness: Reanalysis of linkage data." *Annals of Human Genetics* 46:153–166.

Roberts DF (1983). "Genetic epidemiology." *American Journal of Physical Anthropology* 62:67–70.

Roberts DF (1985). "A definition of genetic epidemiology." In Chakraborty R, Szathmary EJE (eds), *Diseases of Complex Etiology in Small Populations: Ethnic Differences and Research Approaches*. New York, Alan R Liss, pp 9–20.

Roberts DF (1991). "Consanguinity and multiple sclerosis in Orkney." *Genetic Epidemiology* 8:147–152.

Roberts DF, Roberts MJ, Johnston AW (1991). "Genetic epidemiology of Down syndrome in Shetland." *Human Genetics* 87:57–60.

Robertson PE (1983). "Genetic registers." In Emery AEH, Rimoin DL (eds), *Principles and Practice of Medical Genetics*. Vol. 2, Edinburgh, Churchill-Livingstone, pp 1481–1487.

Robinow M, Shaw A (1979). "The McKusick-Kauffman syndrome: Recessively inherited vaginal atresia, hydrometrocolpos, uterovaginal duplications, anorectal anomalies, postaxial polydactyly, and congenital heart disease." *Journal of Pediatrics* 94:776–778.

Rommens JM, Ianuzzi MC, Kerem B, et al (1989). "Identification of the cystic fibrosis gene: Chromosome walking and jumping." *Science* 245:1059–1065.

Rosenberg LE, Fenton WA (1989). "Disorders of propionate and methylmalonate metabolism." In Scriver CR, Beaudet AL, Sly WS, Valle D (eds), *The Metabolic Basis of Inherited Disease*, 6th Ed. New York, McGraw-Hill, pp 821–844.

Rosenthal D, Wender PH, Kety SS, Welner J, Schulsinger F (1971). "The adopted-away offspring of schizophrenics." *American Journal of Psychiatry* 128:307–311.

Rostron J (1978). "On the computation of inbreeding coefficients." *Annals of Human Genetics* 41:469–475.

Rothman KJ (1986). *Modern Epidemiology*. Boston, Little, Brown.

Rothman KJ, Boice JD (1982). *Epidemiologic Analysis with a Programmable Calculator*. Chestnut Hill, MA, Epidemiology Resources.

Rotter J (1983). "Peptic ulcer." In Emery AEH, Rimoin DL (eds), *Principles and Practice of Medical Genetics*, Vol. 2. Edinburgh, Churchill-Livingstone, pp 863–878.

Rotter J, Rimoin DL (1983). "Diabetes mellitus." In Emery AEH, Rimoin DL (eds), *Principles and Practices of Medical Genetics*, Vol. 2. Edinburgh, Churchill-Livingstone, pp 1180–1201.

Rvachev LA, Longini IM (1985). "A mathematical model for the global spread of influenza." *Mathematical Biosciences* 75:3–22.

Rybicki BA, Beaty TH, Cohen BH (1990). "Major gene effects in pulmonary function." *Journal of Clinical Epidemiology* 43:667–675.

Salmond CE, Prior IA, Wessen AF (1989). "Blood pressure patterns and migration: A 14-year cohort study of adult Tokelauans." *American Journal of Epidemiology* 130:37–52.

Sandhoff K, Conzelman E, Neufeld EF, Kaback MM, Suzuki K (1989). "The GM2 gangliosidoses." In Scriver CR, Beaudet AL, Sly WS, Valle D (eds), *The Metabolic Basis of Inherited Disease*, 6th Ed. New York, McGraw-Hill, pp 1807–1842.

Sanghvi LD (1963). "The concept of genetic load: A critique." *American Journal of Human Genetics* 15:298–309.

Sankaranayanan K (1988). "Invited review: Prevalence of genetic and partially genetic diseases in man and the estimation of genetic risks of exposure to ionizing radiation." *American Journal of Human Genetics* 42:651–662.

Santos MCN, Azevedo ES (1981). "Generalized joint hypermobility and black admixture in school children in Bahia, Brazil." *American Journal of Physical Anthropology* 55:43–46.

Sarucci R (1987). "The interactions of tobacco smoking and other agents in cancer etiology." *Epidemiologic Reviews* 9:175–193.

Sattin RW, Rubin GL, Webster LA, et al (1985). " Family history and the risk of breast cancer." *Journal of the American Medical Association* 253:1908–1913.

Scarr S (1982). "Environmental bias in twin studies." *Social Biology* 29:221–229.

Schlesselman JJ (1982). *Case-Control Studies: Design, Conduct, Analysis*. New York, Oxford University Press.

Schlesselman JJ (1985). "Valid selection of subjects in case-control studies." *Journal of Chronic Diseases* 38:549–550.

Schleutermann DA, Bias WB, Murdoch JL, McKusick VA (1969). "Linkage of the loci for the nail-patella syndrome and adenylate kinase." *American Journal of Human Genetics* 21:606–630.

Schmickel RD (1986). "Contiguous gene syndromes: A component of recognizable syndromes." *Journal of Pediatrics* 109:231–241.

Schull WJ, Cobb S (1969). "The intrafamilial transmission of rheumatoid arthritis." *Journal of Chronic Diseases* 22:217–222.

Schull WJ, Hanis CL (1990). "Genetics and public health in the 1990's." *Annual Review of Public Health* 11:105–125.

Schull WJ, Harburg E, Erfurt JC, Schork MA, Rice R (1970). "A family set method for estimating heredity and stress. II. Preliminary results of the genetic methodology in a pilot survey of Negro blood pressure, Detroit, 1966–1967." *Journal of Chronic Diseases* 23:83–92.

Schull WJ, Harburg E, Schork MA, Chakraborty R (1977). "Heredity, stress and blood pressures, a family set method. Epilogue." *Journal of Chronic Diseases* 30:701–704.

Schull WJ, Weiss KM (1980). "Genetic epidemiology: Four strategies." *Epidemiologic Reviews* 2:1–18.

Schulman J, Shaw G, Selvin S (1988). "On "rates" of birth defects." *Teratology* 38:427–429.

Schwartz AG, Boehnke M, Moll PP (1988). "Family risk index as a measure of familial heterogeneity of cancer risk: A population-based study in metropolitan Detroit." *American Journal of Epidemiology* 128:524–535.

Schwartz AG, Kaufmann R, Moll PP (1991). "Heterogeneity of breast cancer risk in families of young breast cancer patients and controls." *American Journal of Epidemiology* 134:1325–1334.

Schwartz CE, Johnson JP, Holycross B, et al (1988). "Detection of submicroscopic deletions in band 17p13 in patients with Miller-Dieker syndrome." *American Journal of Human Genetics* 43:597–604.

Schwartz GG (1990). "Chromosome aberrations." In Hulka BS, Wilcosky TC, Griffith JD (eds), *Biological Markers in Epidemiology*. New York, Oxford University Press, pp. 147–172.

Schwartz S, Roulston D, Cohen MM (1989). "dNORs and meiotic nondisjunction." [Invited Editorial]. *American Journal of Human Genetics* 44:627–630.

Scriver CR, Childs B (1989). *Garrod's Inborn Factors in Disease*. New York, Oxford University Press.

Scriver CR, Kaufman S, Woo SLC (1989). "The hyperphenylalaninemias." In Scriver

CR, Beaudet AL, Sly WS, Valle D (eds), *The Metabolic Basis of Inherited Disease*, 6th Ed. New York, McGraw-Hill, pp 495–546.

Seaquist ER, Goetz FC, Rich S, Barbosa J (1989). "Familial clustering of diabetic kidney disease: Evidence for genetic susceptibility to diabetic nephropathy." *New England Journal of Medicine* 320:1161–1165.

Self SG, Liang KY (1987). "Large sample properties of the maximum likelihood estimator and the likelihood ratio test on the boundary of the parameter space." *Journal of the American Statistical Association* 82:605–610.

Self SG, Prentice RL (1986). "Incorporating random effects into multivariate relative risk regression models." In Mogavkar SH, Prentice RL (eds), *Modern Statistical Methods in Chronic Disease Epidemiology* New York, Wiley, pp. 167–177.

Sherman SL, Takaesu N, Freeman S, Phillips C, et al (1990). "Trisomy 21: association between reduced recombination and non-disjunction." *American Journal of Human Genetics, Supplement* 47:A97.

Shibuya A, Yasunami M, Yoshida A (1989). "Genotypes of alcohol dehydrogenase and aldehyde dehydrogenase loci in Japanese flushers and nonflushers." *Human Genetics* 82:14–16.

Shute NCE, Ewens WJ (1988a). "A resolution of the ascertainment sampling problem. II. Generalizations and numerical results." *American Journal of Human Genetics* 43:374–386.

Shute NCE, Ewens WJ (1988b). "A resolution of the ascertainment sampling problem. III. Pedigrees." *American Journal of Human Genetics* 43:387–395.

Shy CM, Kleinbaum DG, Morgenstern H (1978). "The effect of misclassification of exposure status in epidemiologic studies of air pollution health effects." *Bulletin of the New York Academy of Medicine* 54:1155–1165.

Sigler AT, Lilienfeld AM, Cohen BH, Westlake JE (1965). "Parental age in Down syndrome." *Journal of Pediatrics* 67:631–642.

Sing CF, Boerwinkle E, Moll PP (1985). "Strategies for elucidating phenotypic and genetic heterogeneity of a chronic disease with complex etiology." *Progress in Clinical and Biological Research* 194:36–66.

Sing CF, Boerwinkle E, Moll PP, Templeton AR (1988). "Characterization of genes affecting quantitative traits in humans." In Weir BS, Bisen EJ, Goodman MM, Namkoong G (eds), *Proceedings of the Second International Conference on Quantitative Genetics* Sunderland, MA, Sinauer Associates, pp 250–269.

Sing CF, Moll PP (1989). "Genetics of variability of CHD risk." *International Journal of Epidemiology, Supplement 1* 18:S183–S195.

Sing CH, Skolnick M (eds) (1978). "Genetic analysis of common diseases: Applications to predictive factors in coronary disease. *Progress in Clinical and Biological Research* Vol. 32.

Skoda RC, Gonzalez FJ, Demierre A, Meyer UA (1988). "Two mutant alleles of human cytochrome P-450dbl gene (P450C2D1) associated with genetically deficient metabolism of debrisoquine and other drugs." *Proceedings of the National Academy of Sciences of the United States of America* 85:5240–5243.

Skolnick MH (1980). "The Utah genealogical data base: A resource for genetic epidemiology." In Cairn J, Lyon JL, Skolnick MH (eds), *Banbury Report 4. Cancer Incidence in Defined Populations*. Cold Spring Harbor, NY, Cold Spring Harbor Laboratory, 286–298.

Skolnick MM, Neel JV (1986). "An algorithm for comparing two-dimensional electrophoretic gels, with particular reference to the study of mutation." *Advances in Human Genetics* 15:55–160.

Slamon DJ (1987). "Protooncogenes and human cancers." *New England Journal of Medicine* 317:955–957.

Smith C, Mendell NR (1974). "Recurrence risks from family history and metric traits." *Annals of Human Genetics* 37:275–286.

Smith CAB (1953). "The detection of linkage in human genetics." *Journal of the Royal Statistical Society, Series B* 14:153–192.

Smith CAB (1963). "Testing for heterogeneity of recombination fractions in human genetics." *Annals of Human Genetics* 27:175–182.

Smith CAB (1976). "The use of matrices in calculating mendelian probabilities." *Annal of Human Genetics* 40:37–54.

Smith CAB (1986). "The development of human linkage analysis." *Annals of Human Genetics* 50:293–311.

Smith T (1989). "Vitamins verdict jury still out. *British Medical Journal* 299:529.

Smithells RW, Nevin NC, Seller MJ, et al (1983). "Further experience of vitamin supplementation for prevention of neural tube defect recurrences." *Lancet* 1:1027–1031.

Snow J (1936). "On the mode of communication of cholera." Reproduced in *Snow on Cholera*. New York, Commonwealth Fund.

Sokal RR (1988.) "Genetic, geographic and linguistic distances in Europe." *Proceedings of the National Academy of Sciences of the United States of America* 85:1722–1726.

Sokal RR, Harding RM, Oden NL (1989). "Spatial patterns of human gene frequencies in Europe." *American Journal of Physical Anthropolgy* 80:267–294.

Sokal RR, Menozzi P. (1982). "Spatial autocorrelation of HLA frequencies supports demic diffusion of early farmers." *American Naturalist* 119:1–17.

Sorenson TIA, Nielsen GG, Andersen PK, Teasdale TW (1988). "Genetic and environmental influences on premature death in adult adoptees." *New England Journal of Medicine* 318:727–732.

Spielman RS, Nathanson N (1982). "The genetics of susceptibility to multiple sclerosis." *Epidemiologic Reviews* 4:45–65.

Spinner NB, Eunpu DL, Schmikel RD, et al (1989). "The role of cytologic NOR variants in the etiology of trisomy 21." *American Journal of Human Genetics* 44:631–638.

Stallones RA (1988). "Epidemiology and environmental hazards." In Gordis L (ed), *Epidemiology and Health Risk Assessment*. New York, Oxford University Press, pp 3–10.

Stehbens WE (1985). "The concept of cause in disease." *Journal of Chronic Diseases* 38:945–950.

Stein Z, Hatch M (1987). "Biological markers in reproductive epidemiology: prospects and precautions." *Environmental Health Perspectives* 74:67–75.

Stern C (1973). *Principles of Human Genetics*. 3rd Ed. New York, WH Freeman.

Stolley PD (1983). "Lung cancer in women: 5 years later, situation worse." *New England Journal of Medicine* 309:428–429.

Strabowski SM, Butler MG (1987). "Paternal hydrocarbon exposure in Prader-Willi syndrome." *Lancet* 1:1458.

Strickler SM, Dansky LV, Miller MA, Seni MH, Andermann E, Spielberg SP (1985). "Genetic predisposition to phenytoin-induced birth defects." *Lancet* 2:746–749.

Strom BL (ed) (1989). *Pharmacoepidemiology*. New York, Churchill Livingstone.

Stunkard AJ, Sorenson TI, Hanis C, et al (1986). "An adoption study of human obesity." *New England Journal of Medicine* 314:193–198.

Suarez BK, Van Eerdewegh P (1984). "A comparison of three affected-sib-pair scoring methods to detect HLA-linked disease susceptibility genes." *American Journal of Medical Genetics* 18:135–146.

Susser E, Susser M (1989). "Familial aggregation studies: A note on their epidemiologic properties." *American Journal of Epidemiology* 129:23–30.

Susser M (1985). "Separating heredity and environment." *American Journal of Preventive Medicine* 1:5–23.

Susser M (1991). "What is a cause and how do we know one: A grammar for practical epidemiology." *American Journal of Epidemiology* 133:635–648.

Susser M, Susser E (1987a). "Separating heredity and environment. I. Genetic and environmental indices." In Susser M (eds), *Epidemiology, Health and Society: Selected Papers*. New York, Oxford University Press, pp 103–114.

Susser M, Susser E (1987b). "Separating heredity and environment. II. Research designs and strategies." In Susser M (ed), *Epidemiology, Health and Society: Selected Papers*. New York, Oxford University Press, pp 114–128.

Sutton HE (1988). *An Introduction to Human Genetics*. 4th Ed. San Diego, CA, Harcourt Brace Jovanovich.

Sutton HE, Wagner RP (1985). *Genetics: A Human Concern*. New York, Macmillan.

Suzuki D, Knudston P (1989). *Genetics: The Clash Between the New Genetics and Human Values* Cambridge, MA, Harvard University Press.

Svejgaard A, Jersild C, Nielson LS, et al (1974). "HLA antigens and disease: statistical and genetical considerations." *Tissue Antigens* 4:95–105.

Tatum EL (1959). "A case history of biological research." *Science* 129:1711.

Taylor JA (1989). Oncogenes and their applications in epidemiologic studies. *American Journal of Epidemiology* 130:6–13.

ten Kate LP, Boman H, Daiper SP, Motulsky AG (1982). "Familial aggregation of coronary heart disease and its relation to known genetic risk factors." *American Journal of Cardiologyi* 50:945–953.

Thacker SB, Berkelman RL (1988). "Public health surveillance in the United States." *Epidemiologic Reviews* 10:164–190.

Thomas DC, Siemiatycki R, Dewar J, et al (1985). "The problem of multiple inference in studies designed to generate hypotheses." *American Journal of Epidemiology* 122:1080–1095.

Thomas DS (1988). "Models for exposure-time-resource relationships: Applications to cancer epidemiology." *Annal Review of Public Health* 9:451–482.

Thomas GH (1978). "Screening for genetic disorders: Limitations and pitfalls." In Cohen BH, Lilienfeld AM. Huang PC (ed), *Genetic Issues in Public Health and Medicine* Springfield, IL, CC Thomas, pp 193–205.

Thompson EA (1986). *Pedigree Analysis in Human Genetics*. Baltimore, MD, Johns Hopkins University Press.

Thompson EA (1986). "Genetic epidemiology: A review of the statistical basis." *Statistics in Medicine* 5:291–302.

Tiwari JL, Betuel H, Gebuhrer L, Morton NE (1984). "Genetic Epidemiology of coeliac disease." *Genetic Epidemiology* 1:37–42.

Thompson MW, McInnes RR, Willard HF (1991). *Genetics in Medicine*, 5th Ed. Philadelphia, PA, WB Saunders.

Thomson G (1986). "Determining the mode of inheritance of RFLP-associated diseases using the affected sib-pair method." *American Journal of Human Genetics* 39:207–221.

Thomson G (1988). "HLA disease associations: Models for insulin dependent diabetes mellitus and the study of complex human genetic disorders." *Annual Review of Genetics* 22:31–50.

Tockman MS, Khoury MJ, Cohen BH (1985). "Epidemiology of chronic obstructive pulmonary disease." In Petty T (ed). *Chronic Obstructive Pulmonary Disease*, 2nd Ed. Vol. 28, New York, Marcel-Dekker, pp 43–92.

Tokuhata GK, Lilienfeld AM (1963). "Familial aggregation of lung cancer in humans." *Journal of the National Cancer Institute* 30:289–312.

Torfs CP, van den Berg, J, Oechsli FW, Christianson RE (1990). "Thyroid antibodies as a risk factor for Down syndrome and other trisomies." *American Journal of Human Genetics* 47:727–734.

Trucco M, Dorman JS (1989). "Immunogenetics of insulin-dependent diabetes mellitus in humans." *CRC Critical Reviews in Immunology* 9(3):201–245.

Tsipouras P, Ramirez F (1987). "Genetic disorders of collagen." *Journal of Medical Genetics* 24:2–8.

Uzych L (1986). "Genetic testing and exclusionary practices in the workplace." *Journal of Public Health Policy* 7:37–57.

Valle DL, Mitchell GA (1988). "Inborn errors of metabolism in the molecular age." *Progress in Medical Genetics* 7:100–129.

Vesell ES (1973). "Advances in pharmacogenetics." *Progress in Medical Genetics* 9:291–367.

Vesell ES (1979). "Pharmacogenetics: Multiple interactions between genes and environment as determinant of drug response." *American Journal of Medicine* 66:183–187.

Vogel F (1984). "Clinical consequences of heterozygosity for autosomal recessive diseases." *Clinical Genetic* 25:381–415.

Vogel F, Motulsky AG (1986). *Human Genetics, Problems and Approaches*. 2nd Ed. Berlin, Springer-Verlag.

Vogel F, Rathenberg R (1975). "Spontaneous mutation in man." *Advances in Human Genetics* 6:223–318.

Wagener D, Cavalli-Sforza LL, Barakat R (1978). "Ethnic variation of genetic disease: Roles of drift for recessive lethal genes." *American Journal of Human Genetics* 30:262–270.

Wald NJ, Cuckle HS, Densem JW, et al (1988). "Maternal serum screening for Down syndrome in early pregnancy." *British Medical Journal* 297:883–887.

Wald NJ, Polani PE (1984). "Neural tube defects and vitamins: The need for a randomized clinical trial." *British Journal of Obstetrics and Gynecology* 91:516–523.

Walker AM (1981). "Proportion of disease attributable to the combined effect of two factors." *International Journal of Epidemiology* 10:81–85.

Ward RH (1979). "Genetic epidemiology: Promise or compromise." *Social Biology* 27:87–100.

Ward RH (1990). "Familial aggregation and genetic epidemiology of blood pressure." In Laragh JH, Brenner BM (eds), *Hypertension: Pathophysiology, and Management*. New York, Raven Press, pp 81–100.

Ward RH (1985). "Isolates in transition: A research paradigm in genetic epidemiology." *Progress in Clinical and Biological Research* 194:147–177.

Wasmuth JJ, Hewitt J, Smith B, et al (1988). "A highly polymorphic locus very tightly linked to the Huntington's disease gene." *Nature* 332:734–736.

Watson JD (1990). "The human genome project: past, present and future." *Science* 248:44–49.

Watson JD, Cook-Dugan RM (1991). "Origins of the human genome." *FASEB Journal* 5:8–78.

Watson JD, Tooze J, Kurtz DT (1983). *Recombinant DNA. A Short Course.* New York, Scientific American Books.

Weatherall DJ (1985). "The new genetics and clinical practice." New York, Oxford University Press.

Weeks DE, Lange K (1988). "The affected pedigree-member method of linkage analysis." *American Journal of Human Genetics* 42:315–322.

Weeks DE, Lehner T, Squires-Wheeler E, Kaufmann C, Ott J (1990). "Measuring the inflation of the LOD score due to its maximization over model parameter values in human linkage analysis." *Genetic Epidemiology* 7:237–243.

Weir BS (1990). *Genetic Data Analysis.* Sunderland, MA, Sinauer Associates.

Weiss KM, Chakraborty R, Majumder PP, Smouse P (1982). "Problems in the assessment of relative risks of chronic diseases among biological relatives of affected individuals." *Journal of Chronic Diseases* 35:539–551.

Weiss KM, Ferrell RE, Hanis CL, Styne PN (1984). "Genetics and epidemiology of gallbladder disease in New World native peoples." *American Journal of Human Genetics* 36:1259–1278.

Weiss NS (1986). *Clinical Epidemiology: The Study of the Outcome of Illness.* New York, Oxford University Press.

Weiss NS, Liff JM (1983). "Accounting for the multicausal nature of disease in the design and analysis of epidemiologic studies." *American Journal of Epidemiology* 117:14–18.

Wilcosky TC, Rynard SM (1990). "Sister chromatid exchange." In Hulka BS, Wilcosky TC, Griffith JD (ed), *Biological Markers in Epidemiology.* New York, Oxford University Press, pp 105–124.

Williams RC, Steinberg AG, Knowler WC, Pettitt DJ (1986). "Gm 3;5,13,14 and stated-admixture: Independent estimates of admixture in American Indians." *American Journal of Human Genetics* 39:409–413.

Williams RR (1988). "Nature, nurture and family predisposition." *New England Journal of Medicine* 318:769–771.

Williams RR, Dadone MM, Hunt SC, Jorde LB, Hopkins PN, Smith JB, Oqwen-Ashk, Kuida H (1984). "The genetic epidemiology of hypertension: A review of past studies and current results for 948 persons in 48 Utah pedigrees." In Rao DC, Elston RC, Kuller LH, Feinleib M, Carter C, Havlik R (ed). *Genetic Epidemiology of Coronary Heart Disease: Past, Present and Future.* New York, Alan R. Liss, Inc., pp. 419–442.

Williams RR, Hasstedt SJ, Wilson DE, et al (1986). "Evidence that men with familial hypercholesterolemia can avoid early coronary death: An analysis of 77 gene carriers in four Utah pedigrees." *Journal of the American Medical Association* 255:219–224.

Williams WR, Anderson DE (1984). "Genetic epidemiology of breast cancer; segregation analysis of 200 Danish pedigrees." *Genetic Epidemiology* 1:7–20.

Windham GC, Edmonds LD (1982). "Current trends in the incidence of neural tube defects." *Pediatrics* 70:333–337.

Winsor EJT, Welch JP (1978). "Genetic and demographic aspects of Nova Scotia Niemann-Pick disease (type D)." *American Journal of Human Genetics* 30:530–538.

Wong FL, Rotter JI (1984). "Sample size calculations in segregation analysis." *American Journal of Human Genetics* 36:1279–1297.

Woolf B (1955). "On estimating the relation between blood groups and disease." *Annals of Human Genetics* 19:251–253.

Wramsby H, Fredga K, Liedholm P (1987). "Chromosome analysis of human oocytes recovered from preovulatory follicles in stimulated cycles." *New England Journal of Medicine* 316:121–124.

Wright S (1922). "Coefficients of inbreeding and relationship." *American Naturalist* 56:330–338.

Wright S (1934). "The method of path coefficients." *Annals of Mathematical Statistics* 5:161–215.

Wynder EL (1985). "Applied epidemiology." *American Journal of Epidemiology* 121:781–782.

Yandell DW, Campbell TA, Dayto SH, et al (1989). "Oncogenetic point mutations in the human retinoblastoma gene: Their application to genetic counselling." *New England Journal of Medicine* 321:1689–1695.

Yandell DW, Dryja TP (1989). "Detection of DNA sequence polymorphisms by enzymatic amplification and direct genomic sequencing." *American Journal of Human Genetics* 45:547–555.

Yasuda T, Sato W, Mizuta K, Kishi K (1988). "Genetic polymorphism of human serum ribonuclease I (RNAse I)." *American Journal of Human Genetics* 42:608–614.

Yen S, MacMahon B (1968). "Genetics of anencephaly and spina bifida" *Lancet* 2:623–626.

Yunis JJ (1983). "The chromosomal basis of human neoplasia." *Science* 221:227–236.

Zdeb M (1977). "The probability of developing cancer." *American Journal of Epidemiology* 106:6–16.

Zhou HH, Koshakji RP, Silberstein DJ, Wilkinson GR, Wood AJJ (1989). "Racial differences in drug response. Altered sensitivity to and clearance of propranolol in men of Chinese descent as compared with American whites." *New England Journal of Medicine* 320:565–570.

Index